DOCTORS

DOCTORS

THE LIVES AND WORK OF GPS

Jonathan Gathorne-Hardy

Weidenfeld & Nicolson
LONDON

ISBN 0 297 78382 3

Filmset by Deltatype, Ellesmere Port
Printed in Great Britain by
Butler & Tanner Ltd
Frome and London

IN MEMORY OF MY DEAR FATHER, ANTHONY,
whose life and work I now admire a great deal more,
and with far greater sympathy and understanding.

CONTENTS

INTRODUCTION AND ACKNOWLEDGEMENTS   IX

1 Introductory: The Past   I
2 1890 – 1920   7
3 The Twenties, Thirties and Forties   12
4 The NHS and into the Fifties   22
5 Dr Tom Velling   28
   A Single-handed Practice, South-West London Suburbs
6 Dr James Chathill   32
   A Large West Country Health Centre
7 Dr Anne Uplees   42
   A West Country Urban Practice
8 Sex, Love and Sex Counselling   46
9 Private Practice   51
10 Dr Sam Locking   57
   A Two-doctor Practice, Cumberland
11 Drugs and Drug Companies   64
12 Group Practices and Health Centres   74
13 Money   84
14 Dr Frank Warfield   88
   A South-East Urban Group Practice
15 Social Workers   93
16 Dr David Bilsby   96
   A Lincolnshire Market Town Group Practice
17 Dr Peter Axmouth   109
   A South of England New Town
18 The Consultation   113

viii   CONTENTS

19 Keeping up to Date   130
20 Preventative Medicine   133
21 Fringe Medicine   137
22 The Patients   139
23 An Inner-City Practice: Dr Tim Cerney   150
24 Inner City Problems: Two Slum Practices   167
25 Overseas GPS   184
26 Unemployment   188
27 The Old   190
28 Death   199
29 Euthanasia   206
30 Stress   209
31 Wives and Families   224
32 Why They Became GPS   230
33 A Moral Stance; The Pill, Abortion   236
34 The Characters of the GPS   238
35 Egalitarian Practices   247
36 A Shared Practice: Drs Simon and Janet Kibane   256
37 Women GPS   259
38 An Inducement Practice: Dr Jimmy Colkirk   266
39 The Training of GPS   279
40 The Future of General Practice   294
41 *That* is the Fascination   300

LIST OF DOCTORS   304
SHORT BIBLIOGRAPHY   308

Introduction and Acknowledgements

The aim of this book was primarily to give as vivid and comprehensive a picture as possible of the lives and work of GPs – to record what they did and what was done to them, what their patients were like and what they thought about them, how they got on (or didn't) with their colleagues, to describe what they felt, what they feared, what they enjoyed. To try and convey, in fact, wherever possible using their own words, what it was like to *be* a GP – in the past, but mainly in Britain today.

A secondary aim was to say something about general practice itself. Not about its 'state' – even if the sample of fifty GPs I saw is of some value statistically, it is not really large enough to allow of general judgements (though I do go into most of the important areas). But, gathered as it was from all over England, Scotland and Wales, I did want to give some idea of the extraordinary diversity of general practice. The range is fascinating: from remote Highland inducement practices which, the medicine aside, haven't really changed much in sixty years, to squalid inner-city surgeries, little waiting room steaming and packed out, the over-worked GP not so far removed from the 6d doctor of the 1890s seeing patients one a minute. I would move – another inner-city phenomenon – from some aged, batty figure approaching 100 and still dishing out prescriptions, groping for pulses, peering down throats, to the sterilized hush of an enormous southern health centre, where four, six, eight immensely competent GPs ruled empires thronged with highly trained, dedicated staff, surrounded by glass, computers, and gleaming equipment, in what seemed really mini hospitals – and were sometimes precisely that.

And this is a diversity which neither GPs themselves, nor the students who may become GPs, really know very much about. (Indeed, despite very slowly growing attempts to teach them, most medical students have very little idea what it is like to be a GP.) GPs, like their patients, think that what they are (and the two or three other GPs they happen to have seen) are what general practice *is*. But it is not.

The sample was too small for some purposes; fortunately I didn't have to rely on it alone. There are the two excellent surveys by Anne Cartwright (see short Bibliography) which have gone into general practice very thoroughly. For her last survey, published in 1981 – *General Practice*

Revisited – she wrote to 1,000 GPs and was able to interview 836. I have used her work throughout the book to substantiate, correct, add to or contrast with anything I found myself.

My sample was relatively small. I also suspect it had another defect – it was probably too good. I obtained a large number of my GPs by writing to the medical press; others I met through various forms of introduction. On the whole, one would suppose a GP would be unlikely to write and express willingness to be interviewed if he or she was unconfident or guilty about their competence as a doctor. Similarly, people, whether doctors or not, didn't often suggest I see a doctor because he was useless. Nevertheless I was aware of this drawback and did a good deal of ferreting around to remedy it – with some success. Also, a GP's view of his or her own skill and effectiveness was not always the same as that of an objective observer. And there was always Anne Cartwright – though in this respect I think she may, though to a lesser degree, be open to the same criticism and for the same reason.

But is it in fact possible to define a 'good' GP? Hesse Sachs, working in the Margery Jeffreys unit at the Department of Medical Sociology, Bedford College, did not think so. She had spent seven years doing an in-depth research into general practice. This had not been published when I was writing and with great generosity she gave me a lengthy interview, and her findings enrich the book at several points. But one of the aims of the research was to define a good GP. Hesse Sachs had finally decided, she said, that it wasn't possible to draw up a 'seventeen-point Hippocratic scale. Too many factors, too many variables. I wouldn't spend any more of my life looking for that philosopher's stone.'

There are over 20,000 GPs. I hope I have managed to give some idea of their work and lives, but the subject is simply too large to be fully covered in a single book – at least if it is to be published at anything like an economic price. It wasn't even remotely possible to use all my material. 256 hours of talking, even severely edited, produced over three quarters of a million words of typed interview. Yet further condensation still resulted in a book over 43,000 words too long. I was forced to cut out a great deal. Reluctantly, a section devoted to the GP's relations with consultants went (since this was often illustrated in other sections); so did another on the Royal College of General Practitioners. I had to cut out material which was often of great interest, but of limited application. Thus I lost a description of patient participation (and so lost a long and stimulating discussion with Dr Peter Pritchard) and an account of the curious illnesses which can afflict group practices and health centres. This last has been analysed in a book called *Sick Health Centres*, which I have put in the Bibliography (together with a reference to reading on patient participation.)

I found a good deal of prejudice among British-born doctors against those born overseas. It was difficult to ascertain how accurate this was because overseas doctors are very much under-represented in my sample. I do not think this is altogether my fault. If you exclude Irish-born doctors, overseas doctors constitute 23.1 per cent of the total NHS complement, and 16.2 per cent of GPs. I should, therefore, in a sample of fifty, have included eight overseas GPs. Although none had responded to my letters in the medical press, I managed to find six names and wrote to them a month before I set out across England, Wales and Scotland on the main thrust of my research. Two never answered, two answered a month after I'd returned, one I saw. The sixth answered very late, but I could just have seen her. But most professional writers are dogged by intense money and time anxieties; when it did become possible to see her my own had really gone over the top and had become furies driving me to get on.

I should like to thank Karl Sabbagh, late of the MSD Foundation, for valuable suggestions as to who I should see; Margaret Hammond and the other librarians at the Royal College of General Practitioners for their unstinting help; Dr Ian Battye who read the manuscript and corrected its many errors; and Sandra den Hertog for interpreting, and then typing, tapes often so faint or chaotic my respondents could well have been replying from the moon.

But my main thanks are due to the GPs themselves, whose book this is. Generous with their time though usually hard-pressed, often putting me up for periods of two, three and once five days, allowing me to sit-in on their surgeries and accompany them on their visits – I can do no more than give them my heartfelt gratitude.

And it is these very men and women, whom I should above all thank individually, whose names I undertook not to divulge. Only three of the names in the book are in fact those of the doctors concerned: Dr Lane, from whose excellent *The Diary of a Medical Nobody* I quote, Dr Julian Tudor Hart, and Professor David Morrell. They who I can thank in person must stand in for all the others to whom I have given false names, just as their practices (though obviously of a similar type) are not even remotely near where I place them. To facilitate recognition there is a complete list with short descriptions of all the GPs at the end of the book.

I
INTRODUCTORY: THE PAST

The emergence of the general practitioner, as we would recognize him now, and in large numbers, is extremely muddled. It took place over time and from a number of different, though usually related roots, during the first two thirds of the nineteenth century.

In 1800, the undisputed leaders of the medical profession were the physicians. These had their Royal College, had to have a university degree (usually Oxford or Cambridge), and to have studied physic for five years. They practised in hospitals and, as far as outside work went, restricted themselves almost entirely to the wealthy middle and upper classes – the 'carriage trade'.

Below the physicians came the surgeons. Evolving from the barber surgeons of the middle ages, these had formed the Company of Surgeons in Henry VIII's reign. In 1800, this became the Royal College of Surgeons. Aside from heroic surgery in times of war, and work in charitable hospitals, these, too, largely confined themselves to the well off.

For centuries the poor, the vast mass of the population, received virtually no genuine specialist attention at all. They relied on itinerant quacks, and local 'wise' men or women. These were sometimes the repository of valuable, usually herbal, knowledge: digitalis from foxgloves, aspirin from willow bark, morphine from poppies. More often it was mumbo-jumbo – concocting ghastly potions or slapping on foul poultices.

However, during the eighteenth century, the apothecary's job of making-up and dispensing drugs led naturally to the prescribing and then practising of medicine. By the 1800s three strands had evolved: apothecaries who dispensed; those who both dispensed and practised medicine; and apothecary surgeons who did both medicine and surgery, and now often took the new diploma of the still fairly new Royal College of Surgeons.

By 1814 these last were so numerous that for the first time (as far as I can discover) the term 'general practitioner' – meaning one who practised both medicine and surgery – entered the language. The 'general practitioners throughout England and Wales', said Robert Keirison, are 'so [numerous] that the health of at least nineteen out of every twenty patients is now regulated by them.'

The picture is one of continual if rough and ready upward movement and specialization. As the apothecaries stumbled towards medicine, so the role of *pure* drug dispensers and makers-up became sketchily filled. During the eighteenth century, this began to be taken over by the chemists and druggists, themselves rising from the wholesale drug sellers – the 'drugmen' or 'drugsters' of the seventeenth century.

During the first half of the nineteenth century attempts were made to regulate these haphazard developments; usually attempts by the apothecaries to become more 'medical', while the two 'superior' branches of medicine struggled to remain uncontaminated.

In 1815 the Apothecaries Act pulled them all under the Society of Apothecaries. They had to be over twenty-one, to have received 'five years apprenticeship', testimonials of character and medical knowledge, and they had to make up any medicines prescribed by the physicians.

You could now practise medicine as a 'general practitioner' if you were either a Licentiate of the Society of Apothecaries or a Member of the Royal College of Surgeons or both. (In fact you could still practise medicine provided you didn't *call* yourself apothecary, surgeon or physician. The same is still true in essence today.)

This Act, leaving the surgeons and physicians intact, meant the apothecaries were still very much 'trade'. They were *compelled* to make up medicines for the physicians, and were thus virtually his servants, the licence to practise was simply something they could choose or not, as they liked.

Two court decisions advanced them further. In 1830, an apothecary was allowed to charge fees for attendance as well as supplying medicines. In 1834, he was defined as 'one who professes to judge of internal disease by symptoms and applies himself to cure disease by medicine.'

Throughout this same period the standards of education were gradually raised. Courses of lectures on chemistry, physics and the theory and practice of medicine were instituted, examinations introduced and then refined. More and more schools and hospitals were approved for teaching by the Society of Apothecaries (over 140 before 1830).

One of the most important, but most difficult, areas was that of anatomy, dissection and physiology, since here the knowledge was certain (as it was not elsewhere); but more particularly because this, the area of surgery, was the one foothold the apothecaries could gain on one of the main established branches of medicine. The great problem here was the acute shortage of bodies from which to teach the ever-growing number of students.

By 1820, in the great teaching hospitals, it had become a race between relatives and students. At Bart's, wrote Sir Robert Christian, 'It was no uncommon occurrence that when the operator proceeded with his work the body was sensibly warm, the limbs not yet rigid, the blood in the great vessels fluid and coagulable.'

He remembered his horror as a student when present at the dissection of a man who had died suddenly an hour before. When, with a flourish, the demonstrating surgeon made the first masterly incision, slicing in one go from top to bottom of the sternum, fluid blood gushed in abundance. Young Christian seized the lecturer's wrist; 'Nor was I easily persuaded to let him go when I saw the blood coagulate on the table exactly like living blood.'

This was the period of grave-robbing, since the hospitals and schools paid a good deal of money for a precious, fresh body. Grave-robbing posed problems in law since a dead body was not an object of property. Bridgeman's patent iron coffin was invented. Grave-watchers were often employed until the body had sufficiently decomposed.

In Edinburgh, Robert Knox was a brilliant lecturer and anatomical demonstrator. He paid £2 10s a body (about £64 50p at today's prices) and on 29 November 1827 a man called William Hare suddenly thought of recovering a debt of £4 from a deceased tenant of his by selling the body. This he did and – the grisly tale is well known but still grips – soon realized he'd hit on a simple source of income. He teamed up with a man called Burke and they devised the system of 'burking'. This meant getting their victims drunk and then suffocating them. At least sixteen people were murdered, one of whom was a young girl, beautiful but of easy ways. She was recognized by several students when lying on the dissecting table.

As a result, Burke and Hare were apprehended. Another corpse was found in a box in Knox's rooms and the public outcry ruined his career. Hare escaped death by turning King's Evidence. Burke was hanged. His body, after being cut down, was handed over to the hospitals for the students to dissect.

The Anatomy Act of 1832 recognized that 'a legal supply of bodies was necessary for the proper teaching of medicine'. After this the bodies of those in public institutions who had no known relatives were handed over for anatomy lessons. The Act laid down that afterwards the fragments should be 'decently interred'. (This is still a source of bodies. Each student requires about three quarters of a body. A school with a yearly entry of 100 students will need about seventy-five bodies. A fairly large proportion of these will have willed their bodies for the study of medicine.)

In the 1830s, there were still twenty-one ways of entering the medical profession: eleven universities, nine medical corporations (colleges, royal colleges, and incorporated societies like that of the apothecaries) and on the say-so of the Archbishop of Canterbury.

It would be tedious to trace the rending administrative battles through which these august institutions defended, but slowly lost, their autonomy. But the years after 1850 saw the gradual and final emergence of the general practitioner.

An Act of 1858 created a central governing body – the General Council of Medical Education and Registration. This started a register, which allowed those on it to practise anywhere in Britain. Apart from the physicians, who had their own exam, you still had to become a Licentiate of the Society of

Apothecaries or a Member of the Royal College of Surgeons. In 1879 the SA and RCS combined their exam. Finally, in 1884, the physicians allowed the *hoi polloi* to join them. From then on, and for the next sixty years, the most common qualification for a GP was the conjoint diploma of the two main colleges – Membership of the Royal College of Surgeons, Licentiate of the Royal College of Physicians, MRCS, LRCP.

The physical picture of the apothecary/GP from 1879 on was like this (it was described by W.Rivington in *The Medical Profession*★).

At the bottom was the surgeon-chemist. He did the work of a medical man and carried on the trade of a chemist, but it was this last he depended on – a shop with toothbrushes, soap, nail brushes, hair tonic and so on.

Next came the surgeon-apothecary. They held open surgery, signalled by a red lamp. They did no retail trading, but they would often dispense. They would charge a shilling or so for medicine and advice; and visit for a weekly sum from a penny to a shilling. Dispensing doctors have never entirely disappeared, but as he became grander, the surgeon-apothecary's surgery would go out of sight. Finally he would join the non-dispensing GP of the 1890s. His medicine would be made up by the chemist. He had a brass plate and a surgery in the house. The bulk of his work was visiting, when he charged fees much lower than the grand society physicians. This is a figure common up into the late 1930s and still just recognizable sometimes today.

There are three observations which should be made about, or derived from this extremely sketchy history. The development of the apothecary into the general practitioner was unique to this country. On the Continent, for example, apothecaries remained pure pharmacists.

But this genesis in fact explains some fundamental aspects of general practice, even today. The main point about the apothecaries is that they were not rich. They became doctors in order to earn their living. Already in the eighteenth century, workers were banding together for mutual aid. By 1900 there were some seven million in these Friendly Societies. Part of their contributions were used by the societies to engage a doctor who, in return for a fixed per capita sum a year, would look after the members of the society. Enlightened mass employers often did the same. It was this principle which Lloyd George took over for his Insurance Act of 1911, whereby the breadwinners of families under a certain income had their doctoring paid for (their families continued to rely on the Friendly Societies.) The principle finally became enshrined as the basis of the National Health Service in 1948.

The result of this was that British general practitioners became rooted in local communities with stable registered populations. These populations experienced and learned to value the concept of continuous care through a lifetime. But the doctor, although naturally faced with all the emergencies of illness, also learnt that patients and their health could not be isolated from

★Fawin & Co., Dublin, 1879

home and work and time. The environmental and longitudinal views of medicine have existed in general practice for many years.

Furthermore, the doctor had contracted to provide, initially and until they went beyond his scope, for all the patient's medical needs. As a result, British doctors have remained primary generalists, and have not, as in some countries where there was only a fee system, evolved into primary specialists.

One might note, incidentally, that this particular and peculiar development makes nonsense historically of a criticism often levelled by GPs in private practice against the NHS – that because it is largely based on a capitation fee for each patient, there is no incentive to do good doctoring. The GP gets paid whatever he does. I do not mean there may not be force in the argument, only that if so, the system has been operating over a substantial part of British medicine for 150 years.

The second thing to note about the financial aspect of the apothecary/GP is that depending entirely on low-paying working-class Friendly Society and panel patients (the Lloyd George breadwinners) meant a very low income. There were fairly large numbers of these '6d' doctors, poor themselves, treating only the poor. But there were also very large numbers of GPs who had mixed practices, as now. There are no reliable statistics in this field, but as far as I can judge something like two thirds of the doctors in general practice combined middle- and upper-class patients with poorer ones (in the 1890s it was recognized that a new doctor *carved his reputation* among the poor, and upon this built up a group of wealthier patients) It is clear from interviews that by the 1930s a practice with 10 per cent to 15 per cent of its patients from the wealthier classes would expect to draw over 50 per cent of its income from them. Scales of suggested charges indicate that a similar situation existed at the end of the nineteenth century. It was this that enabled GPs to charge poorer patients fees that were approximately within reach, or accept them for the small per capita payments I've described.

And, clearly, this too weakens, though it does not wholly refute, another attack levelled at the NHS – that because people don't personally and immediately pay the amount towards treatment that would cover its cost, they behave irresponsibly. Subsidized medicine – in this case the rich paying for the poor – has also been a major element in British medicine for over 100 years.

Finally, until well into the twentieth century, really until the end of the 1930s, formal medicine was largely impotent in the face of serious disease. The doctor could reassure the patient and console the relatives, but he was biologically as ineffective, if socially as necessary, as the parson or undertaker.

All occupations are to a considerable extent hereditary. Judges' sons become lawyers, the daughters of teachers take to teaching, plumbers' sons plumb. But the peculiar intensity of doctors' lives, the way this both isolates and elevates their families, the markedly scientific bias of their education (and doctorly bent to their conversation) all, it seems to me, have the effect of intensifying this well attested human tendency. It is not at all unusual to find, at various times, that three quarters of the students at some London teaching hospitals come from the families of doctors or from families that contain doctors. At Marlborough today there is a family which has held a local practice in unbroken line back to 1750. I know of at least two other practices in the south of England which go back to the mid eighteenth century.

This meant that during my interviews – quite by chance, it was no part of my purpose – I sometimes came across echoes of the years when the GP finally emerged: the 1890s and first two decades of this century. It is possible to put some flesh on the bones of our brief historical survey.

The figures given in this and subsequent sections for today's values of sums quoted from the past are based on calculations provided by the Central Statistical Office. This is a notoriously difficult and risky task, however, and the results, say the CSO, should only be regarded as impressionistic.

2
1890 – 1920

DR WASING (eighty-nine): 'I remember of course as a small boy there were no motor cars. My father used to go round in a brougham with a chap with a top hat. In fact, my father always wore a top hat and frock coat. Oh yes. And as a little boy I used to go round in the brougham with him you see.

'Going round the town with a brougham of course was a much slower business, and also when my father first started, although he looked after poor patients, there was no panel or anything, it was all private or there was a certain amount of what was known as "clubs", but which the National Health unfortunately – Bevan – destroyed, the Friendly Societies. They were first rate things. It was a cruel thing he did to abolish those Friendly Societies.'

Dr Veryan had a practice in the south of England. It was one of the areas I mentioned where another practice in the little market town went directly back to the 1760s. Dr Veryan remarked as we passed it that older inhabitants had refused to go into their new general hospital because it had incorporated the old workhouse.

DR VERYAN: 'The building, you saw it, was 1792 – but the workhouse system went on till 1928. They hated it, really dreaded it. I remember about ten years ago talking to two ninety-year-olds. They were saying their mother was left with a little cottage, two up and one down. There were ten children and their father died of TB at the age of forty-three, leaving the youngest child of about six months.

'The mother took in washing – she washed it in the boiler in the corner, and the woman next door did the ironing. She said they lived on an absolute pittance. They had to call on parish relief, this was 1890 I suppose, and what she said was that the overseer from here came round – they were allowed a dole of two pounds of bread from one of the shops in the town – they were allowed a certain amount of bread for each child in the family and a slightly smaller amount for mum – and they got 6d a week for every child under twelve. Everybody over twelve had to work.

'The only alternative, when their father died, was to go into the workhouse but then they would be separated from their mother – the boys would anyway. You know the song, "We've Been Together Now for Forty Years", you realize that that was sung when they were being parted to go to the workhouse.'

DR WYRE (Northern country practice – 1912): 'He was the fourteenth child, so they suddenly had to take to working and he was put into medicine and he married just after he qualified and went on a sunny day to this dotty little village in the Cheviots called Glanton and bought the practice for £36 or whatever, and then a year or two later moved down to the bottom of the hill to the market town, Anneck, and stayed there for the next sixty years practising very happily by himself. He started off on a horse, doing his rounds in the hills, this being 1912. The horse threw him in no time on to a stone yard and broke all his teeth, so he then imported the first motorbike that was seen in the neighbourhood, and finally the first car which, of course, broke down on every journey and was usually brought back towed by one of the farm carthorses who were patrolling the roads.

'Really in medicine at that time there was nothing – no medicines had any value. The odd specifics which were of course valuable, like quinine for malaria obviously, which didn't come into the practice. Digitalis – yes. There are some. But for most diseases – nothing. They used the most elaborate mixtures, all herbs. Sometimes heavy metals which the chemist would compound up. My father used a lot of mortars, the powders all ground up with a little gum, and then there were the relevant pill rollers. Tablets hadn't come in then.

'They were always being got up at night. They were always turning out – in the early days turning out on horses and clopping up the lane. They really worked very hard. The breakfast and lunch gaps were peppered with patients coming into the house to his surgery, so every time we sat down to eat, father would have to disappear. They treated the patients with almost patronizing roughness, dismissed pretty briefly, while they clutched their forelocks and went off. The miners used to come in – there were seats in the waiting room but they never sat on them, they always sat on their hunkers, as they said – they didn't have any seats at home. And after a few exchanges in broad Northumbrian, they went away with a prescription because, of course, Lloyd George's panel system had come in just about . . . It was 1912 I think – just almost after father had started. So to some extent he was a panel doctor, although most of his practice was farmers, farm labourers who weren't in on that.

'He enjoyed the life, he enjoyed it very much, even though he had so little interest in medicine itself. He liked country people. He liked knowing about whose parsnips weren't going well.

'He went on, I think, until he was about eighty-eight – late eighties. And then he stopped on a cold day – Northumberland is pretty bleak and winters go on for ever. He'd got a bit of flu or something, or he got asthma badly, and the neighbouring GP said, "I'll look after your practice", and father handed him the practice over and then rather regretted it of course when the sun came out and he wanted something to get him out of the house.

'He was toughish. But anyway, he had a home help to help him cooking – his hands got a bit shaky. The home help went on holiday and he went into hospital and then suddenly after the four days were up, the home help was back, he was going back and he was caught at the bottom of the stairs. "I can't think why I'm wheezing. I must have got some fluid in my lungs," tapping himself, you know, the self-diagnosing doctor, and the other doctor said, "I suppose you have. You'd better go upstairs." And he went upstairs and died slowly as the fluid level crept up. The GP tapped him and it was half an inch higher and at that rate it would be another twenty-four hours so the doctor rang Peter and me and we turned up and he died a few hours later. But he was very comfortable.'

DR STANE (The Orkneys and Shetlands, 1910): 'At night, in a motor boat – an emergency up in the Islands, somebody very ill, you had to get in a motor boat or rowing boat, four men rowing. When you think of it – the old doctor there, who I remember so well – never had a car in his life, in my boyhood day there. I can see him still in his knickerbockers and gaiters up there, a great big walking stick, a pipe, and a hat on. Time after time we've been to those islands there in an open sailing boat before motors came. By God, they were tough people, they were. Now they've got a helicopter.'

I learned about Dr Quainton with some excitement. He was ninety-four *and still practising!* This surely argued at least some clearness of mind. In one jump, I could hear at first hand an account of general practice in 1910. (I had a subsidiary interest in old GPs hanging on and clogging up the inner cities.)

I was met at the door by an incredibly old figure, bent double over two sticks. He had a few grey hairs, still, round a brown skull spotted with age, a quavery voice; but the eyes were alert enough.

He gestured me into the adjoining consulting room. It was large and dusty, with two long windows hung with slightly tattered dark blue velvet curtains looking on to what was still a smart street. There was a fireplace with a large marble mantelpiece covered in photographs. Above it, a massive oil painting of the Charge of the Light Brigade. Between the windows was an old desk and a leather swivel chair, flanked along the wall by a large sofa. There was another large sofa at the back of the room, covered in pale brown velvet; perhaps for examinations. It was all dusty and crowded, but a fine big old room.

I wandered about, taking all this in and wondering what was keeping Dr Quainton. But, as from the side I saw his hands appearing through the door, I realized it was the actual process of getting into the room that was occupying him. Hands were followed by sticks, arms and legs, and very, very slowly Dr Quainton hove into view. There was a good deal of muddle while we decided where I was to sit. Finally I sat at his desk while he subsided into the sofa.

I realized quite soon I had come too late. The marbles had begun to roll. His memory had more or less gone, as had his hearing, and I have extracted what little pith there was from a long, rambling interview. He'd been doctor to one of the kings before he became king, but I couldn't pin down if it was George V or VI. The tape is punctuated by my yelled questions.

When it was over, I let myself out. Dr Quainton waved feebly from the sofa, too weak to get up. He said he *was* still practising, on old patients who remembered him. The DHSS, who must have been desperate, had removed him from the NHS the year before, on the pretext that he could not do 'visits night and day as required'. It seemed academic somehow.

DR QUAINTON: 'I first started practising in 1912. It's much simpler now. Then there were all those drugs. Today we always write an antibiotic or something like that: just penicillin, one three times a day. Or twice a day.

'It's so much simpler. The difference between the two, now, wait, I've got to sort this out; the difference between the two is that it was all done clinically. In those days we didn't use the laboratory or the X-ray to the extent they use it today. Now you go to a hospital and complain about anything in your stomach, they do a barium meal and take a picture.

'I was in the Navy in the first war and then I was in the Army, during the wars. I spent five years in Mexico. I was in charge of a hospital in Mexico, Tampeco, and then I was in Mexico City for four years, practising medicine. Then I came back here and I've been very successful ever since. As you can see by where I live. I never expected to live as long as this. I'm ninety-four – nearly ninety five.'

From the mid twenties on the testimony is increasingly abundant, and from then until today there are themes we can follow: the introduction and results of the NHS; the near collapse of general practice in the early sixties leading to the Doctors' Charter of 1966*; the growth of group practice and health centres; the changes in medicine; the increase in women GPs; vocational training, and so on.

But a total chronological approach isn't really possible or appropriate. For one thing, a vigorous GP of seventy-five still working could have begun to

*The 'Charter for the Family Doctor Service' was worked out by Dr (later Sir) James Cameron, then Chairman of the BMA's General Medical Services Committee, and his colleagues one hectic weekend at Brighton in 1965. It stated that general practice must remain a family doctor service; that the GP must have adequate time for each patient; be able to keep up to date; must have complete clinical freedom; have adequate well-equipped premises; have all the diagnostic, social service and ancillary aids he needs; be encouraged to acquire additional skills in special fields; be adequately paid by a method acceptable to him and which encourages him to do his best for his patients; have a working day which leaves him some leisure.

This has formed the basis in principle for all subsequent improvement in the GP service, from the massive reforms accepted by GPs in June 1966 to those as recent as 1982, when GP training became mandatory.

practise in 1935. The tale of his life cuts through our period in one swoop. We shall meet several such. The enormous variety of practice in Britain often makes a nonsense of history. Given the changes in medicine and therefore disease, a practice in the remote north of Scotland is much the same, the tempo is much the same as it was in 1930; a rich private practice in London or Edinburgh is much as it was in 1950; inner-city violence and squalor are not new. And there are too many aspects of doctors' lives which are timeless, and where it is more interesting to compare what they say together: their experiences of and reaction to birth and death; how they cope with the stress of their lives, and the nature of that stress; their feelings about their patients, and many more.

But I hope that as they talk and talk, often late into the night, as you meet doctors who dislike their job and doctors who love it, as you discover the nature of their so different practices, as you sit in on their consultations, follow them on visits or race through the night in response to some panic call, there will gradually emerge for you, as there did for me, a sense of what it is like to be a GP, of what their lives are like.

Nevertheless, I shall start in the late 1920s and 1930s. There is a continuity between that period and the twenty or thirty years before that, which we have just glanced at; there is a corresponding continuity forward into the 1950s. Medicine changed, but styles of doctoring, patterns of visiting and other things, lingered on. And quite apart from the fascination of the past, there are aspects of general practice in those decades it is salutary to be reminded of. To recall the poverty and suffering that still existed then; how recent and how dramatic are the benefits of improved housing, drainage and water supply and the chemo-therapy revolution of the late forties and fifties; but above all, perhaps, how, often unable to cure, doctors devoted themselves selflessly to succouring their patients, how long and hard and late they worked, and how close, as a result, the bonds with their patients became.

3
THE TWENTIES, THIRTIES AND FORTIES

Glasgow in the Twenties

DR STANE: 'I qualified in the winter of '26 – '27, that's right. It was a slum practice, actually, and that was an eye opener, in the East End of Glasgow. It was terrible, terrible. It nearly killed me.

'In the Gorbals, actually, and Bridgetown. And the man who I was assistant to was also the police surgeon for the Gorbals district, so I was assistant police surgeon at the same time. And believe you me, on a Saturday night after a Celtic and Rangers match you didn't have to look far for trouble.

'And one of the awful things, that was the time of that awful drink, you know, red Biddy – have you ever heard of red Biddy? It was cheap red wine and methylated spirits. They were knocked out in no time, and we used to pump their stomachs out.

'And the odd thing was, in the morning when I gave them a drink of water, the water flushed out the alcohol *tanned into* the wall of their stomachs and they'd be drunk at once, just for a short while. But the tragedy was a lot got blind with it. It went to their eyes.

'I remember one drunk. He refused to leave when I was at his wife's confinement. I went into the other three 'houses' on the landing and told the women. He got the beating of his life.

'Yes, you see, that was the terrible state of affairs. So many people lived in one-room tenements. Four doors on each floor, with a one-room "house". This is a God's honest fact. They were eleven storeys high; there was one lavatory in the passage. They were born, slept and died in these places. One room.

'Bigger families went to bed in relays. Eight in the bed and sixteen on their feet. And that's where they lived and died. And I have actually seen, in some of these places, not a lot, but I have actually seen it; I've seen a coffin on a table with a body in it and the remains of the breakfast round about. This was in 1927 – fifty years ago . . . fifty-five. You just can't believe it, but it's quite true. Quite true.

'You'd do a confinement on the floor, on a pallet of straw many slept on, with a chamber pot to wash your instruments.

'It was hard work, I will say. I've seen ninety in his surgery – doing them three at a time at the end. But he put as much as he could on his assistant. I never had one day off – perhaps a half. Everything was tram-car or walk. At night, walking through the slums of the Gorbals; it was scaring because it was the time of the razor slashing gangs. They'd slash from ear to mouth. I was never attacked, *never*. You had your little black bag in your hand and it would take you anywhere. Us and the lassies of the Salvation Army.

'The mortality of the kids was sky high. Frightful. They died from what they called green diarrhoea – gastroenteritis. There was no hospital for them. They died in the summer. And the mortality from lobar-pneumonia (pneumonia in one lobe of a lung) was about 43 per cent. As high as that.

'I stuck it as long as I could, then I left. It sickened you, made you very Bolshie.'

A Country Practice – Late Twenties and Thirties

After Glasgow, Dr Stane went to two country practices. The relief in his voice was palpable as he went on to describe this. He was, at eighty-one, of medium height, bald, very alert, modest, humorous. Although he had been in Lincolnshire for fifty years he still had a marked Scots accent. He had been born in the Orkneys, had run away to sea when he was fifteen and a half to fight in the First World War. 'They'd take anything on two legs *then*.' His grandfather had been captain of one of the last clippers and his father had also been in the Navy. The house was hung with purchases from the Far East: lacquer panels, figurines, a large bronze incense burner in the hall. A spacious, comfortable house, very tidy and neat.

The first of his country practices was in Fife.

DR STANE: 'And then I went to a country practice, where it was so different it wasn't true. I was there for six months, and the old chap when I went there, he still kept a pony and trap, and a very nice nag for the country practice in the hills, where there's no roads. And much of your stuff you'd carry in your pockets, or in the saddle-bags; it was awfully nice actually – in the good weather. And there was the doctor's *man* who looked after everything.

'That was family doctoring at its best, there's no doubt about it, it was. You knew them all. The old man I was with, he was quite old, he'd started and done all his practice in the area. He'd brought the young ones on to earth, he'd tended the old people, he'd tended the children's children, and so on.

'Anyway, I came here [the Lincolnshire practice] and he says, "You come here on six months' approbation with a view to partnership." So I was there, with the six months nearly up, and I said, "Look here, what does the partnership cost?" This was in 1931. It staggered me. He said £3,000. (About £57,000 by today's values.) I didn't have a bean in the world. "Well," I said, "that's curtains as far as I'm concerned. I haven't got it. I'll just have to back out quietly." And it was the biggest compliment I'd ever had paid in my life. "Well," he said, "I like you, and I've seen your work and it's very, very good

and you're just exactly what we want, and I'll guarantee you at the bank."
Very nice, my God, yes, that's what he did. And I got married in the
meantime, and my wife helped tremendously, because a doctor's wife can.
She had nothing to offer, I mean financially, because her father had been
killed in the First World War. He was a farmer actually.'

The Diseases

DR STANE: 'The pony and trap had just gone from the practice. We all had
cars, but the roads of course were more empty. You went round to the
various villages, where in many there weren't telephone boxes and in one the
local postmistress used to take messages and wasn't she a card? I used to go
there and ask if there were any messages for me. "Oh, so-and-so", the name,
"came in the small hours of the morning and wanted me to send for you. I
said, 'You go home. I will not phone the man at this hour. You'd have crazed
the life out of him.' "

'And if it was very cold she wouldn't call me out. She'd refuse to. "What!
Call him out on a night like this? Certainly not." Luckily, no one died.

'But we worked damned hard, let me tell you. We were meant to have a
month's holiday, which I never had. None of us did. If you got away for a
fortnight you were lucky. We had no sort of set half days, you were on call
twenty-four hours a day.

'You got the old lobar-pneumonia – you just don't see it now. It took five
to ten days – the three stages. The invasion of pneumonia – the grey
hepatization, the lung grey and solid. Then it becomes red – a red sputum,
you cough up blood, a haemorrhage into it. Now you watched – a pulse rate
of 120, and a blood pressure less than that, you could write that patient off.
The heart was being poisoned with the pneumonia toxin. You won't find
that in the textbooks, that's an observation. Finally, the crisis. The
temperature fell with a bang, pouring with sweat. Recovery.

'You went, och, twice, three times a day, to see them. Aye, and sometimes
in the middle of the night if there was a crisis near and you gave them
strychnine, camphor and oil – supposed to be a very good stimulus to the
heart and, oh, lots of things. You treated the patient because you couldn't
treat the disease. You'd get their strength up – you did all you could do to
keep them going. And sleep was essential, and then of course you came up
against the thing when they're getting near the end, was it safe to give much
morphia or not? And you could only judge that by the pulse and one thing or
another. Because sleep was essential. And we didn't get all these fancy things
for sleep as we have now. It was usually an injection of morphine et hyoscine,
or something like that. Yes, it made them sleep. And you didn't dare give too
much in case they popped out. It wasn't dead easy. It's a thing you could only
acquire by seeing many cases of it.

'Very few in the surgery. Very few people came to the doctor's house. But people who got ill, you went to see them, you saw them out, you naturally did.

'There were fevers – typhoid, para-typhoid, scarlet fever, diphtheria. The ambulance was drawn by a horse – there was no hurry with a fever.

'Diphtheria – a tremendous mortality. On a par with pneumonia, one third. You'd go two or three times a day. You'd nothing to give them, specific. We used to give them anti-diphthetic serum. I don't know whether it worked. Some got better; a lot died.

'And TB. That's gone in my time. In most of the little villages, you found one or two houses with shelters, for them to sleep outside in, supplied by the county. Any amount of those. I went round them all. Every so often the TB officer came round, to see the dying patients. And the big hospitals had these huge sanatoria, now closed.

'Then came streptomycin PAS, and the rest of it, and TB vanished, just like that. Pneumonia's gone, scarlet fever, diphtheria's gone. All gone. These are the things that took up your time in medicine.

'It meant a lot of work, indeed it did. You were always out – late at night often. I've done forty, fifty visits a day. But we all accepted it. You knew nothing else. We went into medicine knowing that's what life meant. But there was a lot to recommend it, you know. There was, there was indeed. You got to know your patients intimately and they either trusted you or they didn't, and went elsewhere. You knew all the little bits and bobs about their body.

'And of course you were a friend. They came with all manner of problems. Whether little Johnny should go in the police force, or would he make a good doctor or a priest or what have you.

'They didn't mind what you said once you'd got to know them. I remember this old thing who was always getting me out, always ailing. I'd been here many years by this time. I went out once again, and she said, "I don't want to bother you, but every bone in my body is aching." I said, "If I were you, I'd get down on my knees and thank God I wasn't a herring."

'And you were the *family* doctor. You knew them all so well. Life was quieter, no distractions. When I arrived they'd only just given up the pony and trap. The stables were still here. You'd stop and chat as you drove. Always had a cup of tea. I was always having to stop behind the first hedge.'

The Medicines

DR WASING: 'My father, I think it was 1897 he qualified, I qualified in 1928. There was practically no difference in medical knowledge in '28 than there was when my father qualified in '97.

'I remember when I first came to our practice here (in one of the large seaside towns of the South Coast), we had all sorts of harmless liquids we used, which we dispensed. There was Mist Explo. A dilution of yellow picric acid crystals, bright yellow. The crystals used to explode if left in the air. Hence the name – Mist Explosive. Out of 2s 6d a bottle we made 220,000 per cent profit.

'We knew we could do practically nothing. We gave sympathy and reassurance, and the necessary virtue was patience. For congestive heart failure, these old girls I remember, was digitalis washed down with a quarter bottle of champagne. It kept the status quo, but they could only just hobble across the room on swollen legs.'

DR STANE: 'Well, you used your placebos. We had a lot. White aspirins, green aspirins and blue ones. We had a mixture of lactose, you know, milk sugar which was dissolved. Some we put some stuff in it to give it a horrible taste, some we didn't.

'In fact we used no end of stuff, you know. We had long lectures on *Materia Medica*. You don't get these things nowadays. We had every drug from every plant and every weed that grew. What was made from it. We made them in the surgery – your mixtures, your concoctions, your infusions. You name them, they were all there, all used.

'For neurotics we only had a mixture of potassium bromide and valarium. The smell rather reminded you of a cat on the ground. I always felt you must be feeling pretty bad to drink that stuff.

'Did any of those linctuses help? Strychnine in the tonic? I don't know. But, you know, there's such a thing as the *vis medicatrix naturae* – the healing force of nature. Old Sir John Craven always said to us – "Remember, 90 per cent of your patients will get better whether you treat them or not. Never give them anything that may be likely to harm them; 7 per cent or 8 per cent will require a little attention and some skill; 2 per cent are going to die anyway. But the healing force of nature is the one thing you've got to remember." A lot of truth in that.'

DR WASING: 'I shall never forget, and I'm sure no general practitioner of my generation will ever forget, the first time they used what was called M and B in those days, in the case of a roaring pneumonia. It was *dramatic*. We used to call two or three times a day or more, and there was a chap sitting up in bed, panting for his breath, looking blue, temperature of 105, you gave him these things and I'd say, "Give him four of those now and then two every four hours", and you'd call next morning carrying your death certificates with you and you'd have a chap sitting up in bed; he'd have a *profuse* sweat, and he was a good colour, cough was loose, he wasn't panting for breath. *Dramatic*. It's altered since then, but I shall never forget.'

The Operations
Dr Chathill came to the same rural/urban practice as his father in the mid

forties. I saw the operating theatre, in the 100-year-old cottage hospital, where fractures had been set. It was small, clean, with tiled walls and a little sink – like a country vet's theatre. In the middle was a narrow, articulated operating table upon which the patients lay, chunky with its chromium knobs.

DR CHATHILL: 'Times have changed, you know, because my father was saying this chap, his senior partner, his treatment of fractures hadn't changed from the chap who taught him, who learnt his in the Crimean War. He didn't believe in anaesthetics for surgical fractures; he said it was soft and dangerous. And his obstetrics were, well, brutal, to say the least of it. This was in the early twenties, but he lasted until the mid-thirties. He retired about '35.'

Yet the senior partner may have had a point. One of the most dangerous things about operations was still, then, the anaesthetic.

DR STANE: 'Chloroform was the safest one from that point of view – but it was deadly stuff you know. After a big operation they were vomiting for days afterwards, and half of them died from liver poisoning. Of course people wouldn't accept that, but half of them vomited their way out. You gave them a quarter grain of morphine and some atropine to knock them out, and then you gave them the chloroform. And in the process of going from the conscious to the unconscious, they became violent as they were on the table, especially with an alcoholic. Actually, the patients never knew this, we actually tied them down, with a broad belt. If you didn't they would have thrown themselves off.'

DR CHATHILL: 'There was a gauze mask on a metal frame and you dropped the ether on to it. It was quite an art actually, to get someone under. They used to fight like blazes because they thought they were suffocating.
    'Later I was taught to give ether through a machine without pentothal. You had to get exactly the right balance of ether and oxygen so that it put them out quickly with a lot of ether, and then lifted the ether and put in the oxygen before they suffocated themselves. I never killed anybody.'

They did far more, in their little cottage hospitals, than set bones. Dr Stane remembers doing all acute abdominal surgery – appendicectomies, hernias, amputations if necessary, hysterectomies and Caesarian sections. And it was all in the local community. 'What made you careful, put the brakes on, was you knew you'd have to live with it – with a botched job.'
    One of the most unpleasant things in rural areas was osteomyelitis, usually got from a blow, a kick, to the bone. Pus went on and on coming from holes in the bone.

DR STANE: 'You never see it now. I hated doing it. The common thing was the tibia and the femur. You got at the tibia with a chisel and gutted the bone from one end to the other. You dug a channel with a hammer and chisel. This is quite true. Osteomyelitis is in the marrow, you see. You have to chip through the cortex, the heavy outside bone, a channel so wide, and chisel out from one end of the bone to the other.

'The surgeon sucked it out – the pus came out. But you couldn't close the wound. The wound had to be packed. It was a disgusting business, I hated doing it. And of course they were ill for months afterwards and some of them died.'

No wonder they were called doctors' 'surgeries'. But many operations took place in the home, on the kitchen table. This was quite usual with minor cysts and tonsils. But GPs would plunge into fairly major surgery, if circumstances warranted it, in outlying cottages and farmhouses.

DR CHATHILL: 'My father had frightful rows with him [the brutal senior partner] because he insisted on using gas to set broken bones. The major row was when he operated on a thyroid. Someone was dying of it, you did die of thyrotoxicosis in those days. And the senior partner was just leaving him. He didn't know what else to do. So my father – he'd learnt the operation from the inventor, his boss Sir Thomas Dunhill – he got an anaesthetist down from London and he went out on his motorbike, and got the fellow down on the kitchen table and damn well took his thyroid out, which is a thing that only a major unit should even think of tackling now, with blood transfusions. The lot. And the man survived and gave him a car as a present. And when the senior partner came back from his holiday he was absolutely livid and thought he'd taken a liberty with one of his patients.'

DR STANE: 'Yes, tonsils in their homes. On a Sunday morning it was tonsil morning. We went on a tour of the country. Another old chap, we took his eye out in his house. He lived away down on the marshes. I don't think he'd ever been out of there in his life, and he got shingles. I didn't know about it till days afterwards. I had to go and see him and he was still at work. God, those people were tough, they really were as tough as nails. It affected his eye and he got an ulcer – the inside of the eye became infected. And the only thing to do is to take the eye out. And I said, "You can go into hospital to have this done"; "No doctor, you only go into hospital to die, and I'm not going into hospital. If you're going to do it you can come and do it in the house." So I got old Dr Blane that I was talking about, to give the anaesthetic, and took his eye out in the house. Amputated an eye. And then – no district nurse in those days – I had to go out for the first day or two, twice a day, to dress it, seven miles each way. It was all part of the job. And if you're on the road for twelve hours a day, you accepted it.

'Once in Lincoln, I went out with one of the surgeons there to operate in the fens, in a very nice house – a farmer again wouldn't come to the hospital – to do a strangulated hernia in his house. He had a lead from the car for a light. It was all very well done. Dr Bucks, he had a practice as well, a general practitioner surgeon, and a very good man he was.'

DR LANE: 'We were general and orthopaedic surgeons, physicians, obstetricians, gynaecologists and pathologists. We did our own blood transfusions with the antique method of tube and funnel, our own post mortems in primitive conditions and all our maternity in the homes of our patients.'

Money

There seem to have been five grades of patient in the class-conscious thirties, though not every practice would have had all of them. In ascending order, these were:

PARISH: The really poor patient got a note from the Relieving Officer, the dispenser of public funds. This entitled him to free treatment from the parish. Each GP or group took so many. Dr Lane's group of three GPs in a reasonably prosperous West Country practice got £60 a year (about £1,135 at today's values) to see 200 – 300 patients.

CLUB: Members of the working mens' clubs made contracts with GPs to treat wives and children. Typical figures for a year's attendance plus medicine would be, per head, 6s for wives and 3s for children (about £6 and £3 today).

PANEL: Lloyd George's insurance for the breadwinner under an income of £400 (£8000); the Government paid 9s 6d (£8·50) a year.

POOR PRIVATE: These were the poor middle class and desperate working class who had saved. Distinction was made between these four groups and the last group. The poor privates might be greeted politely, and Dr Watts's receptionist/dispenser/assistant would wrap their medicines in white paper. But they were seen in a scruffy back surgery, and hurried through. Dr Lane's dispenser turned her head away when handing non-private patients their medicines as though she might catch some fearful lower class bug.

WELL-OFF PRIVATE: These got the works. The front surgery (if a GP had two). They would, in Dr Watts's case, wait in the dining room among the polished silver and mahogany. Their importance can be judged by the fact that in Dr Lane's practice, and many others, though usually less than 10 per cent numerically, they supplied over half the income. They subsidized the rest of the patients.

One might note a number of things about this state of affairs. The fee system of medicine which prevailed explains the ferocious poaching of patients which was sometimes a feature of general practice then, and which persisted into the fifties and sixties, and which occasionally crops up today. But the competition for patients was a method of keeping doctors on their toes and up to date. It also meant the paying neurotic got more sympathetic attention than they may do today. One doctor told me his practice *depended* on his neurotics, with their regular need for visits and medicine.

£400 a year was about £7,500 at today's (1984) prices, so when doctors talk about collectors after debts they are not always talking about chasing the poverty stricken.

Nevertheless, there was real poverty in the thirties. Even the money for medicines and subscriptions to the clubs could be difficult to find. The wealthy are always healthier than the poor, and the panel, club and poorer privates often required a lot of irritable attention. As a result, the poorer privates often ran up colossal bills. (Most practices had debts of up to – in today's terms – £50,000 when the NHS came in 1948.)

There was no hope of them ever paying these, but in numbers of practices they were regularly sent out nonetheless, often, no doubt, causing considerable anxiety.

There were doctors who relied exclusively on poor patients, and these would not have been very well off. As I remarked earlier, I can find no reliable figures for these. But they were not the majority. If the ten or so elderly GPs I talked to, from whom I select some typical comments below, and the account in Dr Lane's book, are anything like representative, then it is clear a good number of GPs were even better off than they are today.

DR CHATHILL: 'I remember my father's senior partner saying, "Never send in big bills. Send in small bills frequently. Cut and come again." I think they did very nicely.'

DR WASING: 'I'll tell you, when I went into the practice first, in 1931 I think it was, '30 or '31, as assistant to my father, my father said, "I'll pay you £300 a year. And I'll give you a rent-free flat." Well, I'd just married then, and on £300 a year we employed a resident cook general you know, maid. Sherry, a decent sherry, was 3s 6d a bottle, whisky was five bob.'

DR SIMON MARTHAN: 'I got about £2,000 to £3,000 a year. If the collector would come – we had three collectors and they took 10 per cent – and say, "No, doctor, they haven't given me anything for about six or seven weeks" then you'd go and have a talk with them and say "Look here, unless you pay for something, you can't expect me to come and see you and give you medicines." You see, they used to expect you to give medicines as well, for their family.

'For them, it would be 3s 6d a visit with a bottle of medicine. It was fantastic. I always think that 3s 6d a visit was very good. That was in 1925. We didn't have many very, very rich ones. We had some upper middle class. And you found, if you knew a person was an affluent type, then you charged them more – 10s 6d a visit or something like that you see.'

DR STANE: 'The money worried them you see. It actually did. They put off bothering the doctor with a night call until in desperation – about midnight – they'd send. Well, if they couldn't pay we never charged them. Of course we didn't. When I first came here a farm worker in Lincolnshire was paid 28 bob a week. That was the wages. You couldn't charge people on that. In many cases they had Friendly Societies. The Foresters, the Oddfellows, the Royal and Antediluvian Order of Buffalos. The Rational Sick and Burial always amused me. And they paid 1d a week and the doctor got a retainer. So much a quarter. You had to have a whole lot to make anything of it at all.

'But the whole thing has changed. It's had to be because it's been realized that the health of a community is not the business of an individual, it's in charge of the State. It must be. That's not socialism, it's common sense. It must be, and that's how the National Health was started.'

4
THE NHS AND INTO THE FIFTIES

The NHS came in 1948. Although this is not, cannot be, a chronological history – as I explained, the picture will build up haphazardly as the doctors describe their lives – nevertheless some major facets of general practice today are not explicable without reference to the situation after the NHS was set up.

In the first place, GPs are independent operators, each separately *under contract* to the State to provide the service they do. GPs are very keen on their independent contractor status, they get extremely shirty if you mention salaries; partly because they have all the tax advantages of the self-employed. But this independent status also permits the extraordinary freedom and flexibility you find in general practice.

The second thing to bear in mind is what seems to have happened during the fifties. (I say 'seems', because there was no reliable and hard research, like the recent surveys by Anne Cartwright.) In general, GPs appear to have come under increasing strain, leading to a near collapse in the early sixties, the reform worked out between 1964 and 1966 (The Doctors' Charter), and the revival of the last twenty years.

There were three sources of strain. It seems likely that, relieved of financial anxiety, people did come to their doctors in increasing numbers, and that this in turn threw up a good deal of hidden illness. There was some exploitation, but most GPs seem to agree not much.

But people came, more and more, because during the late forties and increasingly in the fifties, the feeling grew that at last *doctors could do something*. It is true that during the twenties and thirties, disease had been on the wane. Mortality from tuberculosis fell from ninety per 1,000 in 1920 to forty per 1,000 by 1950, diphtheria cases from 66,506 in 1921 to 49,432 in 1941. There is no doubt that, over the long term, improvements in living conditions — food, drainage, sewage, water supply, housing – were a more important element than the drug revolution in attacking the diseases that had racked society since before the Middle Ages.

But they were not as dramatic. You will recall Dr Wasing's astonishment and excitement as M and B swept his pneumonia patients to health in the thirties. That figure of 49,432 diphtheria cases in 1941; in 1951 there were 658; in 1962 – fifty-two. By 1960 there were only six TB cases per 100,000. In a few short years, it seemed, scarlet fever, TB, diphtheria, pneumonia, small pox, polio and typhoid were swept away or could be treated like minor upsets. *

The doctors practising then, incidentally, became intoxicated by the pill revolution. It is these GPs who tend to continue wildly prescribing. GPs in their thirties and forties, the post-Thalidomide GPs, are more chary.

But this revolution also began the transformation in the pattern of disease which has been the work of the last thirty years. As the acute died away, people began to live longer, and far more of what remained was the chronic, the diseases and disabilities of old age – heart, arthritis, hypertension and so on.

Also, as the acute faded, people started increasingly coming to the doctor about things which, though they were often allied with or had caused medical problems, were really 'illnesses' due to their psychological, social or familial situation. This is an extremely interesting development and we will explore it more deeply later. For the present, it should just be noted that chronic illnesses and those which are caused by problems of this last sort impose particular and peculiar burdens on GPs, for various reasons. The greatest of these is that they don't easily – with chronic disease often ever – go away. They are not susceptible to the short, sharp, rule-of-thumb therapeutic slash.

Finally, the burdens and unfairnesses of the old system of authoritarian senior partners continued. And so did the pattern of doing a great many home visits, even in the big cities. This latter was partly because the vast extension of car ownership came only slowly, but also because the habits of doctors and patients, in all spheres, rolling now with the momentum of over sixty years, carried them both on deep into the fifties.

A Welsh Rural Practice

Dr Thriplow was fifty-eight (but like a great many GPs looked older); he was bald with a monk's rim of wispy grey hair, rather tanned, with sharp black eyes, quiet voice and a manner humorous and shrewd.

He'd come down west into this deeply rural practice and his voice held pleasing remnants of the North. He talked with great affection of his practice, of their arrival and settling there, and he was a striking example of what I was to observe many times: how a doctor is the one person who can arrive and settle in remote and insular communities and become accepted very quickly indeed; within two or three years, quicker if children are born before this. Their 'doctor' status keeps them forever slightly separate – keeps even native-born figures separate – and so allows strangers quickly into that peculiarly distanced but intimate and vital role.

Branch surgeries, to which he refers, seem to have begun in the nineteenth century when doctors had to cover fairly large areas on horseback. They were by no means only rural. Dr Simon Marthan's predominantly urban practice had three in the thirties. Patients would only walk half a mile or so and if you

* *Office of Health Economics Briefing*, No. 19, September 1982.

didn't have a branch surgery, another doctor would slip in and poach.

Dr Thriplow's family also showed another very common GP characteristic – the resolute denial of any parental influence. Sometimes it was GPs denying their father or mother had any role in their choice of profession. Here it was the children. They said his being a doctor had no bearing *at all* on their choice of career. 'I wouldn't be a doctor for anything.' Yet one daughter was a physiotherapist, one son was going to become a psychologist.

This son – seventeen – to emphasize his independence, also smoked like a chimney.

DR THRIPLOW: 'When I came there was no sanitation, no piped water, no electricity. And no one mentioned a contract. He said, "Right, would you like the job?" No description, no idea of the number of hours you were to do – a brief mention of the cash and that was it. I did all the night calls, most of the surgeries, and almost every weekend on with a young family.

'There was a tiny little waiting room and the surgery – very old-fashioned, big desk. *No* facilities. And sometimes it was hectic. Old Dr Harris would come and sit in on a surgery and we'd have two patients, together, in the same room at the same time. This rather shocked me because we were often talking about fairly intimate things. One of the first innovations I made was that we saw one person at a time in the surgery.

'We had surgeries morning, dinner-time and evening, and Saturday morning and evening, and Sunday morning. Twenty or thirty a surgery, twenty or thirty visits a day. It was quite a revolution when we decided to do away with Sunday surgeries. But when I first came it was a real treadmill. You'd start in the morning and it would literally go on till late at night.

'Plus the branch surgeries of course. In fact we still do them, they're a relic of the old days when transport was desperate. We have them in village halls, and in people's front rooms. No facilities at all. We have one in each a week. One of us goes and we have the equipment we have to have as it were. You can imagine, the little room, there may be a couch, but hardly adequate to examine somebody. The waiting room is usually the main living room and often they will sit and watch television. It's really quite homely. People seem to enjoy coming there. But it's usually a case of routine prescriptions and things, blood pressures, things like that.

'At first it was me and old Dr Harris here. At the other end was Dr Hughes – literally geographically at the two poles of the village. They were the two old doctors. Originally they had been on their own, but it got too much for them as they got older and they took partners, and there was great rivalry, great rivalry.

'Families would be divided because the wife had been with Dr Harris and the husband had been with Dr Hughes and they wouldn't change their loyalties so you'd have two doctors visiting in, say, a flu epidemic. Two doctors would be visiting the household and you'd meet, and sometimes

THE NHS AND INTO THE FIFTIES

you'd speak and sometimes you wouldn't. It was really a ridiculous situation, but these two just really didn't get on. And then a year or two after I had been here there was a great fuss and bother in the Hughes practice and two of their partners split off and formed a third practice then, geographically in the middle of the village. And again there was a great fight for patients and family loyalties were split. So now sometimes you got a family with *three* doctors visiting them.

'Subtle pressures were put on people. "I was at school with you"; "My father knew your father", that was the sort of thing that went on.

'When Dr Harris retired and Dr Hughes retired there was quite a lot of bitterness again. I was a relative newcomer, and I was a non-Welsh-speaking Englishman as well, in a very Welsh-speaking practice. There was a fairly fierce and bitter campaign to take patients from the Harris practice. We were really very lucky, I don't think we lost more than twenty patients, so that they had obviously formed their new loyalties.

'Then we joined the two practices, the ex-Hughes practice and Harris practice, and a lot of these families that had been divided in the old days suddenly found themselves with one set of doctors. Much easier from our point of view.

'The last couple of years Dr Harris didn't really do any work at all, although he still took three quarters of the money. I didn't mind. It was how the old doctors ran things. The same thing was happening to my contemporaries.'

Money and Work

DR ABNEY: 'The money was *abysmal*, absolutely *abysmal*. I came here (large, semi-urban Buckinghamshire practice) in 1955 on thirteen years parity. *Thirteen years*, yes. I got less when I came here than as a trainee. £650 a year. And that went on, you got miniscule increments I think. And then, of course, I got up to eleven years and then suddenly, whoof, the whole thing collapsed and there we were taking partners on at three years parity, and I never got to parity.

'I get on with him. He's a good doctor, very nice bloke – bit toffee-nosed – but you could ask what he thought about something. *But* working your guts out, particularly with a *lot* of obstetrics and getting a thirteenth of what he was, or perhaps at that stage an eighth, well, did nark after a time. His attitude was you could either like it or leave it. He said, "Well, I could get another partner tomorrow." '

A great many doctors confirmed this picture, waiting years for 'parity', that is an equal division of the practice income. Sometimes it was divided as with Dr Abney – a thirteenth share the first year, twelfth the second and so on. Or the new partner would get, say 18 per cent for the first five years, 25 per cent the second five years, then an equal third after that – the senior partner meanwhile keeping all the private patients. Another, a woman, described additional petty humiliations. 'And he introduced me as "My junior partner". After I'd been seventeen years in the practice. And he still wrote my calls in my diary. He used to take his diary and my diary every morning and the senior partner laboriously wrote out all the calls.'

DR TRIMDON (Urban practice in West Scotland): 'They're cheekier now. They throw their weight around a lot more than I've ever thrown my weight around as a junior partner because I wouldn't have got away with it. Things have changed. Now we give it to them after a year – except I get more on the side and I have my seniority payments. That's the only difference.

'And we did far more visits. I used to do – this will be '52, '53 – thirty-two visits a day regularly. I would consult for two hours. I'd do fourteen calls in the morning without driving a mile, maybe six in the same street that you could rattle down and you could do six in forty minutes. So I did my fourteen calls. Went into Smithsons to collect the kids and set off in the afternoon at 2 o'clock and by 5 o'clock I'd done eighteen calls more, and that was my routine.

'When I first came here there were several call houses which meant that patients who wanted the doctor left their calls-equals-messages in this house. So I would go to Jamie's, and there was another at Dunray. They were paid a fiver a year. But there was great kudos about taking the doctor's calls.'

DR CERNEY (Northern industrial practice): 'I was very lucky to be taken in by an elderly Irishman – a very charming man – and we stayed together for a year, which was what was necessary for me in order to get a practice. He's now dead. He drank and smoked an enormous amount. The only time I ever saw him without a cigarette was when he was about to have his bronchoscopy. He was chewing a peppermint and looked very miserable. Poor man. He was very nice. He brought up a family of five in the practice house and lived there for thirty-five years. And I had enormous admiration for him because, like so many of his generation, he was *there*. There was none of this business about being on committees and going here and going there and in the College of GPs, going on the BMA [British Medical Association] or something. He was just in his practice every morning and every evening, day in and day out, week in, week out, year after year. And those sort of people were the backbone of the NHS in the fifties and sixties. And I don't blame them in the smallest degree for using deputizing services when they came along, as overworked and exhausted as they must have been. It must have been extremely difficult – because they were the people who were shaping the Health Service. They coped with this great flood of demand which came in 1948 and nobody knew how big it ought to be, neither patients nor doctors knew what should be expected of this new Health Service – what sort of things one ought to ask of it. I mean, on the one hand there were doctors who hated it and said that patients came along and asked for cotton wool and stuffed cushions with it, you know. And they used dressings and gauze to make net curtains. And at the other end there is the objective fact of the rate of prolapse repairs of women done in the early years of the Health Service, and the rate went zooming up like that and then fell down again in the late fifties. It was purely and simply a backlog of twenty years or so and now the rate has settled down and prolapses are being dealt with as they occur, rather than keeping poor women waiting in wetness and soreness for twenty years to have it done. Those are two extremes, but these were the doctors who had to deal with these contrary forces in setting up the expectations and norms for the National Health Service.'

DR TUDOR HART: 'When water stopped being paid for by the gallon it didn't mean that everybody left the taps running all day just for the sheer joy of having free water, and in the same way in the National Health Service it is simply not true that people enjoy consuming doctors and consuming medicines and so on. I know people talk like that but it is a tiny fraction of people who have that particular form of illness that takes the form of wanting to be ill or needing to be ill, that is in itself an illness. But overwhelmingly people don't want to be ill, they don't like going to the doctor's, even if it is free they are still afraid of going to the doctor – removing the economic barriers doesn't mean we have removed all the barriers, people are frightened of going to the doctor because he may find something and they are socially intimidated by doctors, and there is a long wait and it is inconvenient, and you know there are hundreds of reasons. So it is a system that has functioned on a very advanced social principle, but in extremely backward cultural circumstances. There are feudal social relationships within the Health Service.'

5

DR TOM VELLING
A SINGLE-HANDED PRACTICE, SOUTH-WEST LONDON SUBURBS

I had been intrigued by Dr Velling's letters. His writing was very tall and thin, the crowded letters slanting forwards as though driven across the page by a violent gale. His second letter, although I'd signed mine 'Jonathan G–H' came back 'Dear Friend'. The third was headed 'Memo'. When I rang confirming details he said – a note of disappointment – 'Ah, a man. I wasn't sure what sex you'd be.' He had a strong South African accent.

In appearance and manner he was an eccentric figure. He was in his mid-sixties. Short, charged with what I suspect was a fairly irritable energy, with short spikes of grey hair and a bristly beard like an old hairbrush which he said he'd had six months. He had pale, sensitive, rather feminine hands.

The surgery, in a modern health centre, bustling with chiropodists and nurses, was hung with framed photographs, citations, medals, a single framed, faded invitation from a countess ('the Countess Clarendon', he murmured). 'All these, just as they have been. Makes a talking point, a few of them are gongs, the rest things of interest. I often get a shy youngster, a boy of between seven and twelve, who doesn't want to talk. I can say, "Look at that target there, I can still shoot. There's me at my marriage . . . ".'

He had trained before the war as a revenue clerk, he began, but then suddenly darted to his desk and seized one of the envelopes patients' notes are kept in. 'The cottage industry of medical filing,' he said, trembling with anger. 'This,' he said, 'another GP's patient.' He shook fluttering bits of paper all over the table. 'This is absolute anathema to me. I've been waging a private war. Take one of mine – at random. See, in order. Stapled together. The oldest at the back, folded round so you can see at once.' He then went over to a parcel which he had clearly kept for my arrival. Held it up to show me it was still sealed and had not been surreptitiously filled, by him, with notes made chaotic on purpose. 'Here we have the notes of new patients, sent by the executive committee.' He cut it open and yanked out the brown envelopes. 'Look at this! Just stuffed in. All seriously dislodged. No order or rhyme or reason. I'll take these home. I have plugged this with Professor Drury. And it's recently come through.' Then, looking at another one, 'Just look at this. Half the contents are out of date. I can cull at least a third of this. Then get them in date order. Then *staple* them together. My partner was afraid of the stapler. But I can see no other way of preventing them sliding into disorder.

This is my particular hobby or obsession. Records must be in date order. I can't start *thinking* with a patient unless his records are straight. A lot of practitioners don't realize what they miss. They deal with the thing of the moment. They might as well have no records at all.' All this for the first half hour of our interview, Dr Velling walking up and down, grabbing envelopes, emptying them in front of me, ripping open the parcel from the FPC (Family Practitioner Committee), looking more and more wild.

Eventually he calmed down and began to describe his extremely varied medical career. His father had died when he was small, and his mother, who ran a nursing home in Cape Town, gave him the ambition to become a doctor. He was about to train, when war broke out. But after the war he trained in London, did a year in hospital at Cambridge, then did locums in Lancashire, when he married his wife. He joined the US Air Force for a year in 1954, then went and learnt surgery in Durban. The money was bad, however, so he moved next out to a remote mission hospital in Zululand.

DR VELLING: 'The practice was entirely black, of course. I had 60,000 patients in 400 square miles, at an average height of 4,000 feet, but going down to 400 feet above sea level – in the Tugela Valley. You've seen *Zulu* or *Rourke's Drift*? That sort of area.'

JGH: 'When you say 60,000, do you mean you looked after 60,000?'

DR VELLING: 'No, there were about sixty witch doctors, and they referred cases to me. I ran clinics. Each day I went out, say twenty miles in this direction, twenty miles there, twenty miles in *that* direction – an average of 100 patients a day. They'd come down from the mountains on a donkey, or even wheelbarrow, a three-day journey. We'd make a quick assessment. If it was just pneumonia, you'd give them a long-acting penicillin. A lot of them you'd never see again. They were fifty miles as the crow flies, but by the mountainous path routes – 150 miles.

'But we were after TB. They'd be coughing or spitting blood. You'd get them into hospital and put them on streptomycin and INAH [isoniazid]. After six weeks they'd get impatient and want a witch doctor and an *indava* – a tribal council.

'My policy was – OK, a handful of INAH pills, and come back. They invariably did. A little worse; the cavity bigger, temperature up. All the INAH pills distributed in the hope they'd be aphrodisiacs. So you'd start again, a few steps back.'

Dr Velling here diverged. One of the gongs, he told me, was for an operation he'd invented out there. He'd disliked the way they still dealt with babies stuck in the womb – crushing the skull and pulling the baby out in bits. He'd invented symphysiotomy – a simple, but fairly heroic method of delivering such babies which involved cutting through the symphysis pubis, the cartilage which holds the pelvic girdle together, so allowing it to open. He found afterwards it had also been invented in France in the eighteenth century. It isn't done any more because you can have difficulty walking afterwards. 'Surgery of that sort isn't difficult. You just need a knowledge of anatomy and courage,' he said with some relish. 'You see, I just opened up the pelvic girdle' – chopping gesture – 'difficult to explain.'

In 1961 he came to England. He did locums and various jobs as surgical registrar. Finally, he got offered a partnership fairly near where he was now.

DR VELLING: 'It took a while to dawn on me, but he was working the system – chap called Michaels. He spent all his time seeing private patients, but was using my NHS scrip pads. And leaving me to do *all* the NHS work. He was also cheating BUPA. If a chap came with a hernia, a year's NHS waiting list, he'd examine them, say they were fit for BUPA. He'd get them in once a month to give them injections of iron which they didn't need, and after six months he'd say "Oh, now you've got a hernia." So he'd put on his surgeon's hat and take them to a little private hospital run by some nuns in Kensington and operate. He put in a lot of fake claims. He was finally railed for fourteen, and consideration was given for more and for a minor operation he put down as an appendicectomy. He was actually a meticulous surgeon, but he was a crook. Finally he was fined £8,000 at the Assizes and suspended. He was sixty-nine then. He's dead now.

'But I had smelt a rat and had resigned, and he said I had to get out of the area. But in the meantime I'd bought a house, my son was at public school and I couldn't up-anchor again; so the first month or two my income was 25 quid. I had no patients.

'Fortunately, at that particular moment, just when I was about to pack up, I was offered quite a lucrative partnership fifteen miles from here, starting tomorrow, so I did.

'I worked that for a while, then that partner wasn't getting enough to keep his son at public school. So he bailed out and at that stage it was very, very hard to get a partner, and I had about 6,000 patients. This was the late sixties. I then got a partner, a Nigerian. Well, there was mutual incompatibility – nothing to do with him being black.

'So I was alone again. I reduced my list to 3,500 – the most; and the rest went next door. Well they were most unfair. They were three doctors, with 10,000 patients, and we were on a rota. But it was me one night, then one of them, me one weekend, then one of them. I protested – but they said "You've got one practice and it's one practice against one practice."

'I was on the point then of packing up and going back to South Africa. But the deputizing service then saved me uprooting. And this lady doctor, who incidentally had joined Michaels after I'd left, and had also resigned, she was working up a nice little practice. It grew so big she couldn't cope, so she persuaded me to resign, and come and join her. It was a mistake, a miscalculation. I soon found that she had inherited a very large private practice from Michaels when he was suspended. She was spending so much time seeing private patients that once again I was doing the whole workload.

'Well, it's a longish story, but I set up here, and for the last three years it's been a very, very excellent and happy relationship with this other lady doctor. Sometimes we don't see each other for two weeks.

'And then she told me she was going to try for a clinical assistantship to be near her husband, who is a gynaecologist and has been very ill. I thought it only right she did so. And this morning she told me she'd got it. So now I'm landed back, from today, once again solus, with an over-full list. You know, you can't win sometimes.'

6

Dr James Chathill
A Large West Country Health Centre

Dr Chathill was tall, grey-haired and looked a good ten years older than fifty-two. They lived in a largish, rather nondescript 1920s house on what had become a main road. There was something a bit impersonal about it, a 'drawing room' and a sitting room, but both equally neat and clean.

The Patients

Dr Chathill: 'You know all the children very well indeed, so that they come in chatting happily the whole time you're examining them, and don't yell and get tensed up. I've got several I delivered and I'm looking after their babies now. They're so used to me I'm just part of the furniture.

'It's most important, one of the nicest things of all in practice, that you do know your families terribly well. And it's absolutely vital because you know all their past histories, the hereditary traits going through. I've this boy who got into a panic depression when he went to university. I talked him through it. And now again on his first job. I remember his father doing exactly the same when he was in the Army. He didn't know whether to leave and go into commerce. And he had to come and tell me, the same panic and indecision. And I know that, and I can tell the son and I'll get him through it.

'Patients never leave because they think you've been negligent or given the wrong treatment. It's because they think you haven't listened and therefore don't care. You can be as angry as you like. They don't mind because they think you care. But the moment they think you're not interested, they'll walk right out on you.

'I have a woman who's just changed from one of my partners. He's a bit dogmatic and she's intelligent. A middle-aged civil servant with heart trouble. She can't make him discuss whether it's dangerous or what's causing it. He's got a sort of block with her. He doesn't communicate; you can't sometimes. He just tells her it's all right. So she's moved to me because I'll talk to her.

'I suppose a third of a surgery will be minor psychiatric – depression and so on. I'm practised at it. I don't enjoy it. I haven't the patience for the very difficult ones.

'I mean, I have Mrs O'Grady, a woman of low intelligence who has fits.

She gets paranoid every so often and thinks everyone's getting at her. She shouts out of the window at her neighbours and goes round to the police and her daughter's gone exactly the same way, so there you've got them going like blazes together. The daughter's almost ESN and she's having delusions, she thought she was the Queen of Portsmouth, and they wake each other up at three in the morning and row and it has been known for me to be called to stop their fighting. And you can't shut them up in hospital, they won't go, not quite certifiable, and they won't take pills to make them better or calm them out of paranoia. And they will have been coming to my surgery almost every day, complaining about people and wanting me to write to a solicitor. It goes on and on. And if you have two or three in a surgery all going on and refusing to stop talking and delusions or persecutions, it can be very difficult. They take an enormous amount of time and a lot of emotional strain out of you.

'But the ordinary depressions are terribly common. And they do all seem to come together, at certain times of the year. March or September—everyone seems to get better, but they don't. One will appear, or get much worse, and you think "Oh God, we're going to have the lot now" and sure enough next day they all turn up. Sun spots, world news – it's statistically provable. I don't know why.

'But those you can treat very nicely; can teach them. I've got one charming woman who's cheerful and happy, happily married and family grown up and she lives in a small house, and every now and then she will get an acute depressive attack when she has to kill herself. She has to sleep and the only way she can sleep is by taking whatever drug she can lay her hands on as an overdose, and it comes on very quickly and she's tried to kill herself twice now, and not succeeded each time. Now she's on a permanent fairly low dose of anti-depressant drug which her husband keeps, and she's absolutely fine. But take her off that and three months later she'll try and cut her throat or something. It's completely physical, I'm quite sure. A chemical imbalance which we are learning to correct.

'I had a woman this evening who came and sat down and just burst into tears. That's all, but I know her, I've seen her before. She gets recurrent attacks of depression, then eats and then she gets very fat and then she gets a pain in her tummy and she can't sleep and the neighbours turn rather nasty and her mother starts jeering at her. Well, she doesn't have to tell me all that. I more or less put my hands on her head and said, "Right, we'll start now and you'll get better in a fortnight", and she's gone off happy with a few anti-depressant drugs. And I'll see her every week now until she's better and that's that. One knows them so well now, that you don't have to say much.'

The Diseases: Children

'Abdominal pain with children, especially a baby. They can look very well one moment, and an hour or two later be extremely ill. My father taught me how to examine an abdomen without hurting the child. He was very keen on always feeling *towards* the pain rather than touching it. But there's far more. They don't like moving their legs much if they've got an inflamed appendix so they won't walk comfortably. The pain has a slightly different pattern from other pains, and you get a sort of feel about it. The way they lie, the way their breath smells. Well no – they've had to have had it a very long time because it means they're going rotten inside. You don't get that one now. I think it's one of our main troubles that in the past nobody called you until people were really ill and all the signs were very florid and easy to pick up. Nowadays people expect to be cleared up immediately and one sees illnesses at the outset and it's harder diagnostically.

'So that peritonitis I was telling you about. The doctor who leaves it to the end of his visits or who doesn't care or doesn't think about it at the moment, and the baby dies and everybody says how bloody awful he is. But he may be absolutely conscientious. And particularly with children. The signs are very minimal until they get acutely ill. That is the main worry. 80 per cent of our work is standard, easy, everyday rather dull work, taking blood pressures, listening to chests, advising people and then when you're not thinking nature goes and slips in a real dirty one – a rare illness you may never see again. Cancer in a very young person when you're not expecting it: 200 people have bleeding from piles, and the 201st might have a cancer above the pile, so you've got to examine them all every single time.

'Upper respiratory can be anxious-making, too. Babies and small children, a baby can get tired, breathing very rapidly and if he's got any form of obstruction, unless you're alert to it, he'll look all right one moment, half an hour later he'll be grey and gasping for breath, and then he can die fairly quickly.

'But then asthma is an immensely rewarding job in general practice because it is something you can treat and cure completely yourself without any help from anyone else. And it's a disease which embraces practically the whole family and one can cure it by management of people rather than by drugs. I stop people being frightened by talking to them and explaining how it works, by finding out the cause of the asthma, what food sensitivity or pollen sensitivity, eliminating that, so that you can have a miserable child who's wheezing and coughing all day, can't play, can't go to school, and you can transform that child into something very healthy very easily, and it's most rewarding. In the end they know more about it than me and can cope entirely by themselves. You can do that with most diseases, most long-term diseases.'

Preventative Work

'I think the criteria of a good practice is personal care, the ability to actually diagnose and treat an illness early before it gets dangerous; next, health care, the general preventative care.

'I gave a lecture to one of the local factories on how to prevent heart attack. I thought half a dozen would turn up but I had the entire factory – 300.

'We take people's blood pressure when they come in, which picks up most people. We do cervical smears, we discuss diets, exercise, we try and make people healthier. After thirty-five, I try and get them off the pill. I won't give it to them unless they have their blood pressure taken every six months. It's very rare to get heart trouble on the pill, or blood pressure, but I get about one a year of young women, it shoots up immediately and I have to take them off it.

'You have to force yourself to keep a permanent high standard all the time. You can't start taking short cuts. That's what's worrying me in this practice at the moment – we're getting so busy that one tends to take short cuts just to get through people.

'Possibly if I gave a bit more to other people I'd have more time, but while you're taking their blood pressure you can discuss their way of life, you can discuss their weight, the pill, their smoking habits. You can find out what's worrying them, what's worrying their children or their wife at the same time. So it's not *just* taking blood pressure; it's a quiet check-up on the rest of the family. And while you're taking a cervical smear you're taking damn good care to see that everything else in the pelvis is normal: that they haven't got any cysts or polyps. It takes a lot of training and experience to pick up small things early, and I think it's just that little bit risky leaving somebody half-trained to do that, but a lot of people disagree with me.'

The Old

'We're very strong on the old, they're very, very well looked after. They've got centrally heated flats with a warden, they've got double-glazing, they've got the lot.

'In the old days, when they had an outside privy in the garden, trying to go out in the snow at eighty-five, down to the other end of the garden, twice a night, that soon knocked off the weaklings.

'I remember old Makins, he survived. It was a medieval farmhouse, and it hasn't been modernized. I think they've got a gas cooker now, but when I went down there, when I first came, there was an elderly man and his sister living there and they had dogs and they cooked in a pot over the open fire, and they had a trestle, a big oak table with a trestle on either side, and they had an extremely prosperous farm. And upstairs was a panelled room and the roof was just the tiles. There was nothing underneath it so the snow came through the gap in the roof on to his bed. He had diabetes and pneumonia and he nearly died. They were disgustingly dirty. It hadn't been cleaned, and nobody had been cleaned for ages but he was very, very wealthy. It was entirely due to eccentricity, but his grandmother left it to him and she didn't want it changed, so he didn't change it. And he's still there. He's got air conditioning or something clever in the cow byre, but he's still got exactly the same house and he still lives with his sister in the most appalling squalor. And they smell.

'There was another funny old pair in Gough Lane — that's another medieval or sixteenth-century farmhouse that's now been pulled down – and they never washed at all. And they had this one single room on the ground floor, with bicycles and every sort of junk and an open fire and the granddaughter used to come down once a month and try and tidy them up and wash some of their clothes. And he died of old age, and I had to climb up a ladder to the bedroom with a pencil torch, because my torch had bust, and ferret through about ten layers of bedclothes to see whether I could find the body. I did in the end. More and more layers and finally he emerged, but he had died comfortably in his old age. And I went down and told the old woman that he really had died and she just stood there in the middle, and tears ran down her face leaving white trickles as it washed the dirt away. But that's pretty well gone now, we don't see much of that.'

Death

'People wake up in bed and their husband is dead beside them. There was one old lady round the corner who had a tea party and everybody got up to say good-bye at the end and she just didn't stir. She'd died quietly holding her tea cup on the side of her chair and nobody spotted that she'd died. They were all very old, the guests, and weren't a bit surprised.

'Sometimes they know. I had one, Trevane, I can't remember what he died of – cancer – and he suddenly said, "I'm very pleased, I'm dying now." I said, "Oh, are you?" He said "Yes," and he did. Just fell back like that. It was most bizarre.

'And there was another, not mine, he rang to say he was dying and would leave the front door open. When I arrived he was sitting up in bed, dead. He'd had a heart attack before, and he'd felt one coming on at that moment. I think people know when they do have a fatal one, if it's not too quick for them.

'But if they don't know, I always wait till I'm asked. But they're fairly sure. They don't say, "Am I going to die?", they say, "Am I going to get better?" and I say, "No"; and they say, "Roughly how long?", and I say, "I don't know, but it will be more than a week or two or a day or whatever." And one chats on from there. They say, "What happens?" and I try and explain. They want to discuss the fears and worries of death, so they know what they are facing, in the actual act of dying, beforehand. You're always available to talk, to go out. You take no notice at all of the relatives when they say, "Mother mustn't be told." If mother wants to know, then mother's going to be told. And they're always much happier when they are told. You should do exactly

what the patient guides you to do. Some people refuse to discuss it. They go
on making plans for their recovery and you go along with that.

'That's the last great task of a good GP, of a good practice. The hospices
now say they're the only people who know how to do it, but we've been
doing it for years. The art is dealing with any pain before it arrives, before it
gets a hold, so they never have to call for pills. But it's a great art because of
the masses of drugs one can use. You can tailor the pain-type drugs – heroin
or what have you – so they are always comfortable. You can use steroids,
cortisone so that you stop certain bone pain from secondaries; you stimulate
their appetites so they *feel* well. You can use anti-depressants if necessary, but
it's not often necessary. There's a whole group of things. People should be up
and about and well – or not grisly ill. And you should be always available so if
anybody in the family is frightened or worried you can move in quickly and
discuss it. And to do it properly you need a damn good nursing service as
well. The district nurse is almost more important. They will go in two or
three or four times a day to inject, to clean, to keep them comfortable. And in
the end they just drift away, without pain or fear. Sometimes they die in the
middle of a conversation.

'You can feel sad. But I think you always keep yourself apart — one's
emotions always apart. One does feel very sad, particularly someone young,
or something, but you must keep it away, away from your own emotions.
It's not easy, actually.

'The very old don't give a damn. They really don't mind. And they're not
at all pleased if you try and resuscitate them either — as I did when young. I
got snapped at. They felt they just had to do it all over again.

'And, also, the feeling is they were very interested in what was going on. "I
was just going. I was seeing something." "There was a light, and now you've
got in the way." I've met that two or three times. And this business of being
projected from the body. I had a man who had a cardiac arrest, and described
being forced out of his body and being projected at speed towards a light, and
then he felt a frightful pain in his chest and got dragged back and the light
receded.

'It's difficult to tell if it's just cells fading with lack of oxygen and therefore
you get a light. My impression is there's more than that, that they've actually
seen something, you know, something's going on. There's light and it's airy;
and the feeling of getting away, escaping.'

Calls at Night
'We've been here over twenty years now. That's why I think an answering
machine is wrong. If somebody's in a real state, or there's somebody dying,
or a child suffocating, you get an answering machine to just state your
message after the tone, well they can't do it. They don't know how often
you're going to pick it up. Or it says ring another number and they haven't

another 5p or a pencil. They must have a voice this end, to take charge. It's terribly important. A calm voice when you're in a panic.'

During the night I heard the telephone go at 12.15 and again at 12.45. Each time his measured voice and then the car starting up. The first was a woman vomiting blood, which was easily dealt with; the second was acute heart failure, which meant some morphia and other injections. There was another call at 5.30, a woman with internal bleeding, for which he gave her pain-killing injections and will have her investigated. At one point a deer ran into his car, but wasn't hurt. 'We have a lot of them round here.'

Another call at 7.15. 'A woman rang up, she wanted to chat to one of the partners. At that hour!'

The Health Centre

In the morning Dr Chathill, looking fairly tense and jaded, took me to see his health centre.

This is an important development in general practice during the last twenty years, and we shall look at it again later, but some aspects should be considered now.

The 1966 Act encouraged the formation of large group practices operating either from health centres or practice-owned, custom built premises, for which highly advantageous loan arrangements were provided.

Health centres differ from these in various ways. The concept (which is not new – Cronin describes it in *The Citadel* for instance) is that they should be *centres of health* – that is, contain facilities not just for the doctors and their teams, but for as many other specialists as possible, room for visiting consultants, for lecturers and clinics. They are built and owned by local councils. Sometimes they will have small operating theatres, X-rays, laboratories and so on, and doctors who don't practice in them say this means the GPs are not independent – they are liable to swingeing rates and rents, obstruction and difficulties if they wish to extend or alter, and bad design.

Rates are common to all forms of doctoring premises, and I found no evidence of over-high rents – why should councils wish to impoverish their local practices? The second two criticisms bore more substance. Dr Chathill's practice was engaged in a long-winded argument to get the council to enlarge; but at least they didn't have to pay. The design was 'a bit of a disaster'; yet they had been endlessly consulted and it was clear the same disaster would have occurred whoever paid.

Dr Chathill's health centre had a chiropodist, speech therapist (for children and strokes), there was an eye clinic and consultants came once a week. It had a great deal of equipment; an ECG (electrocardiogram) machine, a peak flow machine, resuscitation equipment, X-ray machine, defibrillator, and each GP had an oxygen set in his car. This is all fairly typical for a big south-of-the-

Trent English health centre. Some of it (the ECG machine for instance) had been given, often equipment had been bought by money from the local community. It is possible for sums of £30,000 or £40,000 to be raised. This is certainly admirable, but doctors where it happens boast how much more generous and community-minded their areas are than other districts, which is nonsense. The generosity (a pound or two per head, with an occasional £500 – £1,000 from someone rich) is clearly not without self-interest, since anyone may need a defibrillator or oxygen. When communities don't raise money it is because several practices in different buildings look after them and it is impossible to separate and organize the different practice populations.

Dr Chathill and his six partners were the only practice looking after the 16,000 local population. The health centre was a large, light, airy one-storey complex. Each GP had his own consulting room with its own waiting area; the large central waiting area was also an art gallery (not uncommon); nurses and patients and consultants moved down corridors to and fro to treatment rooms – it was like a mini-hospital.

And this is another criticism of health centres – they are too 'hospitaloid' – too impersonal, intimidating, clean, efficient.

It is impossible to say. Patients are no help. Whether it is one cramped waiting room with benches, forty full, an hour's wait because the inner city GP has no appointment system, a converted Victorian rectory for a three-GP group, or something more like an airport, patients almost invariably prefer what they've got. Certainly I've seen centres which seemed rather cold, with flashing lights or intercom summoning the patients, the hush of a hospital.

But friendliness is to do with people not premises. Dr Chathill's centre was bustling, alive, human and humorous. From the nurses' office, I heard an elderly white-haired woman being helped down the corridor by her older husband. She'd been washing her hair and suddenly her hearing had gone 'quite blank'. The doctor had sent her to be syringed. 'Just go down to the door on the left. I'm a bit busy at the moment.' The couple went tottering down. One of the district nurses I'd been talking to said she'd seen Mrs Derby. Another one came in rather nervously, it was her first week 'on the district' – 'I'm not allowed to be let loose on the population yet.' I could hear the old woman being syringed. Baby talk, 'Back you come. That's it – let's take a peep.' Nurses 'popping' in and out, for coffee, chat. More syringing. 'One more time my love.' The trainee nurse looked like a softer, more worried Billie Jean King. She said she'd seen Mrs Derby. An older nurse had seen her too – 'Oops! You didn't give her *another* blanket bath?' Laughter.

The 1966 Act also encouraged the concept of the primary health *team*: doctor plus health visitor, district nurse and so on. The local authorities supply these and also social workers. But the Act allowed each GP to employ two additional workers, the Government paying 70 per cent of their salaries. A seven-man practice can in theory, therefore, employ fourteen more staff –

receptionists, chiropodist, dietician, whatever they like.

GPs often say they are less intimately joined to their patients than in the past and for many this is undoubtedly true. But, aside from births, the intimacy has not been entirely lost; it has instead been spread into the team. Health visitors and nurses it is now who go into homes, doing vaccinations, seeing the children, taking out stitches, dressing wounds.

Dr Chathill agreed these were an essential avenue into patients – the more effective as they were often the same class, and were *women* as well.

DR CHATHILL: 'The health visitor or nurse will often say what the real problem is. She'll come to me and say, "Did you know Mrs W had an illegitimate baby which aborted, and that's why she keeps on coming in fussing about this pregnancy?"; or "Mrs H's old man is drinking again – she won't admit it but I smelt it on his breath when I went in" and then you know why Mrs H keeps on coming to the surgery with aches and pains.'

DISTRICT NURSE: 'We do everything on the district. Make teas, cook breakfasts, light fires, run round the shops for 10 pences. It's nice on the district. They tell us, the nurses, a lot more than they probably will anybody else. Their little problems, things that are bothering them.

'We go on till we're sixty and then we're retired. I started in a hospital but I've been on the district thirteen years, and I certainly wouldn't go back. It's a freer life. You're not asking if you can go to lunch or coffee. It's a different aspect. There's nobody else. Just you. You do the lot, the lifting, the washing. You can spend an hour or one and a half hours with a patient.

'It's more heartbreaking than in hospitals. In hospitals it's so cold and calculating and they are all nice and clean. But you go into the houses sometimes and it's really tragic. When you walk in for the first time . . . Well, really. I have stood there and nearly cried. The filth they live in. Meagre, isn't it? One room. Especially in homes. No heating, terrible. Lonely; you get used to it.

'And incontinence. You can almost walk about in it. In hospitals you never meet this, because they're so clean. They don't realize the problems. They shove them out. Like our poor Mr Marsh.

'He's a diabetic. He collects rubbish. He goes round all these tips and brings home 'No waiting' signs and old tins, boots, hats, cookers, the lot. His room was just literally piled high with all this junk. But nobody checked he had a cooker or some sort of heating, even a frying pan. He had nothing.

'But then the Social Services did provide him with some stuff and one of us nurses gave him dinner every Christmas. Made sure he was all right. But the Social Services cleared him out because they thought it was dangerous. They left him with nothing, absolutely nothing.

'He was that upset. He's never forgotten it. But he's worse now! He got a whole new lot! Shoes, boots . . . He's a comic really. We tease him. He's about sixty-two I think. Somewhere there. It's sad isn't it, really? It's his way of life and we can't change it. He has to climb over all this stuff to get to his little cooker in the corner. How he does it, I don't know, and how he ever gets to the toilet . . . the mind boggles! But he loves us going.

'Oh the doctors get irritable. Patients get you irritable sometimes. Especially if you're feeling unwell yourself and you have problems which you have, when you get a mouthful of abuse from the patient. You stand there and take it because you can't retaliate. You go outside and say, "You'll never guess what so-and-so's just said." It's nice that we all get on. We have a cup of coffee and a cigarette and a laugh. And if it's sad and your mind goes over and over it, sometimes we discuss it over the telephone when it's been bothering us.'

7

DR ANNE UPLEES
A WEST COUNTRY URBAN PRACTICE

Dr Uplees' house was in the old part of a large West Country river-sea town – one of several high, elegant, wealthy houses. It was surrounded by antique shops, estate agents, one or two smart restaurants. A pricey area – the estate agents' windows showed £90,000, £110,000.

The surgery was only ten minutes away, but the change to rows of suburban semis and council estates was quite dramatic.

Dr Uplees was about forty-three. She seemed a bit mousey and subdued; only gradually did I realize she was a rebellious character, potentially anarchic. She started by confirming and elaborating on the nature of the practice.

DR ANNE UPLEES: 'Yes, lower middle class mostly. Also a lot of immigrants. Not West Indians; Asians or East Africans. They pose problems, the Asians. They're used to private medicine basically. He came with a sore throat and I said "That looks awful. Here's some penicillin. Yes, have a week off work." You'd think that would be enough, but he kept on – "It's too much pain, oh such pain." Eventually I said, "For goodness' sake, I've given you pills, a week off work, just stop going on about it."

'I have enormous respect for the way they've altered the business life of this country, even locally. The English people have imitated them in a way that wouldn't have happened and some of them are absolutely charming, but I don't like their endless fussing trivia.

'I didn't drift into medicine. I knew from the age of four I wanted to be a doctor. I was interested in how the body worked. I used, older, to read *The Modern Home Doctor* behind a chair. It probably had a chapter on sex in it. But I certainly wasn't a scientist – I did English and History. But I found medical school perfectly easy. I remember I came bottom in biochemistry, and the lecturer went on. Next term, I didn't go to one lecture, it was so boring. But I took heed of his words, and I sat down with a book at 7 o'clock and ate five milligrams of amphetamine – it was easy to get hold of – and read the book a few times, got up next morning and was top of the exam.

'That was the trouble, they didn't teach you anything except things you could learn from books anyway. They didn't teach you that people had feelings and adolescents don't know everything – they don't teach you about people and it's rotten for the patients. We only had one question on psychiatry, so we got taught very little. It was a bad training. Perhaps they're taught better now.

'Yet they must have chosen well. Of the six girls in our year, I have five children, so does another, two have four, and one has two. We're all still working. I've never found it any problem at all – really not. I've always had a mother's help, and now a cleaning lady. I've always had a full load and it used to be much heavier in the days when we did eighteen visits a day. But now it's none, or two or three. I can take the children to school, pick them up, do the shopping, arrange the odd day off.

'No, I don't miss seeing them in their homes. It doesn't really make any difference. It makes a lot of difference how they're behaving as a family, but you won't see that by going to visit. One person in the home, the husband, won't be there, will he? You get as much a picture of what the home is like from what a patient says as from actually seeing it.

'Some you get to know very well indeed. Some hardly at all. I think you get what you're interested in. I have a girl I see once a week who's just done her 'A' levels. Through her late childhood and adolescence she was always taking overdoses and cutting her wrists and being in care, and what have you. She doesn't have a father – dead. I don't do much. I just listen to her and chat and anytime I say anything remotely resembling interpretation, she says "No, no, it's nothing like that." But now she's got her 'A' levels and is going to do law.

'And I've another, a boy, who rings me up at all hours because he takes Valium and sleeping pills. I'm going to do a rare thing with him, actually, which is actually to take him physically to a hospital out-patients. They might actually have him in hospital for three or four months and get him off drugs. Because if he hasn't slept for two or three weeks he gets into a really awful state.

'I mean, people like him are the people I like best. It may be because I think if I hadn't done medicine, the *idea* of freedom, I would have become quite wild, a drop-out. I don't know what I would have done. I keep seeing myself wandering around.

'There's a lot of trivia, apart from that. I don't mind. I'm not all that interested in medicine. I think I'm more interested in the people. I think there are more interesting families or interesting homes than there are interesting cases. Besides the interesting cases get taken out of your hands.

'It's seldom something walking into the surgery is terribly frightening. Worst are the emergencies. About four months ago they phoned and said there was an emergency – a boy of fifteen can't breathe. So I presumed it was someone who had got a bit anxious and was overbreathing. I did go straight away as they said it was an emergency and I put the small children in the car and when I got there the mother said "His father's upstairs" – a different father, you know, married again. I went up and his father said, "He's just stopped breathing," which he had. Unconscious. He'd had asthma since lunchtime the day before and they hadn't bothered to do anything about it. I knew I hadn't got any drugs so I said to his father, "You breathe into his mouth and I'll thump his chest", which I did and he was all right. His blood gases were the worst in the whole history of the hospital. We were both very lucky. That sort of thing is the worst.

'A GP's life is stressful, but mostly with people's problems. It depends how many you get in a day. Sometimes it just goes on and on and for the fourth person who comes in whose husband has left and expects oceans of sympathy, it can be quite a bother, especially if your own life isn't marvellous. And, if you lose your temper with patients, they accept it. They know I'm not like that really.

'I go home and forget it, nearly always. There was an exception a little while back. A Thursday before a bank holiday, the last patient was a boy the age of one of my sons. He came with his mother and he was as white as a sheet. He looked so ill it was clear he had something absolutely dreadful. He turned out to have acute leukaemia, which is what I'd presumed he had. But I didn't know what to do. There were four days of holiday, so nothing much could be done in hospital. But he was almost too frightened to come in the door, he probably knew he was very ill. To tell them he was seemed unthinkable. In fact I said, "Here's the form and take him in on Tuesday." At least he'd have the weekend. But I did go home and worry about that. Had it been an ordinary Friday I would have sent him in.

'Yes, diagnosis is intuitive sometimes. You simply know. Then there a whole lot of people in a very grey area, people with a whole lot of vague symptoms which are almost certainly nothing. But there are so many of them and the patients complain about them so often, you feel obliged to send them along to have a thorough investigation. But then, I had a little boy who was very sick. "He's vomiting every time before school." I asked if he didn't like school, and she said he'd always loved school. Nothing else. But I was suddenly sure something was up. Not a sign, but I sent him to the paediatrician. He couldn't find anything, but sent him to the child psychiatrist. But he had another appointment with the paediatrician three months later, and this time one of his eyes was all lopsided, and he'd got a terrible tumour. No one had detected it, but I'd felt something.

'But I've got a woman of thirty-three, dying of cancer of the breast. She thought she had a lump. But it was all so huge, a great diffuse mass, less easy to recognize as lumps or a lump. I said I thought it was nothing, but told her to make an appointment. "Say 'lump' and they'll see you next day." It was cancer and she'd developed secondaries in the bone. I wasn't intuitive about her. Maybe it was because I didn't want to think of her death. One can block one's intuition.

'They come with everythng – except perhaps sex. Very little demand. I think generally the English are a bit stoical about sex problems. If they do, it seems to have been going on for years and years already.

'I once went on a sex course. It was awful. Huge film screen with male and female homosexuals having sex. The lecturer laced his talk liberally with words like "fuck", and watched the Indians falling about and crawling off the floor when he did. The idea is to change people's attitudes and not make them fall on the floor when people say "fuck". I wrote to him saying it might have been because I was ten weeks pregnant, and might have felt sick anyway, but the things I liked I still liked, and the one thing I didn't like about sex is seeing it up on a big screen which made me feel sicker. He kept ringing me up and asking me out to dinner, but I didn't go.

'I don't think men resent a woman doctor, though no doubt there are things they don't come about. I think if they are unhappy they're more pleased to see me. They are much less ashamed of being depressed or whatever than with another man, I think.

'Nor do they make passes. Except I had a sort of flasher person not so long ago. He wanted to register. He made a great thing, the receptionist said, of will the lady doctor be here? I can't remember what it was he said was wrong, but it only happened when he had an erection. And he opened his coat and was undoing buttons. I had to really throw him out. It didn't upset me.'

Although this was a very early interview, and I hadn't yet realized how completely I had to efface myself in order to get the clam-tight GPs to open up, Dr Uplees had been unusually frank and stimulating. Yet as the interview continued, I felt more and more depressed. It wasn't until many months, many doctors and many books later that I realized the significance of this reaction.

8
SEX, LOVE AND SEX COUNSELLING

Dr Uplees and another woman GP were the only doctors I talked to who voluntarily brought up these subjects.

As regards doctors sleeping with patients, it is looked on with greater understanding now than in the past. As recently as the early 1960s a GP was struck off because he'd had an affair with a woman long after she had ceased to be his patient and had moved from the district. Older GPs remember they always insisted on a third party being present when they examined a woman – and many still prefer one to be within earshot. And it is still a major fear, especially among GPs from that period, that they will be accused of some sexual misdemeanour by a patient – something which is not all that uncommon – and find it impossible to prove they have done nothing.

But in general this is a sphere where a good many people tend to have highly coloured and exaggerated fantasies about what goes on.

DR BILSBY (Four-doctor Lincolnshire practice): 'No, there again I think that is one thing why I do not like having friends as patients, because it is a completely different situation. It is all such a clinical situation. I have said before and people have said "Ho ho pull the other one, you like listening to their chests," and in fact it is quite different. It isn't a sexual situation at all in fact.'

DR HEINWAY (Large, rich private practice): 'Naturally I was subject to the usual female attacks. Every woman makes a pass at you and thinks you are the one who can give her the famous orgasm. And I see very rapidly I am not sleeping with her; a) it is against medical rules; b) you lose your patient; c) my father told me, "If you sleep with a woman you will pay." '

DR ABNEY (Buckinghamshire rural/urban GP practice): 'Well – you ask me a frank question – yes, occasionally one gets an absolute stunner. One of my partners – we were talking about it a couple of months ago and he was saying about this air hostess – works for BOAC and she's absolutely *fantastic*. I mean, I was just doing a run-of-the-mill afternoon surgery and I saw a strange name and I thought "One of my partner's" and then in came this apparition – absolutely gorgeous. A girl of about thirty. I'm not one for blondes actually, but she was absolutely stunning and I thought, well I see what you mean. And it was quite obvious that she wouldn't have minded in the least bit. But there we are – that was all right.

'No, I've had one. I had to get advice from the Medical Defence Union once because somebody accused me of poking his wife and so I rang up the MDU and a very, very, very charming solicitor there, he said, "Well, have you, doctor?" and I said "No", and he said, "Well, don't worry. We have to ask, you know. You might have done." Anyway, they sent a letter and the envelope almost burst into flames when the letter came out and curiously enough, the girl's father came to me and he said, "Do you know, you've done a fantastic job. My son-in-law, into bed with anything, absolutely," and he said, "he's *reformed* now. He really goes and spends the week with his wife." And I just laughed and said, "Well, I know the reason for that!" '

DR WARFIELD (Five-doctor city practice in the south east): 'Oh hell, yes. I'm just as human as the next bloke. I like women. I have never been tempted in the sense that I would do it because I think the penalties are too great. To squeeze a woman's breasts, a nice attractive girl's breasts who I've got on the couch – you're a BF if you do you know. It's not worth it for £20,000 a year plus. But the answer is yes – tempted. You train yourself not to.'

Dr Jane Edstone, who had a three-doctor practice in the Midlands, was the other GP who talked about this without prompting. She was alone now, but still attractive, and had had a fairly raffish past with three husbands. She had had a long affair with a professional poacher, traces of whose tenure – in the form of nets, snares, empty ferret hutches – still lingered. She talked with compassion and candour.

DR JANE EDSTONE: 'The bane of one's life is when men patients fall in love with you for the wrong reason. It's awfully difficult. You're interested in them as people, as patients and they misinterpret. But then their marriages are probably a bit wonky. They turn to you, and you have to shake them off without destroying their confidence.

'The awful thing is that people think you are very stable. You acquire stability with other people's problems – but you don't, do you? They fall in love with you for the wrong reasons. They think you can "take it"; but the last thing you want to do is "take it". You want to be able to relax and shove your emotions on to someone else. Not the lot – but some. I want someone who treats me as a human being and doesn't have a false idea.

'I'm always falling in love, but then I kick myself and say "No". My morals aren't at all correct, if you like, but I try to avoid being involved with patients.

It happens, or could. But you're set to avoid the situation, so the poor chap doesn't have a chance anyway.

'But, well, I suppose if I fell just head over heels in love with anyone, I'd just say to the GMC [General Medical Council] and all of them – "Stuff it".'

Masters and Johnson, in their pioneering work on sexual inadequacy, wrote, 'A conservative estimate would indicate half the marriages [in America] as either presently sexually dysfunctional or imminently so in the future.' In that country, most medical schools have the subject on their curriculae, and those that don't run courses on it.

There is no reason to suppose that Britain is very different from America as regards sex in marriage; though it is possible that British couples mind less, or at least complain less, about sexual dysfunction.

But there is also a good deal of evidence to the contrary. The problem pages of women's magazines are increasingly preoccupied with whether or not readers can achieve orgasm. Geoffrey Gorer in his *Sex and Marriage in Britain Today* found that there was a 50 per cent greater expectation of successful sex in British marriages in 1970 than in 1950. A psychiatrist I spoke to in London who specializes in impotence among men spoke of 'a hidden army'. (An odd image.) It is likely, therefore – one would expect it – that Britain is moving, or trying to move, in the same direction as America in this respect.

We are not, to any significant extent, being helped by our GPs. The subject is not, as far as I can ascertain, on the curriculum of a single medical school. (Though in some teaching hospitals concerned individuals have set up courses – Guy's, St George's and the Central Middlesex in London, for instance.) And though Dr Uplees was irritated by the doctor who ran courses trying to rectify this, I found that many GPs were themselves irritated, embarrassed, ignorant or managed by some or all of these attitudes, to fend off such patients.

DR YETTS (North London group practice): 'I did very little, virtually none. I don't know whether I didn't do much because I didn't feel comfortable doing it, so people didn't ask, or what.

'But do you need a doctor to sex counsel? I don't think so. We're not trained to sex counsel. I wasn't even trained in contraception at medical school. I picked it up purely by reading. Sex counselling, good heavens!

'After all a doctor, basically, whatever anybody thinks about prevention and all these other things, is trained in the diagnosis and treatment of disease. When it comes to the crunch, what you want from the doctor isn't all this fancy stuff. That's what you pay your doctor for, in the long run. Sex therapy and all the other things are a little gilt on the lily, aren't they?'

DR BLAIRHALL (Home Counties, six-doctor practice): 'One of the most difficult cases, well, impotence in men. You see [long pause, dropping voice] so often the doctor feels impotent too.

'It's the intractability. All the complex, nervous pathways involved. I mean, you've got to have so many things going right to ejaculate just at the right time. I mean, if you start thinking about it, you become impotent.'

DR ABNEY: 'I've chanced my arm. "Where angels fear to tread". Ha ha. It's difficult. I've never been on a course. One tends to give good, homely advice for some problems. Others – well luckily one of the partners is a girl who's keen on this and she's in cahoots with a very bright psychiatrist and they run a sort of psychosexual service and Sally's jolly good at it.

'I haven't done much, in fact only two patients in twenty-five years. And when they come they're usually the difficult ones. Both mine had been virgins in their forties, married twenty years or more.

'One had a bloody great fibroid there and she thought it was an immaculate conception or something. I examined her and thought, "Oh Gawd, she's VI (virgo intacta). Oh Gawd, what do we do now?" "Well," I said, "I think you've got something." I thought she'd got an ovarian cyst actually, but she'd got a fibroid. Anyway, she had a hysterectomy and nothing there had been used at all!

'And the other one, I did try some psychosexual counselling but it was a total disaster and the husband lit off with someone else so I thought, "Well, perhaps I'm not cut out for this." '

DR JANE EDSTONE: 'Very rarely have people found they couldn't talk to me, I hope. I seem to have a lot of men with sexual problems as much as women. I've always got the impression that men are more inclined to come to a woman because men are – not exactly competition – but they're a bit reticent about admitting failure with other men – the same sex. I get men in their forties or sixties. Usually because they're pushing themselves at work, and their marriages have gone a bit stale, and they think it's the end of the world. I just say that there are plenty of other men in the same situation; possibly you can't be all things to all women all the time, and if you just let it rest for a bit, that particular phase passes.

'You can test testosterone levels and if they are subnormal you can give injections, or you can give it by mouth. Either they come to terms with it, their marriage improves or disintegrates. But usually, or quite often, if you go into it, it's an emotional thing. They've really fallen in love with their secretary, or something. It's difficult to know whether to upset a marriage. You try not to upset a marriage that's working.'

And of course, just as GPs, more than any other profession or calling, see the extremes of life – the saddest, the poorest, the strangest, the most exalting – so do they see the extremes in this sphere too, where human beings can be at their most extraordinary.

I can remember my father, who was intrigued by the bizarre, coming back one day and saying he'd had a naval rating in his surgery that morning who'd complained of constipation, with some rather curious symptoms. On examination my father discovered a Gloy pot embedded in his rectum. He'd asked him how it had got there. "I sat on it, sir," said the rating.

In *A Fortunate Man*, his perceptive, moving if rather humourless book about a Welsh GP, John Berger describes another odd encounter. He gives his doctor the name Sassall.

Dr Sassall is called to an old married couple who'd lived in the forest for thirty years. He knew them quite well. They went every year on the Old Folk's annual outing and to the pub every Saturday evening. The husband had worked on the railways. The wife had worked as a maid in the big house.

The man said his wife 'was bleeding from down under'.

Sassall asked her to undress. The man was rather anxious as Sassall stood in the kitchen waiting. At that age, if the wife has to go into hospital, it can be the beginning of the end for both of them. The man took the clock from the mantelpiece and wound it up.

When Sassall went back into the parlour, continues Berger's description, the wife was lying on the ottoman. Her stockings were rolled down and her dress was up. 'She' was a man. He examined her. The trouble was severe piles. Neither she nor the husband nor Sassall referred to the sexual organs which should not have been there. They were ignored.

9
PRIVATE PRACTICE

Dr David Miston

The surgery, in a wealthy Scottish inner-city area, was more like a studio or film set. It was all underground, very clean, very comfortable, very efficient: a hall with reception kiosk, large waiting room in a well, with comfortable banquettes all round where Dr Miston also gave lectures to students.

At the reception, a fairly forbidding thirty-five-year-old in uniform, but at my name she melted. 'I'm Mrs Miston.'

Dr David Miston was busy, so she showed me round the superbly designed surgery: the dispensary and laboratory, where she analysed specimens and dispensed; the X-ray room with its automatic developer which took the film and printed it in two and a half minutes; the physiotherapy room. The fact that there were no windows to the outside, that it was lit entirely by artificial light, gave an intensity; it was like being in a highly equipped, high ranking bunker during a war – the bunker of the General.

Dr Miston had now finished his surgery. He had a journalist from one of the medical papers with him — would I mind if she sat with us so she could bounce a few questions off him from time to time?

He was about forty-four, tall, fit, with a small quick mouth, the lips thin and pulled in; he was intelligent, rapid, determined, with a rather boyish way of throwing back his head. He was a practised interviewee, pausing when my tape ran out, sometimes repeating when he thought he was inaudible. He only had one holiday a year – two weeks at Christmas.

There was also something emotional about him. At one moment his eyes filled with tears. His argument that people are basically kind and that the poor in a private general practice set-up could rely on charity, while not particularly convincing, arose from his own compassionate nature.

Listening to the tapes later, and reflecting on the interview, I realized that Dr Miston, with his mild but passionate Scots voice, was fairly theatrical. Also a number of his statements had in fact been directed at the pretty young journalist and were to impress her with his humanitarianism and idealism. I think both were perfectly genuine but he laid it on a bit thick.

DR MISTON: 'I was an active member of the Labour Party and was brought up in the health service and believed in it totally. In 1974 I went over to the USA. I had honestly believed that the NHS was the best in the world but I saw standards of clinical practice – particularly of general practice – particularly compassionate, particularly concerned, looking after poor people who couldn't afford it and it was way ahead of anything I had dreamt of. The scales fell from my eyes; it was a revelation. And that feeling has continued.

'So – they have no home visits there? A jolly good thing too. The function of home visits is obviously social. There's no clinical value. Old people – fine. The doctors I saw in the States do home visits to the old, the same as I do. But when a patient is ill and asks for a house call you say, "No. The iller you are the better it is for you to come here, to me." Of course it is, because he's got his own diagnostic facilities. He's got his own X-ray unit, he's got his own path. lab. He does the blood test and X-ray immediately and he's got the answer straight away, and he can see at once what's the matter.

'That's one of the principal things wrong with the NHS – no diagnostic facilities. And *that* is what the College [Royal College of General Practitioners] ought to be really scandalized about. Not the sort of things that they do get upset about, which is non-directional counselling techniques or arranging the chairs in your room. Clinical medicine has gone from general practice. There are doctors who argue that because they've got access to the hospital or to the diagnostic facilities therefore it's just the same; what's the difference in having your own? Well, the answer is, look at the hospitals; look at the path. labs and analyse their figures and you will find that the vast majority of GPs simply don't use them. They really have retired intellectually. They are simply prescription and certificate pushers.

'If you don't use your mind, you find in the end you haven't got it. And unless you have reasonable diagnostic facilities either on your premises or pretty well immediately available, you won't use your mind.

'Take Anne Cartwright's figures for the city centres. One in five GPs employs a full-time member of staff, one in three employs a part-timer. Most doctors are single-handed and you've only got to put those figures together to realize that most doctors work with no staff whatever. And most of the population lives in the cities. It's no use the DHSS throwing in some fancy-pants health centre where the district nurses go out ringing the bells on their bicycles in the middle of Oxfordshire. What *matters* is what happens in Barnsley, Manchester, Liverpool, Swansea, Edgbaston . . . This is what matters. This is where the population is. They simply don't live in villages in Oxford. What's happening in Birmingham, Sheffield, Newcastle matters. Whatever the standards of clinical care, it's rubbish. It simply isn't worth having. There's the isolated doctor who's doing good work, or doing his best within the system. But the point I'm making is, the overall contrast that I've seen between here and in the States is that in the States the doctors are clinicians and I found them much more humane.

'Doctors who think that all this clinical rubbish isn't as important as social concerns are arrogant; they're feather-bedded emotionally and philosophically. They don't have to think; they don't have to be answerable. They have to be answerable to a committee but that's a different thing altogether. You should be answerable to your patients. When a patient says to you "I don't like your attitude" it makes a difference whether the patient ever comes back again or not to me, but not in the NHS – they can say "Up yours".

'In other words, the process of being private involves very considerably more than simply making money. It involves running the business which as any businessman in any sphere whatever will tell you, means you have to think of your clients, otherwise you'll lose them. Now supposing I said to any patient – the wealthiest man in the world – "Open your wallet" – what do you think he'd say? He'd say, "Well, fine, but what are you going to give me in exchange?"

'But it's also pride. It's not just money. In face the NHS GP gets a lot of money. Who else gets paid twenty grand for five hours' work a day?

'If you listen to programmes such as *Any Questions*, if there's any criticism of the Health Service, even the solid right-wing audience that they tend to get in *Any Questions* is upstanding and throwing things. The Health Service is inviolate; it is unchallengeable. People feel that it's the only thing between them and terror, bankruptcy, dying and pain. When you present them with evidence that the Health Service costs £260 a year for every single person and that you will still die in pain in the Health Service if you get an idiot, they say, "Oh yes, but my doctor's terribly good", and you say, "Has he got a nurse or a receptionist or a secretary?" They say, "No, but he's so busy always. He does work hard." "How long are his consulting hours?" "He's there from 9 till 10.30 and 5 till 6 and between that he's on his rounds."

'Are you aware that the number of home visits per doctor averages out at one? One. When a doctor is not in his office, he's on his bum, he's not looking after his patients. The reason the place is so busy is because he's doing an eight-hour day in three or four hours. He's crammed them all into the surgery at once, he's been so bloody mean that he won't even start to look after them in a decent way. Imagine a bank running without the manager. Imagine a greengrocer's running without someone to hump the stuff. You would not tolerate that sort of service from any profession other than medicine. If you went to a solicitor and found the place dirty, would you trust his opinion? It's only lives we're talking about; it's not important.

'You think I'm bitter? You're bloody right, I am. I've been the senior partner of one of the largest medical practices in London for a long time. I built it myself and got the other two doctors in and trained them up and we ran the thing together. I got very considerable experience of what the National Health Service does – it doesn't work. The doctors are more interested in their own free time and making money than in the actual clinical care of patients.

'But I don't want to knock the health service on any other grounds than philosophical. What I'm interested in is why did it all happen? We know it's a bloody disaster area but why? What is it that is wrong? And it was when I first started asking myself that question, I realized it was the basic ideas of the health service that were wrong; the concepts. The universality of free care at the time of need, this results in four million pounds a year being spent on appetite suppressants. That's morally wrong. Look at what is spent on Valium, on cough syrups, and so on. It is morally wrong. We should not be spending money on that. We should be spending money on new hospitals, on giving better wages for nurses, and so on.

'Why don't they have free bananas as well as free Valium? Of the two, I think the banana is probably more healthy. Firstly, you're not treating your patients with pills, which you shouldn't do anyway, and secondly, you're not conning people into thinking you're giving them something when you're not. You're not giving them anything constructive when you give them pills. You're not giving them any affection, you're not giving them comfort.

'What would I do? I would take General Practice out of the National Health Service altogether – it would be totally private. I can see a concept which would retain a Health Service for significant disease – for heart attacks or cancer of the breast. All the rest I'd remove. I simply do not see any moral basis for prescribing free Valium any more than free bananas.

'As for the poor, they would be paid for by charity. Not the state. Not insurance – charity. There is in the country a great wealth of compassion. There really is. Poor people would be looked after by people who want to look after poor people. Look at all the hospitals that were built before; it was all voluntary subscription. They were all private hospitals and the National Health Service nationalized them. Now it's doing its best to close them down.

'I'm not saying I'm right. What I'm saying is "Here are some ideas. Come on. Let's challenge them. Give me a criticism of them and I will learn from that." But let it be constructive criticism. And let it see that I am genuinely concerned with the issues we are talking about.'

NHS GPs and Private Medicine

According to Anne Cartwright's 1981 survey, between 0.5 per cent and 2 per cent of patients use private GPs, often in conjunction with NHS GP cover. Pure private practice is, therefore, a minute proportion of our subject and I have not gone into it in any depth.

Nevertheless, there are one or two brief comments that should be made about it. Some doctors are vehemently opposed to private practice and would like to deny anyone using it any of the NHS benefits.

This argument is barely sustainable. The idea of a possibly combined service was written into the Health Service from the start, when Aneurin Bevan spoke of patients making use of the service 'in whole or in part'. Since everyone, private or not, pays their share of the contribution, how can it be equitable to exclude some of them from the benefits on the grounds that they have paid an extra consultation fee to a doctor?

In fact, you are not allowed to be treated privately by a GP and also be on his NHS list and obtain free drugs. Purely private patients have to pay for their own drugs. But people can be on one GP's NHS list and be a private patient with another doctor. The two doctors collude, and the NHS GP will supply free drugs. Questioned about this some years ago, one BMA official said it was 'undesirable' to be treated by two doctors. But another spokesman said it was quite proper for doctor B to ask doctor A for a second opinion and for doctor A to prescribe free drugs. Sometimes one member of a family is NHS, and he or she is the channel for the rest of the family. But even these subterfuges don't really, it seems to me, undermine the argument that everyone has paid towards the Health Service and should be able to enjoy its benefits – whether or not they indulge in acupuncture, vitamin C or private practitioners as well.

Another argument that was advanced to me was that if private medicine flourishes, then it will be used by the people who run the country, who can afford it, and they will have no stimulus to improve NHS medicine. This seems naïve. You might as well argue that because the nation's rulers travel by official Rover or Rolls or helicopter they will have no incentive to improve public transport. Politicians are moved by what gains votes and furthers the interests of their supporters. There are no votes to be gained nor supporters' interests to be enhanced by attacking or diminishing the GP side of the NHS (we are not dealing here with the hospital side, to which different considerations apply), and that is why, though there has been some stringency, the GP set-up has been less seriously affected by the economies of the last four years than any other public sector except the police.

There is, however, one area where the 'governing class' argument might come to apply. Towards the end of 1982 six GPs set up a super private health centre in Harrow backed by Air Call (Holdings) Ltd, to the tune of £550,000. One of the doctors, Doctor Goldsmith (appropriately named) appeared on TV to extol the project: twenty-four hour personal service, centre containing pharmacy, X-rays, minor op. facilities, nursery, physiotherapist; 'reasonable' fees – £65 per annum, £5.10p a visit, extra £22 per annum and free drugs; fifteen minutes a consultation.

It is too early to say whether the centre is a success — though in wealthy, middle-class Harrow, perhaps serving Harrow school later on, I can see it might well be. But suppose, as Goldsmith hinted, a network of these centres appeared in the inner cities? Certainly the unemployed, the pensioners and alcoholics, the drifters could *not* afford those prices. They would remain with the old, single-handed practitioners; the worst cases getting the worst medicine. A two-tier private-v.-NHS set-up might evolve.

But there is no sign that Air Call (Holdings) Ltd have taken this step. Goldsmith talked vaguely of Brixton. I can't see Brixton being exactly a goldmine.

But by far the largest proportion of private practice is mixed in with the NHS.

DR NYEWOOD (Three-doctor Berkshire group practice): 'Out of a total practice income of say £74,000 – £75,000, about £10,000 comes from private. But not all private patients. You do insurance medicals, insurance reports – you get £9 for your report. It mounts up. Perhaps £4,000 a year. The remainder is private patients.'

DR KINSHAM (Inner city health centre): 'I did inherit from my senior partner about 100 patients. We tried, and try to get them to go NHS. I remember, the classic thing was a lady who wanted injections of B12. So I said, "Well, look, I'll do your B12 level to see whether you need it" and she didn't. She was a South African diamond merchant's wife. Jewish. And she said, "Well, look, you're my doctor and I want it," and I said, "I'm your doctor, and I'm not going to give it to you," and she said, "In that case . . . ", and I was delighted not to be her doctor thank you. And that was it.'

DR JANE EDSTONE: 'I think it is a shame it has to be. I very rarely take one and never long term. If I get a woman who, say, is somebody else's and has a feminine complaint and is too embarrassed, I'll see her on a one-off but I don't like doing it.'

Nearly all GPs do insurance medicals and mobility examinations (which is really an item of service payment). About straight private patients, the majority felt like Dr Kinsham and Dr Jane Edstone. The relatively few who have a few are always careful to point out they are 'historical'; somehow not their fault. Some GPs take one or two by way of contrast and novelty.

They are always careful to point out they do not get better treatment, but it is obvious why a few people prefer to remain private. They pay for their drugs, but they get time, politeness, a visit in hospital, seen when they want to be, in their own minds a tiny bit of *cachet*. Anne Cartwright also found that 33 per cent of men and 26 per cent of women would like to have a private doctor if they could afford it.

10

DR SAM LOCKING,
A TWO-DOCTOR PRACTICE, CUMBERLAND

My journeys before Dr Locking, though extensive – GP practices across England from Cornwall to Norfolk, as far south as Bournemouth and into Kent – had all been below the Trent. Dr Locking marked the start of a drive which would end in the Highlands, returning late in November down through the industrial North and the Midlands.

I left Norfolk and drove into Lincolnshire rather late in the afternoon. For a long time it was the same flat route, the same choked, winding roads and flat dreary fields. But as you approach Sheffield the Pennines, like some not very distant storm, start the land rolling. There were one or two mines, then signs with 'South Yorkshire' and 'Derbyshire' and the names of ancient lords – Chesterfield, Rennishaw. The churches were like castles, not the charming little models of Suffolk and Norfolk with their elegant, miniscule tracery.

Sheffield is built, like Rome only more spectacularly, on hills and valleys. You get marvellous views especially, as it was when I arrived, at night – the sweeps and carpets of light.

I had non-doctor business in the morning and left Sheffield some time after lunch. Leeds to the right, Manchester to the left, Huddersfield, Bradford, Keighley and at last out, up into the Yorkshire Dales. The immense expanse of this Black Country, but somehow merging naturally into the Dales, the dry-stone walls looking like threads from the man-made mass continuing out and out, roots into the moors.

It was dark again when I finally arrived at what seemed like a large village where the Lockings lived.

Buxom, kindly, voluble Mrs Locking was flustered by my late arrival and by a fall of soot from the Rayburn – the wind had been strong as I'd come over the darkening fells – but very welcoming. Sam wasn't back yet, she said. He'd gone racing at Newcastle. She didn't know if he'd gone punting or as a bookie. Some days he ran a book with a friend of his. We could tell which when he came in; if he was smart, he'd have been punting, if scruffy, book-making.

It dawned on me as we chatted and I helped clean up the kitchen that Newcastle must have been nearly 100 miles away.

Sam arrived about half an hour later. He'd clearly been book-making. He was short, fairly tubby, with short, distrait, thinning hair, a sweet smile with hopeless teeth; he looked a bit like Hugh Lofting's Dr Dolittle. He was fifty-four but looked about sixty, his accent a pleasant mixture of the North and Norfolk. He'd had a bad day. Punters simply weren't splashing out. You couldn't lay off bets if people wouldn't take them.

We had supper. (Under my glass was a mat – 'Betaloc SA – dealing simply with Hypertension.' The house, in many small particulars, had been furnished by the drug companies.) Then Sam and I went into the large, attractive drawing room, hung with fine eighteenth- and nineteenth-century water colours, and began to talk.

DR LOCKING: 'When I'd been here three months the chap who took me on told me he was going with another woman and I can assure you, Jonny, this practice takes a hell of a lot of time to get to know people and I was just literally thrown in at the deep end. I came here fully expecting to be the junior partner for twenty-five years and I'd only been in the place five minutes and he said he was slinging his hook, so there I had to go through all the rigmarole of getting in somebody. Luckily I got somebody who's stayed the course.

'So within two years of qualifying I was a senior partner. I had a meteoric rise, if you like, to the high echelons of general practice, faster than I expected. I'd only done eighteen months in a town practice. Very sudden. Quite pleasant, but very *sudden*. I'd still got a lot to learn, even when I was senior partner.

'It was bewildering really. You know, the important thing with a practice like here if you come for the first time, you've got to get to know all the different relationships with people, because they're all related and half of them have got nicknames. And I'm still learning things and finding such people are related. Perhaps people that I don't often see, they always come as a surprise. I'm learning all the time about the actual content of the family history of the people. Very interesting it is.

'And I intend to stay. I'll be a doctor till I'm seventy-five, eighty. That's my intention at the moment. Because you see, I *enjoy* it. I can't say that I'm dedicated, no way. But you see, I have a wonderful relationship with them all. They all seem to like me. When I put up for Parish Council I got in by a large majority. I got in by about . . . I got a tremendous lot of votes anyway, I absolutely pissed in to put it bluntly.'

JGH: 'They knew where you were immediately, when I asked up in the village.'

DR LOCKING: 'Did they? Good . . . Yes . . . It's a *town*, not a village. A town, I always understood when I was brought up, should have 1,000 inhabitants and when I was putting up for Parish Council I knew exactly who was on the electoral roll because I went through it like a bloody toothcomb and it's under 1,000 but it's still a town, so take that how you like.

'It's a very large area – 400 square miles. Coming down to the southern aspect of the practice, it goes as far as Clawthorpe Fell. That's a very, very horrible road over there – it's rather like being on the moon.

'It was the custom when I first came here, fewer telephones, especially out on the Fell farms, if they wanted him to call, they would always put out a duster, by which sign the doctor knew he had to call. The vet has a red duster, or red flag usually.

'We get some fearful winters. But the funny thing is when we get a lot of snow the work is never as hard. They don't get flu and things because they can't get to the various things that are going on. You know, they can't get to the WI or they can't get to the various functions, because they're snowed in, so everybody stays fairly healthy; but when you get a mild winter you get a busy winter.

'We don't have branch surgeries, but I carry a lot. I'm like a travelling shop: a wide spectrum of antibiotics, cough and stomach medicines, ointments ranging from piles to cortisone cream. And my emergency bag. I don't often have to use it, but it's *there* if I need it. I do sometimes stitch away from surgery, but we encourage them to come in. Or they'll ring after hours and come into the house. In summer, I'll do two or three stitchings a day.

'Now my friend in Scotland, who's a single-handed practice, hardly does a stitch from one year's end to another. But he has a hospital nine miles away. The fact that we've got a hospital thirty-seven miles from here, of course, I suppose makes us self-reliant to a certain extent. You know, you sort of feel you've sort of got to cope with things. I mean, you're more involved with things that are going on than a town doctor. A town doctor isn't really a proper doctor.

'If you look at the map you'll see we're surrounded by mountain ranges so in the past when communications were not what they are today, and transport wasn't what it is, you got a very close community. So there's an awful lot of inbreeding. I wouldn't say there's so much, say, madness as you'd get fifty or sixty years ago. There's a fair bit of depression and certainly you do see where insanity can run in families. Here's just been a very recent sad case of a young man who hanged himself in a barn. It happened when I was off and my partner was on call and I was up racing at Wetherby. And this has highlighted the fact that this lad's mother and his father's mother hanged themselves, and I think another of his grandmothers, on his mother's side, and an uncle or great uncle hanged himself. So it does run in families.

'But more particularly, the things that come to mind are blood pressures – hypertension – and diabetes. These two to my mind stick out. If I see people with any bizarre symptoms, his father's brother was a diabetic, I'll probably grunt to them, "You've got sugar int' family. Bring me some urine." Which they'll do and I'll test it. It's interesting, very interesting.

'You'd think – country folk, healthy. But whether it's the inbreeding, also the diet, they're very *un*healthy. They need a lot of doctoring; they do. A tremendous lot.'

Sam Locking described his workload. Two surgeries a day except Saturday, which was emergencies only, and Tuesday afternoons. Twelve to twenty people a surgery, and a good many visits, with long drives. There were no appointments and people clearly called at the house at any odd time – 'Is doctor in?' Tuesday afternoon was market day and surgery ran from one till four, packed out. Farmers came in from the auctions, wives from the outlying farms in to do the shopping. 'I usually chat, perhaps nine tenths, about things other than their ailments and it comes out in the wash as it were. Winter, they often come into our waiting room to keep bloody warm.'

He went on to explain it was still a very close-knit, closed-in community.

'But I've woven my way into it. I'm a good mixer. I can just switch on 'doctor'. Then I can go and see my race-course friends and mix in. And I like them. I regard them as equals. Some of them call me Sam. We are geographically and intellectually isolated and you have to make your friends in the local community or go without. And I intend to retire here. It behoves me to get on. I've always been one for looking to the future. When I was at medical school I wasn't very bright but I always made friends with the younger ones, those in the year below, because I knew then I could always fit in with them. I knew I'd never catch the buggers up in the year ahead – you know what I mean? I was always *paving the way*.

'You get quite close. I've had one or two friends that I've been quite pally with and they've popped their clogs. I've rather taken it as a matter of course. You could get quite involved and, you know, upset.

'But I'm lucky in that the dispensary is in my consulting room. The partner and the receptionist have to sort of barge in during consultations, and although it might be a bit embarrassing for the patient, it often saves me being *involved*, if you understand. You know, it's very easy to *break it up* at the point you've had enough.

'Now the dispensary. Very good. I don't have any money worries now. In fact, we get quite a lot of free drug dinners actually. We go out at least twice a month on a drug dinner. These aren't your in-and-out town lunches. These are proper dinner jobs, plenty of wine, you know. You assemble at – it's always the same – you assemble at 7.30, dinner at 8. There might be a short film or a talk for a quarter of an hour which is the object of the exercise; then a slap-up dinner. It's a good do.

'Where was I? How did I get on to that? Oh money, yes. We weren't dispensing when I first came here; I rather introduced it. We were an inducement practice – a sort of GPs on National Assistance. I didn't really like that set-up. So I started dispensing and 800 of our patients get their medicine from us. I educated my boy at public school from what I made on drugs really. In fact last year they were both at school. It cost me seven grand a year.

'But over the years there's been one big change. The summers. They've encouraged people to come in bloody droves to the Fells. And it brings in its wake an extra workload of holiday people. Honestly, it can be like Morecambe or Blackpool. You get the whole spectrum. Ankles, cuts. We get old ladies breaking down in buses – coach tours, you know. You have to go and do a consultation with a full audience of the bus passengers. You have to be a bit of a showman, really, because you feel that you're putting on an act for *them*, never mind attending to the patient. You sort of feel you've got to let the audience feel the patient is getting his pound of flesh, you know.

'But these townees, they must really piss their doctors around because they come for the most *trifling* complaints. We don't mind; we get 3 or 4 quid for every one we do, but it is rather robbing the Government. Some of them are all right, you meet some nice people, but some are a right bloody pain, and you think to yourself, by God. You feel sorry for their doctor, you know.

'But you get bad things too. In fact we were sitting here just like this watching the television. There's pot-holes near here and it said work had been going on all day to recover these bodies. And I thought, "Well, if it's been going on all day and they haven't called me in . . ." and damn me, about five minutes after that the bloody phone went and I had to go.

'I had to be lowered down. It was a bit frightening. But plenty of people to lower me. You're very much the VIP of a situation like that. I rather tend to lap it up [laughing].

'But that upset me, did that. There were at least three, three in wetsuits, two on the stretcher sides of the ambulance and one in the passageway, dead, all in their wetsuits. A most grotesque sight, you know. Like batmen. In their suits all three lay parallel, you know. One in the well, and the others on the sides. They'd drowned.

'Road accidents are worse. That's what I dislike most. Did you come in on that horrible winding road off the Fell there? Well it was just before you descended the steep corner, someone was coming very fast and the car just went off the road and just bounded and bounded for . . . well, it must have been for nearly a quarter of a mile and these bodies scattered all over . . . four of them. One old lady was killed outright and there were three others. God, they were all unconscious. Scattered bodies. It was a right carry on. We had all the police. They even called police off the motorway. All you can do is just to sort of put in air-ways and dispatch them as quick as you can.'

We talked some more, but Sam Locking seemed to be getting restless. When Mrs Locking came in, he got up and said he had something to attend to.

Mrs Locking stayed to chat to me. She said he'd be working in the surgery. He pretended the practice didn't worry him, but it did more than he let on. He often got up like that and went off to write consultants' letters or something.

Sam was away an hour working. When he came back we managed a bit more medical talk.

'When I first came they tried to make me doctor them in the street. I soon put a stop to that. There's that tendency to try and corner you. You know the old trick at cocktail parties – this is going up the social ladder a bit, the sort of middle-class range. They try it on. And I can't stand that. I can't stand that, being bloody cornered. I don't want to talk doctoring when I'm out, normally. If anyone stops me in the street and says "Will you lay a bet?" or "I've got a good thing for you", or "How did you get on at so-and-so the other day?", well, I'll stop and talk to them as long as they like. That's the conversation I want. I don't want to hear about their bloody kids' rashes. You sod off.

'Keeping up to date? I suppose so. But I have quite a good relationship with consultants. If I get stuck I just ring them up and ask them. Easy way of doing it.'

But it was clear he was losing interest. Whenever we left medical subjects he visibly brightened, though he perked up when I asked him about his early life.

'I was always going to be a parson. I'd always dreamed that I was going to be a parson. I think I'd have been a bishop now if I'd been a parson.

'But in fact I never really worked until I was thirty-five. I was a bit of a playboy quite honestly. You could stay at Trinity College, Dublin for ever, if you could afford it. I didn't have money, but I used to sort of fiddle what I wanted. A sort of entrepreneur. Buying and selling antiques; going across the border with cameras and that sort of thing.'

JGH: 'Do you mean smuggling?'

DR LOCKING: 'You could call it that.'

After that we abandoned medicine and discovered a shared interest in Johnson and Pepys. I found this kindly, humorous, slightly eccentric man was cultivated and well read. We chatted about Boswell and the Thrales, and he described building up his collection of Rowlandsons and water-colours. Eventually I went to bed, while Sam Locking rang his GP friend in Scotland, who he thought I should see.

The towels in the bathroom had been supplied by Fabrol; by my bed was a glass – Altacite PLUS. I filled it with Chianti from a bottle in my suitcase. Knowing the alcohol statistics of doctors, this was not something I had expected would be necessary. But to my surprise, all the doctors I visited were virtually teetotal. This evening, for instance, I'd had two tiny glasses of Mateus Rosé.

The next morning the Lockings were going on holiday. There was time only for a brief chat, during which I learnt, however, that he had not gone to work the previous evening. He'd felt a cold coming on and had gone to have brandy and lemon with their neighbours the Joneses. He'd found you could drink large quantities of brandy and lemon without getting sloshed. It occurred to me that what might be happening was that the doctors and I were each drinking secretly and separately.

Before they left they said I could certainly stay on and write up some notes. I waved goodbye, watching them drive off – Sam puffing at his pipe, Sue Locking chatting away – then went up to the study. The leather blotter said, 'Rythmodan in DISOPYRAMIDE from Roussell (100 mg capsules) for the treatment of cardiac arrhythmias'. I'd finished my tapes and was anxious, among other things, to get down a last, vivid glimpse Sam Locking had given me of his practice and himself just before they left.

'A bus load arrived and I was called to this old lady who'd fainted. When I got there I found she was dead. The trouble with this town is there's no mortuary. I knew it would upset them all if I said she was dead. I got them to strap her into the passenger seat next to me. Her son in the back (I told him). We drove round to the police station – it simply looked as if she were asleep. People kept on coming up to chat. I had to get rid of them. Old Jock Thomas came up. He's the biggest gossip in the place. "What's up with her?" he said. "She's asleep," I said. (Poor chap in the back!) "What you sitting there for then?" "Bugger off, Jock," I said. Do you know, we were there an hour waiting for the ambulance. The things you do!'

DRUGS AND DRUG COMPANIES

The subject of GPs, their prescribing and the activity of the drug companies has had and continues to get an enormous amount of attention.

The cost of pharmaceutical products is not just the biggest in the NHS GP bill, it is larger than all the others put together – salaries, health centres, nurses, health visitors, the lot. It was £1,400 million in 1983. We can't just ignore so expensive a part of our subject.

But you do not often hear what the doctors themselves think of the drug reps or of the various ways these astronomical costs could be reduced. Perhaps, therefore, the best way through this area is to hear what the GPs say; commenting as we go but commenting, in view of the media attention, briefly.

The Reps and Their Activities

DR ANNE UPLEES: 'I think the reps that come and sit in the surgery for ten minutes are just as useful as seeing a film for ten minutes and having lunch. Some know what they're talking about, some don't. But you do get to hear of any worthwhile new drugs through the reps coming.'

DR TELSCOMBE (Large East Anglian group practice): 'They're programmed to spout something – but I use them. I get out my *Mims Companion*, which lists all the drugs made by each company, and I'll say, "I had a lot of trouble with that one the other day, can you find out so-and-so." You know, problems. And Winthrop are very useful for producing goodies. I said yesterday, "I want a notice for the car park asking patients not to park there if they're not attending surgery." In a month's time I'll have some nicely produced stickers we can use.'

DR BLAIRHALL: 'When I was very busy in the sixties I said, "I'm going to stop seeing drug reps," and I haven't seen a drug rep in the surgery for sixteen years. But latterly, drug reps have been holding luncheon meetings at a very nice establishment on the river there and the trainee and I go on Wednesdays and Thursdays when there's a drug lunch. And I find them quite useful to find out about what drugs are being marketed. I also find it a marvellous point of

contact with our opposition practice and there's two or three of them *always*
go and if I didn't go I would hardly meet them.'

DR ABNEY: 'I see the drug reps. The ones that come here are people that
mostly know what they're talking about. There again, the drug companies
are tending to send round dishy birds now – this is a new thing. There's one
from Aylesford, she's fantastic. She almost asks you – she leaves her address
and for 50 quid I should think you'd be there. "I've got a very nice flat," she
says, "right on the London Road," and I said "Oh yes?" But she's just a
come-on I'm sure. She just appeals to our baser instincts. Some of them are
useless, but there are old friends who've been coming here for a long time. I
see them because we have a natter and they leave their latest guff and they
clear off.'

DR TRIMDON: 'They've proved if they send reps the sales go up, you see. And
I think it's true to say, if you see a rep, in the next two or three days as long as
it's in your mind, you'll probably write out two or three scrips. And you
might forget to go back to your old faithful and just carry on.'

GPs, that is to say, are relaxed about the drug companies; they see the reps to
learn about new drugs, to get surgery stickers, see their colleagues, have
dinners, because the reps are attractive and so on. They are also all vaguely
aware that it works.

This, of course, is the nub – as Dr Trimdon was aware. And it has been
proved abundantly. In a recent TV programme, largely concerned with the
American firm Eli Lilly, the makers of Opren, the vast sums disbursed were
described. Probably more was spent, individually, on consultants. But
consultants are a way of getting at GPs – who will ask their advice, and take
their imprimatur on the drug given to a returned patient as evidence of its
efficacy. But large sums were spent on GPs themselves. One rep, out of a force
of seventy, spent £300 in four days wining and dining GPs – aside from the the
usual flood of trivia.

'Lilly wouldn't spend a dollar,' said the ex-sales director, 'if they were not
certain of getting three times the money back.' It has been shown that once a
GP is convinced he will go on prescribing a drug for years.

One result of this is that a good number of GPs prescribe far too much.
This will come as no surprise to anyone who has accompanied these GPs on
their visits and observed, not just the abandoned, but sometimes almost wild
way they rip off scrip sheets, or leave vast piles of signed pads for nurses and
sisters to issue repeat prescriptions.

There are reasons other than promotional pressure for GPs to over-
prescribe. As we know, the bottle of medicine was for decades the tradition.
Both doctor and patient feel something has been done. A prescription is often

a way of getting out of a more time-consuming analysis and treatment. It is a way of cutting short the consultation – or more. Dr Nyewood – 'It's a nice way of getting rid of the patient; you scribble something out and rip the thing off the pad. The ripping off is really the "Fuck off".'

Patients are perfectly well aware of this (two thirds of all patients leave a surgery with a prescription). Cartwright found that 52 per cent would like less prescribing, and that three times as many thought this than in 1964. 38 per cent would have preferred a ten-minute discussion. This seems to be particularly true of GPs dealing with the old, and *Pulse* recently described an experiment where in the London Borough of Newham the drug prescription in old people's homes was strictly monitored and as a result halved. The homes were transformed.

But there is no doubt that the major measurable force to over-prescribe is drug company promotion. Drug companies have time and again tested two groups of GPs, one subject to promotion, the other not. Group 1 invariably prescribes, not just the drug promoted, but *more* than the other group. This really brings us to the case against the pharmaceutical companies.

The Case against the Pharmaceutical Companies

The argument of Inglis and other critics is, quite briefly, on two fronts.

The first is that, in their anxiety to recoup money invested, drug companies ignore adverse reactions to drugs developed till the last possible moment – the results are cases like Opren and Thalidomide. And that even when finally, virtually by force, they are prevented from marketing them in the West they will continue to do so in the Third World. I don't really want to go into this. It is to do with the morality or otherwise of certain companies, which is not our concern.

One should, however, have some idea of the sums of money involved. To develop, test and market a new drug can be very expensive. The usual development period is about ten years. Sums of £50 or £100 million are not unusual. If something goes wrong, this is a lot of money and time to have wasted. But if it goes well, conversely, a lot of money can be made. In 1981 the top ten drug companies had an £18,000 million turnover. Their profit margins were 17 per cent higher than other top companies. (When Inglis wrote in 1964 he quoted figures of 21.4 per cent compared to 11 per cent.)

But the morality or immorality of certain drug companies is just a consequence of the commercial orientation which dictates their activities – and which is the main thrust of the criticism. Opren and Thalidomide have had two effects on the pharmaceutical industry: a large increase in time-consuming statutory checks and tests; and a reluctance among research scientists to pursue often brilliant hunches because the results of failure are so dire. This has severely discouraged primary research, from which totally new products might emerge. Instead they have concentrated on 'me too' drugs. These are minute variations on established drugs, just different enough to get a different patent and a slice of the existing market. Inglis estimated 70 per cent of American research went on this type of thing, while only 1 per cent went on primary research.

The result has been and continues to be an absolutely ridiculous proliferation of new drugs – very few of which are in any significant way different from their cousins. Most common diseases have fifty or sixty related remedies. Opren was the twentieth anti-arthritic agent – and quite unnecessary. Several drug companies use computers to churn out new names. Neither the public nor GPs can possibly keep track and are therefore totally dependent on the drug companies, their various promotions and the papers like *Pulse* and the *Practitioner* which they finance. And that is why, although the large companies do spend many millions researching and manufacturing these 'me too' drugs, the figures are dwarfed by what they spend on selling and promotion.

What can, or should be done?

Generic Prescribing and Other Solutions

One solution often proposed is generic prescribing. This means prescribing the basic formula from which the 'me too' varieties have evolved, and which are nearly always very much cheaper and usually just as effective as the developed varieties. Dr Kinsham was involved in a pilot scheme in London which supplied the generic names of five drugs to fifty GPs – Nitrazepam rather than Mogodon, Indomethacin rather than Indocid and so on. It was calculated that this would save the NHS £100 million a year. They saved £250,000 doing the study alone, which was much more than it actually cost to set up.

But GPs have mixed feelings about this, about other solutions – and about the drug industry generally.

DR COLKIRK (Highland inducement practice): 'Tagamet is £75 for 500; Zantac, the new one from Glaxo, is more – £27 for sixty. One scheme is that it would deter people if you put the price on them; and it *would* deter some of my anxious, conscientious little old ladies. But that idea has against it precisely that – it *would* deter and the point of the NHS was that that sort of anxiety should go.

'But these things are good. The argument for using something like that or Zantac, is that it cures the pain of stomach ulcers very effectively, and it keeps the patient out of hospital. The other way to cure the pain is to operate. Now operations, and stays in hospital, are so expensive that even these incredibly expensive drugs are far cheaper. So that when politicians say the drug bill is ridiculous – it's getting out of hand, they don't realize how much hospital time that is saving. I've got two patients on these drugs who would certainly have required operations long before now if they hadn't got these drugs.'

DR BILSBY: 'The point is generic drugs are given names to describe what they *are*, you *can't* shorten them. Whereas the trade names are short and easy to write down. I mean, Slow K. You can't really prescribe potassium chloride coated in slow release core in 600 milligrams, or something like that, you know it's much easier to say Slow K'.

DR TELSCOMBE: 'In some people there really are differences. I have one patient who takes a blood pressure tablet, Aldomet, and when I tried to put him on Methyl Dopa, the generic equivalent, he reacted most peculiarly. He couldn't take it at all, so we had to go back to the trade product again.'

DR WARFIELD: 'I would like to see the patients pay for their non-essential drugs. This would cut out a lot of demands for rubbish that we unfortunately have to perpetuate in the interests of good personal relationships.

'As for generic, well, it's all very well, but the profits of the pharmaceutical companies are going to dive and we are dependent on them to produce new and valuable drugs.

'I mean, there are damn good drugs. Take Zantac and Tagamet – one is SK & F, the other is Glaxo. This has revolutionized the treatment of peptic ulcers. It cost about £50 – £100 million to develop, and that's a lot of money to recoup, but it has revolutionised the treatment of hiatus hernia and peptic ulcers on a scale that is unbelievable. Take the pill. It's also caused a lot of problems I might say, but that's by the by. Some of the new modern drugs are unbelievable by my standard of twenty years ago. Some of the newer hypertensive agents are incredibly effective, and incredibly good. People would have died years ago without treatments like these. I've got a patient who's lived twenty years after her blood pressure reached a level which, when I was a student, would have been regarded as a death warrant within two years. The pharmaceutical houses have produced some astonishing drugs over the years. Not every pharmaceutical company, not every year, but when they do hit a winner, it's a 100 million quids' worth.

One of the things that is going to happen in the future is anti-viral drugs which will be very important. But it's going to be development on a massive scale; and there's all this genetic engineering producing new drugs from hormones, which at the moment we can't produce synthetically. So all these things require vast amounts of research by pharmaceutical industries. The answer is, I have mixed feelings about prescribing generic stuff. It would save a lot of money, but equally well might put the pharmaceutical industries in jeopardy and therefore jeopardize any further progress in treatment of diseases.'

In an article in the *Guardian* in March 1983 Professor Shuster of the University of Newcastle on Tyne proposed a radical solution to the problem.

First, he argued, if there are to be new drugs, there will be some that, after long trials *on the public*, will eventually show up as doing damage. The public now has a totally unrealistic view of how safe the introduction of new drugs can be. Testing standards are far higher than, for example, they are in the motor industry or for the production of quick-setting concrete. But against the damage, the public should see what it is like to have the disease. Often you are better off with the side effects. This is arguably true of Eraldin for instance.

He might have gone on, as did an *Office of Health Economics Briefing* (No.19, September 1982) to argue that damage done by a few specific drugs should be set against the good done by the generalized many. From five drugs alone – Intal for asthma, Betablockers for angina, Zyloric for gout, Indocid for arthritis, Aldomet for blood pressure – has come the rather cumbersome but nonetheless impressive concept of 200 million years of worldwide patient benefit. 250,000 children's lives have been saved in Britain alone since 1940 by the development of vaccines, penicillin etc. 'No one would argue that such a ratio (as opposed to 500) makes the Thalidomide disaster "acceptable" in any sense', says the paper. But in fact that is precisely what it *is* arguing, as a later quote makes clear: 'Clearly it would have been unacceptable to have foregone all pharmaceutical innovation in the twentieth century even to have avoided the price paid by the Thalidomide victims.'

So first (though he does not make this crystal clear) Professor Shuster would like less stringent, more 'realistic' regulations as regards testing.

But the most convincing part of his argument is to follow. The root of the problem is the commercial base of the companies. This dictates the need to a) recoup on investment b) make sufficiently large profits to create new products, as Dr Warfield rightly noted.

Suppose, says Shuster, you have a bright idea for treating eczema (he is a professor of dermatology). But after several years of development and promising tests you find that after it has gone public and contrary to expectations, the drug is really no better than its rivals. Should you just scrap it and the £25 million you've spent? Clearly, says Professor Shuster, you should. But a commercial company can't possibly do that. It would soon go bust for one thing. You recoup your investment by advertising and promotion and, though you didn't do what you'd hoped, at least you've earned enough to start again with something else.

The fact is it is simply frivolous to suggest a solution which can't work. If by some miracle all GPs and consultants started generic prescribing all that would happen is that drug companies would raise the price of generic drugs to the height necessary for them to make the profits they now obtain on their 'me too' varieties. They would also raise the prices on those 'me too' varieties sufficiently different to still be necessary. And to maintain profitability there would also, no doubt, be a dramatic shift of spending away from speculative research and 'fringe' activities like ads in *Pulse*, post-graduate teaching and the like.

The only real solution is to remove the intense pressure for commercial profitability which is at the bottom of the whole thing. The industry would then be able to look at sickness and disease and decide where new drugs were *needed*, not where they would be most profitable.

Professor Shuster looks first at nationalization, but rejects it because this would not really remove the commercial base. This is further intensified because the major pharmaceutical companies are international and have to compete on equal terms with each other. And in fact this would really be little different from what happens now. The vast drug bill is as large as it is because the Government concedes to drug companies the need for a 25 per cent profit margin. They are, that is to say, *already* subsidizing the companies. All that would happen is the companies would not need to waste money on unnecessary research and invention.

The final alternative is subsidy. Government money taking the place of commercial profit gained by excessive promotion and unnecessary 'me too' research and drugs.

For an instant, light dawns – to be replaced almost immediately by gloom. Because, the brute fact is – would any government do it? It is totally alien to the ideology of the present administration. It is difficult to say what other governments might do, but given the priority likely to be given to unemployment over the next decade or more, such an expensive reform would come low.

A reform which won't be accepted is as frivolous as one which won't work. As to his first suggestion, which is again logically impeccable, I can only say that cars and quick-setting cement are all very well, but there is something peculiarly horrifying in medicines which are meant to heal turning out to maim. I think it would be very difficult to overturn the choice that has been made here.

It looks as if we will have the present situation for some time. Piecemeal improvements will take place. As the chemo-intoxicated fifties GPs retire, over-prescribing will improve. In fact as far as tranquillizers go, this has happened – down by a third since the mid-seventies. (The total of *all* prescriptions has dropped 7 per cent in the last six years.) Raising prescription charges, incidentally, can be counter-productive. GPs just prescribe in bulk so that poor patients don't have to go so often. Cartwright suggests that doctors should ask patients if they'd *like* a prescription. They'd be surprised at the number who'd say no. Prices need not be marked on containers, to protect Dr Colkirk's nervous and conscientious patients. But it's GPs not patients who need to be reminded of the costs. Perhaps chemists should be instructed not to dispense a prescription unless the GP had marked the cost on it.

As for chemists, one GP, concerned with the problem of variable quality among generic drugs, said it should be left to them. The doctor should specify what he wants generically – say tetracyline, 250 milligrams – and the chemist should dispense the cheapest and most reliable brand. This is within his competence. The trouble is, it is entirely in the chemist's interest to dispense the most expensive drug possible.

As we shall see, the chemist is an extremely important side-kick to the GP. It is in any case, interesting to look for a moment into one of those obscure lives. And it is also a way into a further and deeper look at other adjuncts to GPs – their groups and health centres, their nurses, midwives and health visitors, their partners, the way they order their working lives.

Mr Poyle, the Chemist

Mr Poyle, about forty-four, whose shop was near the Three Elms surgery in the Lincolnshire town we shall shortly visit, was tall and military, with black hair cut short. Very much a product of Boots' training, I felt. He was obliging and eager, and had a measured, rather soporific way of speaking. He had a very blue chin and cheeks and I could see the hairs on his chest poking above his neat shirt collar and blue tie.

MR POYLE: 'You do three years getting a university degree, then a year's practical training under a qualified pharmacist, and Boots is pretty much the obvious choice, as they will take on young graduates, whereas a small private pharmacist won't. I got on quite well with Boots for about ten years trolling around the country. There are forty branches in a Boots territory so you get a lot of experience, and then your own shop. But you never know where and I was on the promotion list, my wife and I sweating once again where would the call take us – outer Hebrides, Liverpool or wherever, and suddenly we realized this could go on *ad infinitum*. At that stage we realized home life was more important, so we upped and came to Lincolnshire, where we had the chance of buying our way in.

'Financing a pharmacy is very difficult. You would expect to pay £20,000 for even a small pharmacy for goodwill, fixtures and fittings; and a further £20,000 to stock the place. I was very lucky and we borrowed the money from one of my wife's relatives.

'Well, most pharmacists would agree that that is their profession and dispensing is the name of the game – but it is difficult to make a living out of the NHS side alone. Chemists' shops have already had perfume and the like and we're always searching – we've just started on wine and beer-making.

'My pharmacy is a prime example of being away from the town centre and near the surgery. In fact there's been a pharmacy here for 150 years, and the Three Elms surgery for 100 years, so we're traditionally close and I get about

80 per cent of prescriptions from them. We're very close. They like to know what I'm having distribution problems over. I can give advice of what is available in a range – I'm thinking particularly of surgical appliances. I stock what I know are each doctor's particular favourites and so on.

'One problem we don't have here which I've had in the cities and that is the addict. You have the choice whether to take a registered addict on your books or not. The procedure is very strict. They are only allowed them at certain times and if they don't fit in with your hours it can be difficult. I have had some very nice middle-class ones, very respectable, who come in and you wouldn't know. But you get the hippy type who can be quite vociferous. They've been known to come in first thing in the morning because they've nowhere to sleep and sit in the shop till 10 o'clock, the time for their drug. One doesn't want such people there for hour after hour. There was one nasty incident, my day off, this young addict came in late in the evening after 10 and asked if she – it was a girl – could have her supply and was told no. But she made an excuse so they rang the local hospital and the houseman on duty answered no, don't dispense. When this young addict was told she went absolutely berserk and started grabbing bottles of mixture and hurling everything round the shop, causing several hundreds of pounds' damage to fixtures and fittings. And when she appeared in court the next day the consultant just said he wasn't responsible, she hadn't had her fix, and we didn't get a penny out of them for damages.

'The other addicts are of a different nature, who are on cough mixtures and the like – with a lot of codeine and ephedrine. And they build up tolerance and take more and more, and they take a whole bottle of cough mixture in one go and two pints of beer, get a high mood out of it way beyond the two teaspoonfuls. And we're responsible for that. You can't buy those things in the supermarket. But you can usually spot someone who is hooked on these soft drugs. They tend either to be very scruffily dressed, a rather glazed expression, a high look, or else the other sort is a bit too respectable, very polite and talkative and it's "yes sir, no sir, three bags full sir", "I've got an auntie with a cough and cold", "I broke the bottle yesterday", all sorts of excuses. You soon notice and refuse and perhaps give your colleagues a ring.

'Of course generic prescribing would save the NHS a great deal of money. I'm for it. You see we are paid a flat 40p for dispensing, and then 10 per cent remuneration on the cost of the drug. Now if the drug is an expensive £100, I get £10 for 10 per cent and 40p for dispensing which is £10.40p. But if, say it is a generic one of 40p, I get 40p for dispensing and 4p added at 10 per cent, which is a total of 44p. So the profit margin is much greater, over 50 per cent, with the cheap one.'

JGH: 'Yes, but it is a great deal nicer to get £10.40p than 44p?'

MR POYLE: 'Being that the amount of work is usually the same, that is true, one makes more in cash terms dispensing the expensive item. That is correct.

'As to your question on mistakes – usually it's the receptionist who can't read the doctor's writing. The GPs make a slip, they're only human, and then you ring up and politely ask. You have one or two where the strengths are just nonsense – but so bad no one in their right mind would dispense. A decimal point in the wrong position can make a tremendous difference to the strength.'

Mr Poyle was more fortunate than the average. A survey of chemists – or pharmacies as they prefer to be called – reported in *Pulse*, September 1982, showed an average in eighteen days of 2,101 prescriptions; 1.86 per cent were queried – most of which, three quarters, to correct omission of dose, strength and so on. There were, out of the 2,000-odd, forty-six overdose, forty-nine illegible, eighty-nine wrong medicine or it didn't exist, and 226 'gibberish'. As there are about 350 million prescriptions a year, the total *number* of overdose prescriptions is quite high, gibberish even higher. Since the court decision in the case of Dr David Jackson, chemists are now legally responsible for ensuring GPs' prescriptions are not dangerous.

But the relationship between them is a simple one, mutually beneficial – and GPs invariably said it was satisfactory.

The only time there is serious friction is when a GP suddenly starts to dispense himself. This he can legally do if there is not a chemist within one mile of the surgery. Dr Locking ran into some trouble with the local chemist. She was coming to the end of her career and was anxious that she might not get a good price. However, Dr Locking and his partner didn't, as they put it, 'go *all out* on the dispensing'. The old chemist got a good price, and when the new man came in they made an amiable arrangement to split the business. Fairly amiable, anyway. 'Obviously he'd rather we *didn't* dispense.'

12
GROUP PRACTICES AND HEALTH CENTRES

We saw earlier that one aim of the Doctor's Charter was to encourage the primary health care *team* – operating either from health centres or from group practices in their own premises.

This move was successful, and the inducements it produced continue to operate. Cartwright's survey shows that in 1965 there were twenty-eight centres with 215 GPs; in 1977 there were 731 centres with 3,800 GPs (nearly a fifth of the total). As regards partnerships, in the same period patients with a single-handed practitioner had fallen from 45 per cent to 25 per cent. Cartwright says that single-handed practice is on the way out. There is the same increase in 'the team': secretaries and receptionists have increased two and a half times, nurses seven times since 1964.

Statistics reveal trends. They hide variety – and much else.

Variety extends even to the renting and use of health centres – seen as monolithic (and by many GPs not in them, quite erroneously, as rabidly left-wing). When Dr Abney and his partners moved into their health centre one partner – 'a loner' – stayed on in the surgery in the middle of the town, though sharing the centre's facilities, paying his share of the rent and so on. Conversely, it is not unusual to find a single-handed practitioner in a health centre, surrounded by groups, sharing everything but quite distinct, perhaps still doing his own night calls.

The facilities for groups buying or building their own premises are extremely advantageous, varying slightly by area. In Lincolnshire, for example, once it has been approved by the FPC (Family Practitioner Committee – responsible for GPs within a certain area – usually a county), a third of the cost is granted at once. And a high proportion of the remainder, plus the interest on what are often large sums, is reclaimed from the Government over several years. As a result, in that county, eighty practices own their own premises.

But there are endless variations on this too. Dr Nyewood's group premises belongs to the Parish Council. £10,000 was raised by the community ('The Brownies had a sponsored silence'), the council borrowed the rest and is being repaid by the practice with a rent of £10,000 a year. Dr Nyewood, who was inclined to complain, complained about this too. But since the Government reimbursed the practice 70 per cent and since the practice income for him and his two partners was £75,000 approximately, it didn't seem too bad.

One interesting result of this is that GPs are now about to return, partly at least, to the pre-war custom of buying their way into practices – though the whole development is so new no one seems to have quite faced up to this. But each partner pays a fair proportion of his salary while the group is paying for the premises. This share will appreciate and when he retires the incoming partner will presumably have to take out a loan and pay him back. Dr Telscombe said it wasn't at all the same, since you weren't paying for the 'goodwill' (which is not allowed). This seems rather academic when you are having to find £5,000 or £10,000 or whatever it is. Besides, you can't use your share of the property for a pub or to sleep in. It is of value only to a doctor, and to him because it is part of a thriving practice. That 'thriving practice' element is the goodwill.

But when it comes to how they run their groups, who their patients are, the stresses involved, the differences become as many as the GPs involved.

DR THIRIPLOW: 'Initially we kept very much to our own patients, but now we see each other's patients without any distinction; though patients can choose. Often if you start seeing someone through an illness you'll see them till the end. With three it was as close and personal as with one. But it's hard with five. Sometimes you don't see a patient for years on end.'

DR KERRIS: 'We share our patients equally. There can be tension with your own patients – you feel yourself stuck with them. But if you *share* a patient, there can be tensions round that. I mean we don't slag each other off; don't say "Bloody hell, did Dr Nick do that?" But there can be things that need discussing. I remember with slimming tablets, with my Puritan upbringing I wouldn't prescribe them. Whereas Nick was more liberal. But we talked that out. We don't have radically different views about minor tranquillizers or anti-depressants or things.'

DR WARFIELD: 'Patients have a choice. They can either wait to see who they want, or be seen then and there by whoever is free. But we try and share the work equally, otherwise it makes for irritation. The younger people don't mind who they see. The older ones do mind but usually we can accommodate this because they often have continuing problems and we can organize repeat appointments. But we don't like patients chopping about, especially in the same illness; we will not have that under any circumstances.

'But you have to keep absolutely full, up to date notes for it to work. In fact we're culling the notes at the moment. You know, Mrs Bloggs had a baby twenty years ago and is now menopausal; that has no relevance any more so into the waste-paper basket. Well no, not in fact. We burn them. With the exception of my trainee who culled the notes and threw one into the waste-paper basket; that evening my partner picked it up blowing up the path. "Dr Johnson, thank you for your letter about – (patient's name, family two streets away) who is out in the Persian Gulf and was indiscreet enough to acquire gonorrhoea." '

DR CHATHILL: 'We have our own patients, but when you've known someone for years, you tend to chat to them. You get very used to them. You can therefore miss things. Then you go on holiday or are away, a partner sees him – and picks things up.'

DR YETTS: 'Health centres are only impersonal if you don't know anything about making them personal. We each took our own list of patients. We also split the office so we each had our own receptionist, so she got to know my patients as well as I – better than I very often – and she could sort out lots of problems. And when a patient joined they were given a leaflet with the name of the doctor, receptionist, nurse, district nurse and health visitor. So they got five names to relate to instead of thirty. We were little tiny practices, in that we only, normally, saw our own patients, with our own receptionist – but all the back-up.

'That's the special thing, I think, about general practice. That's why it's different from hospital medicine or from abroad. It's "my doctor". You might not see him for twenty years but he's "my doctor". This is why we built up having our own patients. For "my doctor". '

Over the country as a whole, Cartwright found that, in groups, 50 per cent of patients usually saw their own doctor (as compared to 85 per cent with single-handed practices). In health centres they were slightly more likely to see another doctor than elsewhere (33 per cent compared to 22 per cent). But, as regards the feared breakdown of family doctoring, there had in fact been an increase in the whole family having the same doctor – 85 per cent did, compared to 77 per cent.

But, you might ask, what do the patients prefer, what do they make of it? The baffling thing is that here, as practically everywhere else, patients seem to like what they get. In fact there is a perfectly sound reason for this. But it is baffling for researchers, as indeed I found, because it means it is often difficult to find what they feel about anything in any large number – though, of course, individual reaction you do get. In this context, Cartwright did find that health centre patients were marginally more critical about the time and care taken in examination and found their doctors less easy to talk to (though this may be because health centres have more overseas doctors than elsewhere). But they still saw the doctor as a personal friend as much as other patients; and the extra facilities made them feel their GPs had a wider scope. As for other patients, Cartwright found, as did I, that they were largely content.

Appointments

DR TELSCOMBE: 'I book in eighteen patients a surgery, with spaces for four more. Those four are sacrosanct till the morning in question, so that people who are ill can ring up and get one. What tends to happen, someone rings up and the girl says "no spaces, but if you ring in the morning I'll be able to fit you in" which isn't quite the idea but I understand the hassles.

'I like to think I won't turn anyone away. If they insist, and refuse the offer – just one offer – of another day, then the girls have instructions to phone me and say "will you see an extra?". The record's been thirty-six in the morning surgery.'

Dr Telscombe can stand in for all the rest. All the group and health centre practices I saw, except one, had appointment systems, and this is the national trend. Since 1964 appointment systems have multiplied from 15 per cent to 75 per cent. Those that have them say they are quicker, and this is quite true. At all the time spans from under ten minutes up to half an hour, Cartwright found appointment systems were markedly shorter.

But Hesse Sachs, whose research was at much greater depth, made an interesting discovery here. It wasn't the actual amount of time waited that mattered. In one practice she studied the patients waited half an hour and thought it fine; while in another practice patients who waited a quarter of an hour thought it outrageous. What mattered was the average time for the practice and when that was exceeded by a significant amount the patients complained. As usual, patients preferred whatever system obtained in their practice.

It is usually single-handed practices where you still find the massed waiting system – partly, no doubt, because this saves on staff. But these doctors also say that they will see any patient the same day, whereas appointment system doctors won't – and this too is borne out by research. This is one area where patients do complain (though usually about receptionists).

Another interesting observation was made here, this time by Cartwright. Delays in being given appointments seem to be due to the personality of the doctor. These same doctors were those whose patients waited longest in the surgery, and were also those who complained they had a higher proportion of trivial complaints. The suggestion is that these doctors are alienated from their patients, and the various delays are designed to block them off – which they succeed in doing.

But it is clear that the pious statements made by appointment doctors about 'slotting in' and the like are frequently false. Nor is this surprising. GPs made many other enlightening observations about other aspects of their partnerships, but it is clear from the first two doctors below that the appointment system is largely for the benefit of doctors, not patients. Not that there is necessarily anything wrong with this. It often makes them function better – as these observations also make clear.

DR WARFIELD: 'Appointments let in even loads. Now we don't have a peak on Monday morning. That used to be a dreadful business. Now we simply will not see repeat consultations on Monday, are you with me? The other thing we've done with workloads is not to see elderly people or kids under school age in the evening when you're getting tired. We virtually refuse old people and people not working. I explain – it will benefit you and benefit us. There's nothing more boring than a short morning surgery, you're finished at 10, nothing to do till past 11 or 12. And then find you're facing a bulging evening surgery which you start early and go on and on and by the time you've finished you're absolutely flaked.'

DR BLAIRHALL: 'The biggest fear a doctor has is that he's going to miss something. The pressure of work with a non-appointment surgery of thirty or forty people, one after the other. And you got the last one out and you thought "Oh my God, what have I missed today?" But I've not had that fear since we went on to the appointment system because I'm not doing any less work, but it's handed out in an orderly fashion at a regular rate so that you've got as much time as you want for every patient. A waiting room full of people, waiting to come through to one doctor, through that door, is like a head of steam. That's gone with appointment systems.'

DOCTOR'S WIFE: 'They come to me with problems. Like, say they can't get an appointment within three days. I tell them the quickest answer to that one is to say, well all right, if you can't give me an appointment could the doctor come and visit, and you'll find the receptionist will get you in sometime.'

DR TELSCOMBE: 'We have a buzzer, but I prefer to go and get them. It's quite useful because you see somebody and think "Heavens, I forgot to ring up about their X-ray", or forgot to organize anything, and have time to do it before their turn comes.

'I have a white chair. Sometimes if you have a patient who can't see very well, and you have a dark chair, he'll miss it and fall on the floor.

'I'm far more ready to see people now than I was ten years ago. If I'm reading here of an afternoon and someone comes – my afternoon off – I would have told the receptionist to make an appointment. Now I let them in. It's like letting someone come in front of you in a traffic jam. You feel so good, so relaxed.'

Dr Nyewood commented that after they'd moved into their brand new parish-owned premises, his consultation rate soared. And had continued at that rate.

MRS NYEWOOD: 'But quite honestly, they used to be standing in the tiny waiting room and they would think, "Oh Christ!" You know, "I'd rather go home to bed." '

DR NYEWOOD: 'I thought there was quite a lot to be said for having a scruffy, disgusting and really rather loathsome surgery, a real black hole.'

MRS NYEWOOD: 'You've been much happier. You can't keep away from it.'

DR NYEWOOD: 'It's certainly nicer for me reading the *Lancet* or something, which doesn't often happen. But the point I was making is that the important side of general practice is that it should not be too clinical. It shouldn't be too perfect, it shouldn't be white coats and endless washing of hands and this sort of thing, because you mustn't make people feel alienated. They have got to feel, "Poor old doctor in a scruffy and filthy dirty suit, cigarette stains on his fingers, I bet he is longing for a large gin," this sort of thing. These are the things that should be going through a patient's mind.'

DR VERYAN: 'I think one of the good things about a health centre is that there's competition to keep up to date. You daren't let yourself down in front of your colleagues.'

DR BLAIRHALL: 'If a doctor offers twice as many appointments in a week, in three months the patients will fill them. We made the mistake when we went from three to four doctors, to reduce the load, of offering a third more appointments. Within three months they were all being taken. Now that we're going from four to five, we're going to offer the same number of appointments but spread over five doctors. One time the senior partner died and one doctor was seriously ill. We were 300 appointments adrift, and we found that in three months' time the patients adjusted to what was available. Same thing applies to the doctor's use of hospital facilities. For eighteen months we had a series of useless locums and the number of patients referred for eye appointments plummeted. You can't use a service that's not there.'

DR WHEATACRE: 'One battle we lost in our final battle with the Medical Officer of Health and all of them, was we wanted to have two common rooms: one for us, and one for the receptionists and nurses and health visitors. We knew very well that you couldn't, with large numbers, with thirty people in the room, hope to achieve anything. We failed in that, and for the first two months we couldn't discuss anything. We'd retreat to one room and make the rules and so on. And then it occurred to some of us – we'd have the common room *now*, from 11.30 till 12.30; our receptionists are in till 11.30; and district nurses and others come in at 12.30. So we have an hour and that's fine and we can talk. But the idea that you can have the whole primary health team talking and collaborating is absolute rubbish, and it's obvious that it's rubbish.'

Dr John Wheatacre was seventy-five, and not as remotely crusty as he may sound here (though it is interesting to compare what he says with some of the egalitarian practice beliefs). He looked about sixty, got up at five every morning and we shall meet him again because he made general practice vivid and fascinating in a way no one else I spoke to was quite able to equal.

GPs and Their Partners

DR MISTON: 'The major reason why general practice and group practice doesn't work is because you have to have more in common with a partner than you do with a wife. You have to have the same friends. If somebody treats your friends as his enemies or nuisances it becomes a bit tedious. And one does like different types of people, and if he says "That terrible Mrs Smith" and I think she's lovely, that does put the hackles up a bit. Secondly, you have to have the same clinical standards. If your partner treats diabetes with aspirin, you've got a problem. Thirdly, your attitude towards finance has to be the same, particularly in terms of investment and improving the premises and improving the services, because you can only do that at the expense of take-home pay, whether it's in private or National Health Service. It becomes an overall philosophical approach as to what is your *life* – as to which is more important to you, my work or my friend. Money I spend on this or money I spend on that. You have to have the same standards, the same number of hours per day. You can easily do everybody else's work and get the same bread at the end of it. You have to have the same sharpness of mind. If someone's a bit thick, you may have to carry the can; or if somebody's amazingly bright you get shoved to the end of the shelf.

'Then you've got to put up with partnership wives. The wife says, "I'm not going to put up with a husband who stays out till 7 o'clock. I didn't marry him for that. We've got children and what's more it's important to pay for them to go to private school." The chap then is caught between his loyalty to you as a partner and his loyalty to his wife and home. It doesn't work and it never will.' (Dr Miston had left his NHS practice and now had a lucrative private practice in Scotland.)

Dr Harriet Lynsford was in a three-doctor Yorkshire practice. She was tough, depressed and slightly off-hand, aged about fifty. Her hair had been blonde but was going grey, and she had clearly been very attractive. Indeed was still, but she was tired when I talked to her.

DR HARRIET LYNSFORD: 'Well, it was tricky. Very tricky. You see I actually had an affair for five years with this twenty-year-older senior partner. Well, it was fine at first, except he got me into drinking too much. We used to drink a bottle of fizzy wine every afternoon, or perhaps a bit more. And then another one after surgery. Oh yes – a bottle a day is too much for most women. They can certainly be damaged by it – a lot are.

'It got extremely tricky when I got fed up with it and he didn't. He was very unfair and quite threatening. And of course the staff couldn't understand his shouting and swearing at me. Emotional explosions in the surgery. He kept saying "I don't know if I can go on working here", and I felt he really meant "I don't know if *you* can go on working here." I felt my job was slightly under threat. We ended up moderately friendly. He's left now.'

Fragment from a Practice Meeting

The problem in this particular practice was that there were seven doctors and they only had four bleeps. Therefore if a doctor was needed urgently, three doctors were always unavailable. (Bleeps were passed round in rotation.) There was the usual practice meeting to discuss various things, finally this came up. There was quick agreement among the six junior partners to buy three more bleeps.

SENIOR PARTNER: 'Two more.'

DR X: 'Why not three?'

SENIOR PARTNER: 'I don't need one. I'm always available.'

DR Y [who dislikes the senior partner and has been brooding about this, among other things, for about a year]: 'What do you mean, you're always available?'

SENIOR PARTNER: 'What I say. I can always be got hold of.'

DR Y (exploding): 'You're bloody well *not* always available. It used to be quite impossible to get hold of you on Tuesday afternoons. Now it's Thursday afternoons as well. You're the laughing stock of the practice. "Where's Dr Z?" "Not available." It's monstrous.'

SENIOR PARTNER: 'That's quite unfair. I take the dog to the common for half an hour. I don't need a bleep.'

DR Y: 'You need a bleep more than anyone else.'

SENIOR PARTNER: 'I am not going to have a bleep. Any more business?'

*   *   *

DR COLKIRK: 'Have you come across *partnership agreements*? The terms, laid out and signed, solicitor, the lot? It wasn't too bad over the last number of years, but with this glut of doctors at the moment, we're beginning to hear of a lot of nasty arrangements among doctors. Like an established principal taking on an assistant with a view to partnership, and then never proceeding to the partnership. Leading the guy along the garden path for a couple of years and then when the guy says "Well, what about this partnership?" "What partnership?" So the guy leaves after two years, and he gets another sucker for two years. And the reason it happens is that they never have proper partnership agreements; it's a word-of-mouth arrangement and doctors tend to trust each other until proved otherwise.

'I'm on this Committee, and there was this Jamaican GP. He'd taken two Indians in succession up the garden path and dropped them. The third chap was a white man, Seventh Day Adventist or something, very powerful religious evangelical type, a church of his creed was there so he was anxious to stay. And when he didn't get the partnership he complained. But the Jamaican just yanked in another Indian. But the evangelical type just opened up in the same building and the chances are the Jamaican will lose all his patients to him as he's white.'

DR BILSBY'S WIFE, JANET BILSBY: 'Every wife thinks her husband's carrying the entire practice. That's just automatic.'

DR NYEWOOD: 'I mean, when old Geoffrey's away, quite honestly it doesn't make the slightest bit of difference – I mustn't say that too loudly – but if he was away for a whole *month* – I might just notice. I suppose. There it is.'

DR WHEATACRE: 'It's very hard for everyone to see the same number. To actually *do* it. They say, "I know you're only seeing so many this morning, but it's old Mrs So-and-so" or "It's that interesting girl", you know. You can't stick to it. We don't even try to stick to it. We each have our own patients and we can do what we like. We're having a count at the moment of how many patients each doctor's seeing, because *two* doctors are thought – and I think rightly – by the younger partners, not to be doing their share and so there's a census going on. But, you see, you can't even it out. The fast worker will do more – happily. We do our own surgery count but some of us start early and some start late. But one woman partner sees remarkably few people. She, to some extent, is a bit lazy. She's terribly interested in photography. We've always said before that OK, we're not going to try and share it out equally; it's inefficient. It's far better to see six of your own than one of somebody else's. It's not only pleasanter, it's more efficient. You know your own neurotics, but other people, it's not so easy. "I've got a terrible pain . . ." Am I *missing* something here?

'I'm against the count but the new younger partner's feeling a bit exploited and insists on having it. It'll probably have a good effect. She might come in a bit earlier.'

This situation can only arise because many practices are extremely relaxed about doctors' lists. One partner may well have 3,500 (the maximum) technically on his list, but he may never see 1,400 of them during his entire practising life; they will have become spread amongst his partners. In his turn he will be seeing patients which technically belong to the other partners in the practice. One might note in passing that Dr Wheatacre was the practice 'conciliator'. Hesse Sachs found that nearly all practices (as do most organizations) had a leader and a conciliator, this last often but by no means always a woman GP. Sometimes both roles were combined. Sometimes two doctors shared a role.

Another solution a good number of practices adopted was simply to remain totally separate individuals, often hardly seeing each other for days on end. 'A general practice is more of an arboretum than a pine forest,' said Dr Telscombe. 'Individual specimens rather than a number of the same.' It was virtually impossible for this practice to have a practice meeting or to decide on anything together, like choosing the colour of paint to re-do the reception area, at all, and Dr Telscombe just went ahead on his own. We shall go into this more deeply when we come to stress and see how GPs in a practice support each other – or rather, as is the case usually, don't support each other.

In fact I found very few practices where the doctors were what you might call great friends. They could meet socially, they were friendly, but it was an office relationship – as you might expect.

But it was essential, as we've just seen, for people to feel the work was fairly apportioned, or not mind if it wasn't. And the other area it was essential to get right was the sharing of the practice income – the area, that is to say, of money.

DR JANE EDSTONE: 'About £26,000 before tax. I should think I take home £19,000 net.'

DR TRIMDON: 'Not as much as my colleagues down south. I make what 22, 23 thousand up here. I bet they're on 30, 33. So I think, therefore, we're spending more time on our patients. We do more for them. I've had patients wander in and they'll say "Examined? You don't expect me to be examined down there?" '

DR CHATHILL: 'I suppose about £30,000 per annum. We work harder than most GPs. We work damned hard.'

DR WHEATACRE: 'We're *incredibly* well paid for doing something really, even if you don't like it terribly much, you can skip through surgery and get off to the golf course, and other things.'

DR ABNEY: 'I'm perfectly happy with the money I make. I think I probably get overpaid if you really asked me to be honest. But I think I earn it. Because I'm not a worrier, but I do worry about patients and this is what I'm paid for.

'One of our partners is a big money-maker but he does this on the side. It's [whispering] amusement machines. He owns some and they absolutely make a fortune. He drives round on Saturday and collects the money and repairs them.'

When the NHS was set up the system of payment was basically a capitation system with a very limited number of 'items of service' payments, via a pool. This was a certain sum of money set aside each year which had to be shared among the 21,000 or so GPs. It was highly unsatisfactory. Sometimes the pool ran out. Sometimes there was some left and each GP got sent £10 or whatever it was. It meant GPs didn't get paid more for doing more for a patient, and the only way they could make 'a decent income' was to take a full list (then 4,000) which was killing. GPs' pay was fundamental to the malaise in the late fifties and early sixties.

The Charter swept all this away, especially the hated pool. It was replaced by a practice allowance, at present £7,000 (and in certain circumstances you get a supplementary allowance of £1,200), a more generous capitation fee, and 'items of service' payments. Each year the Government Review Body decides what the average gross take-home pay of GPs should be after practice expenses and adjusts all these charges accordingly. In 1982 it was £18,990.

When you ask about 'items of service' GPs talk vaguely about 'vaccinations and immunizations' as though there were about half a dozen.

Pulse and the *General Practitioner*, the free GP magazines (laughingly called 'medical comics') supported by drug ads, are obsessed by money, and large chunks of their space are devoted to it each week. Once a month *Pulse* does an updating of 'items of service' in the *Blue Book*, the GPs money bible. The updating for August 1982 contained 179 items of which vaccinations and immunizations were, oddly enough, among the cheapest – £1.75p for initial doses, £2.50p for final doses. Six other items, taken at random, were: cervical smear – £5; temporary resident cover of two weeks – £5.85p; night visit between 11 p.m. and 7 a.m. – £11.80p; seat belt exemption examinations and report – £19; miscarriage £24; a colliery visit underground – £41 the first one and a half hours, £15 each subsequent hour.

It was calculated then that if he really worked at 'items of service' each GP could increase his income by £6,000 a year. But, as Dr Kinsham pointed out, the paperwork involved would be ghastly, and a great many GPs can't be bothered. 'GPs are not terribly interested in all the effort of maximizing their income. They'd rather minimize their work than maximize their income, I think you'll find.'

£18,990 was a projected *average*. I met one GP earning (taking home) £34,000; but in a large practice in the South, with, say, thirty or forty private patients, some factories and a hospital appointment it is not difficult to get over £45,000 – though you'd have to work hard. The poorest GP, if that's the word (excluding the egalitarian practices) was in the remote Highlands of Scotland, an inducement practice where he took home £12,000. But GPs can also charge a good deal to tax: if they run two cars a tax allowance is made for one and a quarter; telephone and so on. Practices, or GPs, can also increase their income by £3,000 a year by taking a trainee GP, though this is not, or not meant to be, a sinecure. All the practices I saw shared the practice income equally, partners reaching parity in one to three years. But they had all heard of those where the money was not shared equally – where, say, the senior partner kept all the private work and his seniority increments. When this happened, you almost invariably got trouble.

Seniority payments are part of the extremely cushioned way GPs coast into what is often quite an active old age. They come after seven years as a GP (£1,450), fourteen years (£2,475) and twenty-one years (£3,920). On retirement they get a lump sum, which is a year and a half's salary, and a pension which depends on years of service. But it is possible to buy years by taking a slightly smaller annual salary and typically a doctor retiring at sixty could have brought his total years of service up to forty. The pension is usually about one third the annual gross salary and it is index-linked. 'I'm told the BMA negotiators tried it on years ago not expecting anything,' said Dr Wheatacre gleefully, 'and to their astonishment they got it. Index-linked.' Dr Blairhall, retiring at sixty, having bought a total of forty years, investing his lump sum, and having saved as well, reckoned his income would remain the same after retirement as before.

He was not going to do what a good many GPs do. It is possible to 'retire' for twenty-four hours in order to qualify for your pension. You then return and work part time. If you worked full time they'd stop your pension. But it is possible to keep most of your pension and bring your income up to what it was before by your part-time work, normally about a half load.

There are several other aspects of group practice we should know, particularly relations with figures other than the GP – social workers, consultants, midwives, receptionists. But I think these are best approached through three individual doctors and practices, the last of which will carry us through to the very heart of general practice – the consultation and the GP's relations with his patients.

But before then we should just imprint a typical day, a typical week. This could be repeated *ad infinitum* by each doctor. They are all different, but also, like life, all the same. Some variant you could have found in 1900, 1920 and 1950, some variant on the round of surgeries, visits, special duties and every so often (or all the time) on duty for emergencies during the day and the night. It is against this archetypal pattern that all we have seen, all that we will see, is played.

'My week is, we start at half past eight, I do a surgery on Monday morning, half past 8 to, well, quarter to 11, something like that. Ante-natal clinic 3 till 4, surgery from 4 till 7. Visits – there's always a lot of visits on Monday, and then I'm on call on Monday night, which means all the night calls for the practice, 21,000. Another surgery at half past 8 till 11 on Tuesday, and then I do an afternoon one on Tuesday, which is 2 till about 5, and then I'm off early on Tuesday evening, but having worked for forty-eight hours virtually solidly – no, thirty-six hours. And then Wednesday I have a nice surgery where I can please myself. I start at 9. I'll see any patients that want to be seen on that morning, but if I've got some special long cases or insurances or something that I want to do especially, I can fit those in on Wednesday morning, and then I'm free at about 1.

'I do early visits on Thursday, dental anaesthetics for an hour on Thursday morning; surgery from half past 10 till 12, or just after, and then Thursday afternoon I have two industrial commitments which I fit in. I'm the MO [Medical Officer] for Sainsburys. I do Thursday evening surgery from 4 till, what, sort of sevenish. Friday I do morning surgery, half past 8 till half past 10, 11. That varies. I mean, sometimes you finish at half past 10. We have a post-grad session every Friday at the hospital – very efficient. You go up there, you have a quick lunch, get up there at about half past 12, meeting starts at quarter to 1, out by quarter to 2, and back here by 2 or 4. I do alternate Fridays. I do an early one, one Friday and a late one the next Friday. So I'm doing two and a half evening surgeries a week – three one week and two the next. And then Saturday we run rotas. We have, out of the eight of us, four in on Saturdays. Two doing surgery and two doing visits and then we work a rota for the weekends, so with the senior partner out of it, by agreement, I do one full weekend on in seven. And that's a real grind. You are on absolutely full bore the whole time. We've got back-up. You know, we've got a second on, but you try not to call him out. I mean, he's on the phone anyway. And you're going like the clappers the whole time. And that's the week.'

Dr Frank Warfield
A South-East Urban Group Practice

The surgery was in an ugly but large and solidly built Edwardian house of grey granite on the main Maidstone road leading out of the town.

Now mostly converted for surgery work, it had once been the home of the pre-war single-handed GP who'd run the practice. This is very common, and you can somehow still sense the old dining room beneath the waiting room, the kitchen where the two receptionists tick off appointments and deal with arrivals, the downstairs cloakroom which was now a treatment room. It was perfectly comfortable, adequately clean (plastic flowers could have done with a dust), and extremely well-equipped – one of the few with a computer. But it was nothing like a health centre. The waiting room had wooden chairs all round the walls, a few health notices, piles of old *Woman's Owns, Woman's Realms*. The GPs' consulting rooms were off down the corridors; each patient was told when to go by the receptionist.

Dr Warfield was fifty, with a strong, sensual face, his cleft chin tucked in under his lower lip, cheerful, extrovert, brisk. He moved about a lot, thrusting his hands into his pockets and jingling change, tipping himself back in his chair and thumping his feet down on top of his desk, taking off his watch and pulling the elastic metal strap in and out like a small metal concertina. He had a very rapid delivery, the words running together, talking straight, blunt, a trace of Yorkshire. At the same time he was clearly kind, and odd expressions of compassion, even tenderness would suddenly alter what was a faintly porcine appearance. I think, like many GPs, he was a good deal more sensitive than he wanted to seem.

DR WARFIELD: 'The idea of doing medicine attracted me I suppose simply because I hoped one would earn a reasonable income, and have a reasonable standing. My uncle was Professor of Public Health in Maidstone, but, when I said I wanted to do medicine he said, "No, I wouldn't do that lad." In fact nobody said "Jolly good idea."

'Certainly not my father. My father was a butcher; a very good butcher but he could hardly write his name in fact. He left the children entirely to my mother. He was very often a man of very few words. I think he was intensely proud when I qualified but he wasn't the sort of chap that would flatter his children. My mother was a different kettle of fish altogether. In fact, they were so unlike it wasn't true. She was more intelligent. She came from a different background. Her brother was the professor. She made sure we all got to the grammar school by giving us a jolly good push and encouragement and a good clout and a kick up the arse where necessary.

'I always had a slight inferiority complex about my academic achievements. I never had any setbacks but I always had to bash the books fairly hard, harder than some, so I decided I wasn't really consultant material. I was probably wrong. I could have done psychiatry without any difficulty. But anyway – that meant general practice.

'Well, when I came out of the Army I applied for this job in this very house. I was very lucky. There were 100 applicants, but the only reason I got the job was I was the first to be sent for as I was local, and I took my wife with me. And when the daughter opened the door she said, "Hello! Fancy seeing you, Rachel!" They were in the same form at school. "You knew my daughter at school?" he asked. "That makes a lot of difference." So I started here.

'Well, he retired within one year, and I took a partner whom I'd known when doing obstetrics at South Mead and the practice grew fairly rapidly and then we needed a third. So I bought another house, and we began to take this one over more and more. We started with only the ground floor – the two of us sharing a consulting room. Then I built a little thing out here for the reception area. Then we moved upstairs – got a part-time, two consulting rooms upstairs. Now we've just acquired a fifth. And a trainee.

'We've got a few ones, fair smattering of twos, much bigger proportions of threes, fours and fives equally divided. If you have all one class that's bloody boring. If they're all social class five that's soul destroying. If they're all social class one, it's damn hard work. Harder work because their demands are different, but equally taxing on one's nervous energy. I'll give you an example. Mrs Bloggs brings in John with a sore throat – social class one. "What do you think the germ is, doctor? What sort of a germ is it in the throat? How can we prevent it? Should he really have an antibiotic this time? Do you think the time has come when he might need an ear, nose and throat opinion?" Right, social class four comes in. I say "Good morning Mrs Smith." "I think he's got a sore throat again, doctor. Have a look." "Yes, he's got a sore throat, Mrs Smith. He'd better have some tablets. He'll be better in two or three days." "Right, thank you very much doctor, sorry to have bothered you. Goodbye."

'Easier. But social class four will have a whole tangle of personal problems, family problems.

'When I said I could have been a psychiatrist I simply meant it doesn't require much intellect. I used to think that psychotherapy was bosh but in fact all GPs have to practise it on a simple level. "Well, Mrs Smith, that little lump in your breast is nothing more than a small gland. If that's what's been worrying you, go away and forget about it." Obviously you get more complicated problems – marital or bereavement problems – and these require talking about for a while, for five or ten minutes, a weekly basis. But I will not go in for twenty-minute sessions of psychotherapy. Nobody has proved that at the end of the day it improves the outcome. So there comes a time when you have to drop the act and say, "No more psychotherapy, Mrs Smith", otherwise you'll breed a practice of doctor-dependent patients and that's what we don't want.

'In fact in general terms we will not let patients tell us what we're going to do. We will not tolerate people who cause us a great deal of difficulties and muck us about. On the whole we've got a fairly well trained practice who don't give us a *tremendous* headache.

'There's five of us with 9,800 patients. But don't forget the two females are part-timers. Which is all they can possibly do. It is a myth that women keep perpetuating, female medics, that they can in fact hold down a full-time job and a marriage and family. Absolute bosh. They really cannot. I have watched, it has been as much as Lucy Burke can do to manage a part-time commitment with two kids. She is constantly chasing her tail and this is something you shouldn't have to do in general practice. Can't attend meetings and so on at such and such a time; got to collect the kids from school. You know, you name it, all the problems involved. She just never has time to sit on her arse and contemplate, she never has time to read a journal, which I think is very important. You've got to read the *Journal* to keep up.

'Mistakes? God Almighty! Of course I make mistakes. You can't be a GP and not make mistakes. There are mistakes of management you'll make occasionally. You will certainly make diagnostic mistakes simply because things just simply don't add up. There are certain fundamentals you simply mustn't make mistakes on – drug interactions or giving drugs that are contra-indicated in certain conditions or of no proven value and so on.

'I think probably the commonest thing, without doubt, is missing when people have coronaries and they present in an atypical fashion. The difficulty is you've got to be very careful that you don't diagnose every chest pain as a coronary or you're going to cripple a lot of people psychologically by labelling them as having heart disease. It's a mistake you must avoid at all costs. And in doing that you're inevitably going to miss the odd coronary patient who has had a coronary.

'The worst cases are the long standing chronic psychiatric problems that have come back and back and back. I've got one patient who has been twice a week for twenty years with no change in her condition. She's had a fair smattering of organic diseases as well, mind you, but it's been very highly coloured by her personality and acute chronic anxiety. An inability to cope with even common illnesses.

'But there are a certain number of conditions which are not amenable to any treatment. I've got several patients who've had the same problem for twenty years. The truth is, nothing can be done for them. Twenty years ago I found it frustrating. I was there to cure them and that I hadn't done it was failure. Now I just accept it and realize my limitations.

'I get on very well with the consultants round here. One or two stick in my gullet for various reasons. Well, one in particular. He's a grasping, greedy sod and I think we a had a major row over a patient – a lad who was run over by a bus who – they had to amputate part of his pelvis both ways – he nearly died, he was in the unit for weeks. He had 150 pints of blood, he had massive skin grafting done; an absolute wreck, a horrific wreck. He had to have a colostomy, he had to have a urethrostomy, his bladder had been ruptured, his pelvis was smashed to pieces and he had both legs off. Now, he was sent home eventually. I'd been to see him. This was an occasion when a consultant should have picked up the phone. He knew me well enough socially to say, "Look, Frank, I'm sending this lad home. I'll put you in the picture and tell you what's on the file." We didn't even get a discharge letter. I was so furious I sent him a letter that simply blasted him. In fact, I've had several goes with him.

'But the rest are good. One highly insensitive physician. The consultant geriatrician is damn good. He'll come and do a domiciliary within two days, or take them in if the home's no good. Health visitors not much cop. They don't like soiling their hands with work. As for the social workers – poof, not much help.

'What? Too highly trained? No, just no bloody good. They're not interested in social work, many of them. They're interested in changing the political philosophy of this country and that's not what social work is all about. They should *not* try to change society through policies and politics involving their work and that's where you've got what 'social work' is all about in my opinion. A lot of left-wing trendies sat with gym shoes and dirty army greatcoats on and these are the sort of people who are seeing patients and patients are horrified and even what I call respectable working-class social class fours and fives, cannot believe it when the social worker turns up with long greasy hair, dirty nails, an army greatcoat on, and gym shoes.

'And another thing, they are not medically trained. A lot of social problems are mixed with medical ones and you have to know both. We have a fair understanding of social work, but not vice versa. And they won't be taught under any circumstances. And, they will argue about compulsory orders. I've had patients so overtly potty you don't need any qualifications to see they're dangerous. I had one severely manic woman who was literally ripping the psychiatrist to pieces before our eyes. I said to the social worker, "That's the sort of thing that happens when you refuse to sign a compulsory order." He'd been discussing the patient's "liberty". It's pathetic.

'They will never leave a card with their name and address. "Who came?" "A social worker." "Who?" "I don't know!" So you've no bloody idea who it is. I have to ring up. I can eventually trace them but it's extremely irritating.

'Another thing they don't do, for instance; they see a patient and they never let us damn well know the outcome. It's so bad that a social worker can ring me up and say, "I don't think I know you, Dr Warfield," even though I've been here twenty-two blasted years. The social workers' department – principal offices for this town – is literally across the road here in the shopping precinct. I say, "Well, if you look out of your bloody window, you can see me in my effing consulting room." '

To have interviewed in depth everyone concerned with GPs – social workers, consultants in each speciality, dozens of the primary health care team, scores of patients – to have read the literature about them as well as about doctors, would have taken years, if not decades. Accounts of all these people, therefore, are always from the GP's point of view and as such will no doubt often be unfair.

But if the GPs I spoke to are anything like representative (and Hesse Sachs found exactly the same thing) then there is something very wrong between these two groups which seriously, sometimes totally, undermines what they do together. Out of the fifty-odd doctors I saw, only three had satisfactory relationships with social workers.

Indeed, personally, they often praised them. Dr Kerris said, 'There's a very, very, very good team here. They are absolutely brilliant. And it's terribly difficult because they are just under absolutely stunning pressure. They've got just a hell of a lot of work and nobody thanks them for it.'

Nevertheless, Kerris went on to criticize the system. The trouble was you could never talk to an individual concerned with the case, in authority. Some elderly person you were concerned with vanished into the social work allocation system. 'If all the social workers are busy then your little old lady might still be waiting, so you ring up and ask what's happening and talk to a *different* duty officer.'

This was compounded because in most cases either the social workers or else their leaders and usually both were situated literally miles away. In Dr Abney's case, forty-five miles. 'But I mean, to arrange a meeting on Saturday when I was on call anyway and darting round here, there and everywhere, with someone coming over from *Aylesbury* – *well*! Laughable.' Dr Thriplow described how patients went berserk occasionally, and how you needed a social worker to certify them, and again they were forty miles away. 'It's no joke sitting for two hours with a demented, potential homicidal maniac. Whereas, before we had a local one and you'd ring up and he was a big tough chap and we never had any trouble because it was all on a personal basis.'

In fact, it was while talking to Dr Thriplow that I was given a simple demonstration of how hopeless the present system is. We were just about to discuss one of his cases, when by chance the social worker concerned, a young man of twenty-seven, turned up. It was about an old woman. Dr Thriplow explained in careful detail how she lived alone in this icy cold house, how she'd hardly lasted the winter, pipes had burst, when you went in it was *freezing* and it simply wouldn't do. The shop next door was now willing to buy her house – he knew them and didn't think they'd cheat her. The problem was, where should she go? He thought an old people's bungalow. Could she manage, asked the social worker, did the little town *have* any sheltered accommodation? It gradually became clear that, well-meaning as he was, he knew absolutely nothing about any part of the situation. He'd been trying to get her into an old people's home. Dr Thriplow didn't favour this. She couldn't speak Welsh, and many in the home did. Also, she was independent, she was coping well enough on her own. Winter was the danger. She'd have quite a bit of money when she'd sold the house – some thousands – and would be able to afford sheltered accommodation. In fact, by the end the social worker had really abandoned any inter-personal role – the real work in such a situation, talking to the neighbours, persuading the old lady and so on – and left all that to the doctor. He would do all he could to get the appropriate accommodation, giving up his plan for the old people's home.

'The people from the shop next door phoned – Shopper Evans – because they couldn't get in touch with her. Why don't you have a word with them?' Seeing the social worker's face, he added quickly, 'Well, I'm going round there anyway. I'll have a word with them.'

He turned to me. 'This is a social problem, not a medical one.' The house had been like a *fridge*. This was because she was, to put it mildly, thrifty. He described this at some length and it sounded fairly mad. 'There's a step ladder to the electricity meter so she can run up and down to count the units.'

My own feeling was that, with such a temperament, the idea of selling her house just to fritter all the money away on either an old people's home (£90 a week while funds lasted, then free) or sheltered accommodation would horrify her and she'd rather stay in her fridge-like house, where no doubt she'd die next winter. 'People have that right', said Dr Thriplow mildly.

The two questions are, are there insuperable barriers preventing GPs and social workers co-operating, and if there are not, can they administratively work together from the same premises dealing with the same people, and if they can, does it work?

Some doctors thought they'd never get on. Dr Trimdon said the Social Work Act of 1968 had given social workers a number of statutory powers to do with the old, the mentally ill and deprived children. These they regarded as far more important (especially the last, since cases got such publicity). But their powers, which put them on a par with GPs (who they regarded as agents they could use or not, as they liked), irritated GPs, who felt jealous.

Dr Yetts said the subject was so immense there was a book in it (there *is* a book on it – *Social Work and General Medical Practice – Collaboration or Conflict?*, by June Huntington*). He said that general practice is a mature profession. Social work is young, insecure and can be compared to teenagers.

* Allen & Unwin, 1981.

There is the ambivalence of wanting to be independent and not wanting to be, which comes over as resentment.

As to each practice having a social worker, they'd tried it for years and it was quite impossible. 'You can't employ an equal' is how they feel. 'We got absolutely no co-operation.' But I see from the notes that Dr Yetts speaks of the social worker 'turning up' at the Health Centre for weekly meetings – not, therefore, working from it. Also, 'different' social workers turning up, which obviates the whole thing.

In fact, social workers can be attached to practices, and when this happens it works very well. The three practices that had excellent relations had all done this. Hesse Sachs found the same.

I spoke to the social workers. One said GPs were hopeless in a great many ways. They never had the guts to give evidence in cases putting children into care – pleading (I could see their point) patient relations.

A second said she thought a 'patch' system was being introduced. This is not quite the same. The populations don't coincide, the social worker is not based on the surgery or health centre (though this last is not essential). However, if it is indeed being introduced it is with staggering slowness. Meanwhile, a lot of highly trained, dedicated young men and women are a great deal less effective than they might be. And a lot of stress and irritation is put on a group of people who have more than enough of it anyway.

16

Dr David Bilsby
A Lincolnshire Market Town Group
Practice

I drove across Suffolk and Norfolk to King's Lynn and then on into Lincolnshire, where Dr Bilsby lived. Mist covered both counties, so the vast flatness of Norfolk was confined, circumscribed. At one point I saw a line of men in a beet field. They were standing motionless, bowed, with bent heads. Through the grey mist they looked like a line of prisoners-of-war. I had spent much of my childhood in East Anglia. Did they still pull the beet by hand, and then fling it up into the carts with those wide, curved, long-pronged forks with bobbles at the end of the prongs? On and on across the flat county, the little fourteenth- and fifteenth- and sixteenth-century churches looming up out of the mist, more numerous than pubs. How vast village England still was. I noticed two district nurses getting into their car in a lay-by. In the woods the leaves were still on the trees – yellow, green-yellow, brown-paper brown, russet. A good autumn. Out in the flatness they were blown bare – branches tangled and black.

As I came into Lincolnshire, the names became more and more fen-like – names with dyke, marsh, fen itself tacked on to the end.

The Three Elms surgery was set into the old wall of the little Lincolnshire market town. It, too, was in a converted house but had been the surgery for 100 years. There were three full-time GPs, one woman part time. Downstairs, a waiting room and district nurses' room. Then up some steep winding stairs, which in fact brought one to street level, and to the small reception window. I went through a door beside this and was at once – Dr Bilsby had warned them – absorbed and involved into the tremendous bustle and activity of the nerve centre.

Three blue-coated receptionists hurrying about, two answering the blinking lights on the little switchboard.

'Can I help you? . . . and the address? What is it he's got?'

'Yes, it will be some time today.'

'Yes, it will be 6.30 this evening.'

To each other, 'Well, he's cried wolf too often. One of these days it's going to be too late for him.'

Back and forth, getting the patients' record folders from the five tin files. Mrs Jones, to me, 'It's the fat ones you've got to beware of.' She was the head receptionist, the practice manager. She hurried about, enjoying it. 'We're going to keep fit this morning.'

Now the doctors arrived to collect their pile of record cards and to go to their surgeries.

David Bilsby is energetic, strong, thirty-five, bearded with a soft Lincolnshire accent. He is the youngest of the partners, kind and, I've already gathered, the most popular with the staff. It sounded as if he was almost too gentle, put upon. (That night he had to go out to a mother who rang because her child had a sore throat. When he got there, the child was asleep.) But after I'd seen him with his patients I realized this was not so. He was kind, certainly, but brisk and didn't waste time. He was quite able to distance himself.

He explained he'd cut down his surgery that morning, he'd three visits to do, some telephone and paperwork and abandoned me to the bustle. This carried on throughout the morning, slightly diminishing, but not much. I helped put prescriptions into record envelopes – the form EC5 – breaking off from time to time to conduct my own 'surgery'. First came the midwife. She had a restless, smiling, humorous manner, throw-away, but gradually this went as her descriptions took wing. She was about twenty-seven, with a strong, good-looking face, high cheekbones, small even teeth, a fine figure; on her feet big, clumping boots. Her hair was in braids. Oatmeal complexion.

MIDWIFE: 'I used to do a lot of work on farms. I always liked delivering the animals, but you can't be a midwife to animals. So I did my training, which I didn't like much. They teach you all these different ways, everybody something different, and you store it all up. And then in the hospital they interfere a lot. I don't like staying in the same place too much. The only real way to do it is on the district, and with a GP unit. It's nice really – we deliver on our own up there – the GP comes if he can get there, but otherwise we just have our own staff. We don't have anyone else breathing down our necks.

'Now I have a child of my own – ten months. I have a child-minder looks after her. That gives you an insight. It's exactly how you think it is. Well, you learn how it feels, how it hurts. They think we none of us have babies you see, and we don't know what we're talking about. It helps for them to realize we do know a little bit.

'You look back at the end of a delivery and you think, did I do that right or you sometimes think you could have done better. I had my first still birth yesterday, it wasn't a very nice experience. I think she suspected it, but it was the poor husband I was sorry for, standing there watching it all. But if you've been doing it for three years it is quite lucky this is the first. Before I had my baby I seemed to have nothing but frights, the babies' hearts were all stopping. I think that is one thing I have appreciated, you value the value of the baby more. You know, a lot of these babies are not really wanted or planned or anything. They don't seem to care much about them after they are born. But we do have quite a few middle class people who plan their babies, they really want them and they want to enjoy the pregnancy and the delivery, and they breast feed them, and well, they are a pleasure to deliver. It's not just getting it over like a good many of them, is it? And I like to be flexible and go along with their wishes. Music, you know. It could be a Boyer delivery, that's about as far as we go. We don't go so far as to put them under water, do we?

'We always have the fathers in. And here they're very good and they stay for forceps and everything. Occasionally one is a bit squeamish, aren't they? And it could be any class, no difference there.

'The one with the still birth, I tried to warn him, but we weren't completely sure. Then she was ready to push, the pains were absolutely terrible, and suddenly the waters went and meconium just squirted everywhere – that is the baby has his bowels opened before it is born and that is a bad sign, very distressing. I was pretty certain then.

'He stayed. He needed her, she needed him, didn't she? I think it was easy for him to appreciate it as well, what had happened. Then he stood there and tried to cover it in case she looked suddenly, you see. The doctor still hadn't arrived and I said the husband had better tell her. The policy in hospitals now is that they are quite in favour of patients holding still births, you know whatever it is, whether abnormality or whatever. They always used to take them away and they never saw them and they always regretted it. So I wrapped it, all its lips were red and it wasn't really a very nice sight, and I gave it to her, and she had a little cry and then they took it away. They didn't want to see it again and she kept crying during the day, but she is very perky today, I have got to go and see her tonight actually. That was one where I had to be flexible really, because I didn't know what was to come, and I was really relying on the GP to do the dirty work for me.

'The recent one I had that was absolutely normal was one I went out to first thing in the morning. The ambulance arrived just the same time as me and I thought – oh, poaching again. I looked into it when I got there and they had already gone in, so I rushed up to have a look at her and she was ready to have the baby. She was only seventeen, in this tiny room, unmarried living with her boyfriend. So the ambulance men carried her down, just a little girl. The boyfriend came as well, carrying my bag and we came down this road here with flashing lights just in time for a nice normal perfect delivery. He stayed. He had a look when the head was nearly there. He said, "Ooh, I think I'm going to cry." He was quite a big chap and I said, "You are not allowed to cry, not until it is over," and the other nurse said, "No, you are not allowed to cry. Oh, all right then." I think it was bringing tears to his eyes because the poor girl was suffering. Oh dear, it is marvellous, oh you get some great times you know, patients are good fun mostly. I had this one girl and she kept kicking her husband and I was a bit nervous at the terrific kicks. So I said let's have her over on her side and deliver her on her side, with somebody holding the offending leg. I went to see her after – the delivery was fine, no worries. And I said, "My God, that was a bit much you with your leg, why were you doing that, by the way?" and she said, "I don't know, I didn't realize I was doing it, but I used to do karate eighteen months ago." It was just as well I didn't get a karate kick, wasn't it? She was lying on the bed and all of a sudden this leg would kick out, kicking her husband. He didn't mind, they don't seem to mind what they get, do they? They feel it's their penance, I think. Great fun. Oh, it can be very rewarding really.'

Dr Bilsby had now finished his surgery, and we set off for his first visit. We went via the GP ward in the hospital, where the GPs could deliver or oversee the delivery of people in the practice. GPs are often a bit sentimental about these, as was the midwife, making them seem almost the same as home deliveries. No doubt it is nice to have your GP present, but they are very definitely hospital wards, neither more nor less 'cosy' (though smaller than some – twelve beds here).

Sister Mullins was small and plump, and couldn't meet your eyes. She liked delivering babies. It was satisfying. She said the mothers had questions, which, even if they felt a bit ashamed of, they badly wanted to know the answers to. Like, 'If I have a lot of heartburn, does that mean the baby will be very hairy?'; 'I'm carrying it well forward, does that mean the baby will be a girl?'; 'If I massage olive oil round here, will it slip out easily?' 'They ask us,' she said, 'they wouldn't ask the doctor.' Bilsby agreed, interested, that he hadn't been asked any of these questions.

As we drove, we talked about the practice. I had read some research that showed sick people were atypical. GPs lived their lives among these and therefore formed a biased view of human nature, based on their experience of this atypical percentage. David thought this wasn't true. 'Most of the people we see are perfectly ordinary people with very minor illnesses – colds, sprains, that sort of thing.' He thought consultants hadn't a clue about the outside world. He'd gone with a consultant to see this old fellow living in a room by himself, covered in newspapers and blankets and about fifteen layers of clothes. 'We must examine him,' said the consultant. And stood there, as if he thought the clothes would be removed miraculously. David had to step forward and get them off.

We were by now completely lost in the coils of a council estate. I wondered what would have happened if it had been an emergency at night. David explained, as we searched, that it was a little girl, about two, who had convulsions whenever her temperature rose. Not epilepsy, though he was giving her Epilim. It wasn't uncommon and she'd probably grow out of it. But it was ticklish, knowing what to say to the mother. She was understandably very worried now whenever the child got a cold; even teething could bring it on. She would bath her in cool water, but it could happen so fast with children. It would almost certainly be all right. Yet children could die of fits.

We eventually found the house, No. 53. Acrylan carpet, the telly off, but Radio Two-type music on the record player. Nappy on the floor, toys, a feeling of slight desolation. The little girl was on her mother's knee, sniffling.

The mother looked about thirty, short hair, tired, her mouth turned down.

She started to explain as soon as we sat down. 'Last night I stayed awake with her all night and kept her cool.'

The doctor examined her. 'She's not been sick at all?' A new manner. He was professional, slightly detached.

'It's her ears and throat. She isn't eating; she's drinking an awful lot.'

That feeling I knew so well with babies and children. They, their problems, *become the only thing that matters*.

The GP examined her; when he looked at her throat she cried. 'All done now,' he said. He wrote out prescriptions – panadol mixture, and more Epilim, while the mother talked. 'She's so active, she picks up infections. I can't remember when she last had a full night's sleep.'

The GP explained he was giving an antibiotic for the ear (antibiotics reassure). Finally, he took the little girl's temperature. It was normal. He was visibly relieved. 'You sponge her.' She laughed. 'I've got used to that now. It's quite a routine in this house now.'

Outside, he said she was in fact about forty, this was her second marriage. The husband would be back next weekend and he was a help. I asked what friends she had. He said her mother lived nearby, but didn't come in; he was vague about friends. I felt he had done what he could and the woman was receding.

On the way back he talked about a research project he was engaged on in psychokinetic phenomena. But it was the scientific side that interested him, the statistics, the probability, possibly physical explanations.

We were to call at the Three Elms surgery for some notes, but here he was trapped by four more unexpected patients. 'I'll do a couple of telephone calls as well,' he said, vanishing.

The reception bustle is in full swing still. The room is warm after the cold November outside. Central heating here; the treatment room next door has a two-bar electric fire. In the corner behind the central table there is a cupboard with an electric kettle, tea, Nescafé, mugs, a tin of Royal Dansk biscuits. Fragrant waves increasingly pulse from this important point.

A pram is brought in and put in the corner for the baby to be watched while the mother attends an ante-natal clinic upstairs. Mrs Jones says, 'They used to leave them outside. That was no good.' A woman comes in who has cut her finger on her bicycle. She holds it up, bloody but not too bad, at the reception window. One of the district nurses takes her next door to the treatment room where I've been intervieweing and, in full view, dresses it. When she's finished, I go in there with Sister Barnes – 'Barnsy' – lively, merry, most senior of the district nurses. We leave the door open.

DISTRICT NURSE: She explained that they were officially on duty from 8.30 to 5.30, but in fact they worked a great deal of unpaid overtime. But she enjoyed the work. She had her own clinic in the surgery for treatment – dressings, injections, ear syringes. Otherwise it was out in the community, 'on the district.' 'We have a lot of responsibility ourselves, but we can always come to the doctors. The freedom of it, the meeting people in their own homes and seeing to not only their treatment, but also the whole of the family is involved, children, parents, the cat and the dog we have to attend to sometimes. In fact, it is all very interesting to deal with, not only nursing.' She described how her family fitted in, her husband, working shifts on a farm, was willing to 'roll up his sleeves and be at the sink'. And all the duties – the cutting of the nails for the old, the bathing of the old, and all the many aids they now had – 'A van with hoists, hoists yes, to lift the patients who are paralysed out of the bed, out of the bath, on to the commode.' Levers, pulleys, cradles, all from the stores. 'Which means several journeys, there and back. We just get paid for the mileage you see, our own car is going to have bumps galore by those careless men and we have to stand that, that's the only thing.' She described the routine of injections for the terminally ill, and how they work it out with the doctor, a big last dose to take them through the night, with tablets to take at the end. One patient had been terminally ill for a year. 'We could never have that again – oh my!' In some surgeries the doctors dictated, but 'here our doctors say "do as you like Barnsy" and I do it.'

BARNSY: 'It's a very, very happy surgery and I think that even the times I've been very down and pressurized with work there's always a laugh here. Why, and we have parties.'

MRS JONES (overhearing as she passes the door and joining in): 'That was a lovely party wasn't it? Everybody just went mad for the evening.'

BARNSY: 'Everybody came in fancy dress. Dr Chamberlain came as Pedro the fisherman; Dr David came as a nurse, if you please.'

MRS JONES: 'Everybody kept asking me what I was going as. I had to go from there at midnight as I was going to Spain so I had to have something I could get off quickly.'

BARNSY: 'She was a baby, a nappy on; she even had a little potty – oh, we had a lot of fun.'

MRS JONES: 'So when he came along and picked me up he just stood there. He didn't know what to do, he didn't know what to say – he was lost for words. I'd got one of those big sugar dummies, a bonnet, a big nappy and a little top.'

BARNSY: 'It was super. She got first prize for that. Dr Ryton came dressed as Robinson Crusoe – parrot on his shoulder, through the traffic lights and all, didn't he?'

David Bilsby now reappeared and we set off on our second visit. He described the way people managed with death and old age – their determination to keep going. The old, old man who had just died, and been looked after by his wife and her ninety-year-old sister. He refused to sleep downstairs, which David hadn't realized until he came to give him a catheter, when he set off up the stairs, 'And at each step he'd stop, he couldn't quite lift his foot to the next step, and the two old ladies bent down and lifted it up and the same thing would happen with the other foot, and repeated fourteen times, all the way up the stairs, these two poor old ladies.'

We were near a second estate and David explained the next problem. This was a man who had epilepsy. His wife had rung, desperate: 'You've got to do something about him, doctor. He's got some disgusting habits. I can't stand it. I'm afraid I shall have another nervous breakdown.' The problem was he was sixty-three. It was very difficult to get someone of that age into hospital round here, just to give her a rest. If he'd been sixty-five it would have been different. (I realized how very important and useful it was for GPs to have access to hospital beds.) Difficult to treat him. He was on phenobarbitone and Epanutin. The drugs made him dizzy, unable to walk; but if the dosage was lowered he had fits.

A small council bungalow. The door was opened by the wife – tiny, in trousers, dyed hair in rollers, very thin, so you could see the scalp, little nervous determined face, mouth quivering as she immediately went into how she couldn't stand it.

We went into the bedroom. Curtains opened. Double bed, a lot of cheap furniture so you could hardly move – make-up on a dresser doing as a dressing table, cupboard. The husband was in bed, very grey, unshaven. Roughening of the skin. He looked to me as if he drank. While the doctor fairly briskly examined him and talked, I could see her across the way, listening behind the living room door. He hadn't had a fit for a month, but very dizzy. Appetite? 'I've had nothing today.' 'Not even a cup of tea?' 'No.' Dr Bilsby took a blood specimen. Man couldn't remember which arm had been taken last. 'I'll get both ready,' laughing. Scrawny arm, pale vein. 'Little prick,' said the GP automatically. The blood unexpectedly thick and dark. Then he looked through his notes. 'You've seen all the GPs.' It was one of the bulging envelopes. 'When did you last work?' 'Four years ago. When the attacks came the doctor's letter said no ladders. That was it, they didn't want to know me. After twenty-two years.' He was bitter. I wondered if the GP could have worded it differently so that he could have kept his job.

GP obviously baffled. (It was clear now how important it was to see the same patient, certainly through one episode.) However, he said he'd get Dr Sawrey out that evening, a doctor who'd already treated him for his epilepsy. Dr Sawrey would get him into hospital.

He explained to the wife what he was doing. She only gathered that he was going to get her husband off her hands for a while and relaxed, the long, broken teeth becoming covered by the thin lips.

In the car he said he hoped Sawrey could get him into hospital. It was possible he needed a complete rethink of his epilepsy treatment, but it would have to be monitored.

I thought of that couple, helping each other end their days, not able to cope really, locked together. 'He has some disgusting habits.' I'd noticed, in a boot beside the bed, a plastic bottle into which he peed. Poor, alone, disliking it all, *hating* it. He looked seventy, set for death as the only real solution.

We returned to the surgery and David Bilsby rang Dr Sawrey, but he was out. It was now the end of the other surgeries and the GPs came in and sat about the reception area, filling out the notes of the case histories, entering prescription details, talking to the nurses and auxiliary nurses. Dr Ryton said 'Basically he's OK. But he's *deaf*. I should yell. He's able to do it himself but he does need a good going over from time to time.'

Mrs Jones takes time out to finish a talk we'd begun earlier in the morning. I had read in the latest Cartwright report that what patients principally disliked was the receptionist asking what was wrong, why did they want to see the doctor? This should be stopped, she said.

PRACTICE MANAGER AND RECEPTIONIST: 'Well, you have to, don't you? How could you tell if it was serious otherwise? Some patients think we try and keep them from the doctor, but we don't. Say it's Thursday, when surgery finishes at 5 o'clock, if they tell you what is wrong and you see they'll ask for a call, it is far better for them to come in to the surgery and the doctor to see them at the end of the ante-natal.

'But you have to protect the doctor a bit – tell a few white lies. Is doctor in? No – signalling all the time for the doctor to keep out of sight. And they try and talk on the telephone, but I say – far better make an appointment and see him face to face.

'People think reception is just sitting at a desk. But you're not just sat there to see the patients and say "Take a seat." There's the paperwork. Drawers of it. Ante-natals, on the first visit the patient has a blood grouping form, cytology form, haematology form, ante-natal record card and envelope. About five forms and a FW8, which she needs to claim for prescriptions. You might have four or five first visits in one ante-natal clinic. There is an awful lot of paperwork there. You don't relax at all. When you have a break mid-morning you go upstairs and shut yourself away for a quarter of an hour and we come down and start again.

'I couldn't do anything else. I couldn't bear to be at home. You get so involved with the patients, it's super. You have got your favourites, like one old girl when she comes in she always insists on giving me 10p shoe leather money, and I always take it, because it offends her if I don't. When we've got 30p we buy a packet of biscuits.'

It was about 12 o'clock and the doctors had finished the last details of their surgeries. There was a feeling of getting it polished off. 'That's done – away,' said Dr Rimpton. It was a battlefield to which the enemy always returned, the dragon's teeth of local illness.

Before we set off on our last visit, David took me round.

They had virtually none of the glossy equipment of the big southern hospital-like health centres – no ECG, no microscope, no age-sex register ('but we have records going back to 1912'), they do a few coils. They had had a spirometer (for measuring breath flow) but it disappeared.

Our last visit was six miles away. The practice was about ten miles across, that is, it was ten miles from the surgery to the most distant patient, so it could be a twenty-mile round trip at night. But most of the patients were in the town itself.

This wasn't Dr Bilsby's patient and he didn't know what was wrong with him. He'd forgotten to bring the notes. He'd had an operation for piles three months ago.

We arrived at a rather fine, if somewhat dilapidated farmhouse. We went in through the kitchen, after getting no answer to our knocks. The house seemed deserted – good, solid furniture, pictures, rugs on the flags. But eventually, after a lot of shouting, a faint voice came from upstairs.

There were more calls before we located him. A strong, virile-looking man of perhaps fifty-five or sixty lying in bed, very short hair round the sides, bald on top of a nut-brown, bony scalp, dark eyes. A gent; with a voluble, clearly anxious explanation. Two weeks ago, having dinner – Dr Voe, the anaesthetist was there actually (I realized this was a hint; one lost on Dr Bilsby) duck in aspic, suddenly – dramatic gesture – completely blocked *here*. He pointed at his stomach, at the top. Then described a night of vomiting, acid stomach, a lot of fluid produced – a colourless jelly. Hadn't thought much of it, just one of those rare seizures. Until yesterday night it happened again. Exactly the same. He'd saved some of the colourless jelly to show Dr Bilsby, who seemed only marginally interested in it.

Dr Bilsby examined him, felt his stomach, stethoscoped, then wrote out two prescriptions. He soothed and reassured. This was very common, you often didn't find a reason. Did he smoke? Yes . . . well, that could be stimulating the glands to over-produce acid. Or spicy foods – avoid these. If it happened again, he might have to have an X-ray and go into it. Start on food gently. 'Tea?' said the man, fussed, having been expounding a theory of alkaline saliva which he'd tried to swallow. 'Coffee?' 'No', said Bilsby, 'start on milky things'. This seemed to calm the man. Bilsby rose briskly and asked him if he wanted a certificate to be off work, as if he were a common labourer (who don't, in any case, any longer require short-term certificates). The man looked a bit non-plussed and said 'No, no'. After a moment he added, in a very gentle reproof, reinforcing his earlier hint, that he had had to postpone an important *business conference* in Buckinghamshire, because of the illness.

In the car, David seemed quite unconcerned. He'd given him stuff to stop him being sick, and something to stop fluid coming up in his throat. He said, rather pleased with his subtlety, 'You noticed how I didn't tell him to stop smoking? He'd have taken no notice. I just introduced it, put it in his mind to think about.' I didn't think the man had actually noticed this. What he had noticed was being taken for a farm labourer instead of a man who had duck in aspic with the anaesthetist, Dr Voe. It also seemed to me that the symptoms were anxiety ones and that David had made no attempt to find out if this was so.

As we drove back he told me that those able to produce poltergeist and psychokinetic phenomena were markedly more prone to epilepsy.

At lunch, David again phoned Dr Sawrey and found he was in Greece. He'd get another doctor to look at the second patient we'd visited but he wouldn't be able to get the sixty-three year-old into hospital. The GP's day is endless little tasks like this – ringing up, being baulked, trying another doctor, another hospital, another department or official, getting back to the patients. Cumulative.

During the afternoon I spoke to the woman part-time GP, the chemist and a lot of patients.

In the evening the Bilsbys had another GP friend to supper. Wine flowed (here at last were doctors with whom I could abandon my surreptitious bedroom swigs), the tape recorder forgotten, and I heard examples of GPs' gossip, among other things. Dr Hamstall was about thirty-nine, forthright, resembled Jimmy Greaves somewhat.

Dinner Talk

They said they neither of them prescribed placebos, but when a patient clearly wanted a prescription, gave a tonic or vitamin solution. Dr Hamstall said that just seeing a patient was a placebo effect. David's wife, Janet, said that lots of patients just came for a shoulder to pour their woes upon.

DR HAMSTALL: 'Do you get much of that, David? I suppose I get the odd one.'

DR BILSBY: 'Oh dozens – I took them over from old Geoff. Dozens. I spend hours listening.'

DR HAMSTALL: 'They expect it. Mine don't.'

DR BILSBY: 'I let them know I'm busier than he was. But I don't know how effective it is – if they come back next month, how much good you did with the last talk.'

DR HAMSTALL: 'I don't mind people who unload once in a while, but on a regular basis I am not going to do it.'

DR BILSBY: 'Well, if one takes a minute, you can give a bit more time to eleven others. Someone with a special problem, you can get them to come back after surgery for as long as necessary.'

DR HAMSTALL: 'Ah . . . the difficult ones.'

DR BILSBY: 'Well, not exactly. But I never know about difficult patients. I mean, some of the allocated ones aren't difficult. They just get a reputation for it. Mrs Harley came with a huge folder. She'd been on every doctor's list in Lincolnshire practically.'

JANET BILSBY: 'She'd had every organ, not essential, actually essential to life, removed.'

DR BILSBY: 'That wasn't entirely her fault either. If you go to those private London surgeons and can pay they'll operate. She had this reputation – a letter from the DHSS saying "Oh yes, we get so fed up with her, when she comes on the phone we put her through to an unused extension." That's the way people handled her in the past. All she wanted was somebody not to say, "Oh you are imagining it," but just to say, "Oh dear, dear, well I hope you feel better soon." That is literally *all* she needed. She was ever such a nice lady. She's in a long-stay hospital the other side of Lincoln and myself and Sister Barnes, who you met, go and see her.'

DR HAMSTALL: 'Yes, but you get some. I remember where one patient absolutely insisted I went, but it was four in the morning. She said she'd had a dry throat for half an hour. I just refused to visit. She removed herself from our list later. I suppose it was a cold.'

DR BILSBY: 'I remember somebody ringing me at two in the morning just to demonstrate his cough because I hadn't prescribed an antibiotic the day before.'

DR HAMSTALL: 'Well, it's very rare but sometimes you have to do something. There was one got me out of bed at 2 o'clock in the morning, supposedly unconscious, but there he was, half-sitting back in his chair, and I thought he was probably messing around. What you do, is hold their hand above their nose and let it drop. If they're unconscious it flops, but if not, it sort of goes over there. Well, I knew then he was messing around so I decided I'd wake him up using more painful methods. I did an external rub which is really very painful if you do it hard enough, rub the knuckle up and down on the sternum and he decided he was awake then. He said he didn't like my attitude. I didn't like his attitude either. Next thing I heard he was down at the accident unit complaining he had been assaulted by his GP.'

DR BILSBY: 'Well, you get GPS too. Especially with drink.'

DR HAMSTALL: 'Yes, it's a common thing with GPS. That's when they go off the rails. A chap, do you remember, his daughter used to drive him around because he was too drunk to drive.'

DR BILSBY: 'Your mother knew him in Devon, didn't she?'

JANET BILSBY: 'Yes, and he had been doing a lot of locums, which is always a sign of trouble, usually drink or drugs.'

DR HAMSTALL: 'The partner before me drank a fearful lot. He rang me up when I was a houseman, and I thought it was a friend of mine pulling a fast one, he was so slurred. I nearly said, "Piss off, Dave." He eventually got dismissed by my present partner when one particular day he nodded off in the surgery, in the middle of seeing a patient. The patient came out to the receptionist and said, "I think the doctor is asleep," and she went in and he couldn't be roused. Snoring.'

DR BILSBY: 'My thing was forgetting. Now I tend to keep spares of everything in the car. Plastic gloves, just think if you want to do a PR (per rectum) and you haven't got a pair of plastic gloves.'

DR HAMSTALL: 'Oh yes, I've turned out without most things, without a prescription pad, that's annoying. Or leaving the bag at the surgery. You look very stupid when you put your ear to your patient's chest because you've forgotten your stethoscope.

'I remember once, my partner told me the wife was odd. I had as usual been drinking too much coffee in the morning. It was opened by a man and I said, "Before I see your wife, could I just use your loo?" So he showed me through to the back and his wife was in the kitchen ironing, but my partner had said she was a bit of a nutter, so I wasn't too surprised. I used their loo and came back and said, "Righty ho, now I'll see your wife," and I found I'd come to the wrong house.'

The next morning, with a slight hangover, the first for weeks, I went to say good-bye to the Three Elms surgery. It was as before, the telephone going, lights winking, patients arriving, all bustle and hustle. It was a happy practice, as Mrs Jones had said, and in some ways more reassuring than the large health centres with all their equipment. I felt almost sad leaving them, missing, for a fleeting instant, the bustle, the noise. I drove back across mist-shrouded Norfolk. What's more dreary, I thought, than a vast damp field of beet under a grey sky. Except to the farmer, for whom it meant money. Or that same farmer, with twelve-bore, walking through it, when it could mean partridges or even a few pheasants whirring up. I saw they did have machines for lifting beet.

17

Dr Peter Axmouth
A South of England New Town

Peter Axmouth, thirty, had his practice in one of those odd phenomena of the seventies and eighties – an 'overspill' town in the south of England below London. Here, apparently quite arbitrarily, a town was being created from virtually nothing, tacked on to a village ('The Old Town'): dual carriage-ways, shopping precincts, miles of carefully different yet identical estates, facilities, developments, amenities, centres, all with vast parkways for the future ten-car family, a mini-Brasilia plonked on to the gentle English countryside. As I drove into this desolate scene I noticed how the planners had skilfully woven their work deep into the fabric of our history – Boadicea Promenade, Saxon Way, Pepys Avenue.

Dr Axmouth didn't comment on the weirdness of his surroundings as we talked in his small but extremely well-equipped purpose-built surgery; I don't think he thought they were weird. Indeed, he said at one point, 'Until it became so nice and big and swish.' He was rather small, with a sharp intelligent face, and small, very white hands. He was a rather subdued, sad person, inhibited – but made a great effort to tell me things.

DR AXMOUTH: 'From public school I went to Cambridge to read veterinary medicine, but changed my mind half-way through the degree course. I didn't seem to fit into the vet school very well. I was a bit more intelligent than some, but more than that, I less and less saw myself as a vet. I certainly wasn't a large animal vet and it seemed more and more a waste of time to be training to treat people's poodles.'

(He took his degree in medicine and then went to a London teaching hospital.) 'I did the statutory house jobs and at the end of that time I would really have liked to try and be a young physician or possibly anaesthetist which was attractive, but wisdom was beginning to seep in and we were beginning to see how jolly fierce the competition was and how jolly long we would have to spend going from hospital to hospital chasing jobs, you know. So having been disappointed in what seemed like one fairly likely job, I went out west, to Exeter.'

Here he began what is now the statutory final training for a GP – two years in hospital and one year attached to two general practices, six months in each. But 'I got out after two years. It was one of the nurses and it didn't work out so I thought it better to be far away. Physical removal is sometimes the best way to go about these things.' He moved to another hospital, met his present wife, another nurse, who was about to come to the 'New Town'. They moved together, and, still undecided whether to become a GP or not, Axmouth took a vacant post of Child Health Officer.

'The doctor goes round the schools, looking at small children and saying "Yes, you're healthy" or "No, you're not healthy", and goes round to clinics looking at babies and saying "Yes, you're a normal baby for six weeks" or, "A normal baby for a year", and it's pretty ineffably boring. After about six months of that I was just about at screaming level when the chap who founded this practice, or his wife to be quite precise, left him and he decided he couldn't carry on and pushed off. And he was looking for a locum to cover the three months of notice that he had to give and someone said, "Why not try Axmouth who's getting bored out of his mind in Child Health?" So he tried me and I did.'

He stayed in fact nine months, while the practice grew from sixty patients to 1,000. New practices of this sort are paid by what amounts to a salary – what they call the Type D allowance. (One might note in passing that GPs become incensed if you suggest a salaried service. In my experience it works perfectly well in practice, with none of the disadvantages they dread.) Unfortunately to qualify as a senior partner getting this allowance you have to have five years' GP experience. Axmouth had an uneasy period while candidates were interviewed, wondering if the new man would keep him on. Fortunately, they got on and he did. Axmouth was now finally committed to general practice.

'I suppose what I like, particularly after hospital medicine, is the freedom and ability to take responsibility. What one doesn't like is it can be very humdrum and boring. Part of it is very trivial, a lot of it – which is not to say unimportant. This may be because it's a New Town, with a lot of young folks and babies. But I think there's an appreciable minority who misuse your services because they come far too often for far too small things.

'You said one of your doctors said it was a bad thing to ring at night and get an Ansaphone giving you another number. I think I can counter that. It's unbelievable the number of calls at outlandish hours with silly questions. At least with an answer machine they get a human voice. When I was a trainee I slept in the surgery when on call. The answer machine would wink, and then, if they really needed it, a little later the night phone would go. It was quite striking how often the answer light would go and then the night telephone would *not* go. It acted as an idiot filter.

'And they expect magical things, as if you could bring their husband back, which you can't. And the odd one really enjoys the catharsis and just goes on and on. This can be frustrating, especially if you're busy. I've found it very difficult to bring that sort of thing to an end without offending or ruining the effect of what I've said. And you get no training in that at all. You certainly can't learn from books. Some go into it far more, with videos and looking at themselves doing it and that sort of thing. I suppose a good trainer or consultant in your past. I remember Hugh Jolly was brilliant at carrying on a consultation with a worried, tearful mum, psychotherapy sort of thing with an enormous pack of audience. I don't know what it's like to be on the receiving end as mum with babe and this sea of faces.' Peter Axmouth went on to say how his wife was under great pressure 'on the district' in a rougher end of the town and how he had to support her. 'It sometimes seems like the final turn of the screw after a hard day.'

'Not that I dislike medicine *all* that violently and intensely. But I see the horizons could have been broader somewhere else. But it's all might-have-been. I'm a technical sort of chap. I could have been a reasonable photographer, even if it's fairly lowly. Or an administrator. When we're endlessly discussing this practice with the development corporation I can see myself in their seat. The seat of power.

'I don't come from an upper-middle-class family; I come from a very much lower-middle-class family and went to public school on a scholarship and my maternal grandfather was a carpenter in the days when carpenters actually knew how to work with wood; my other grandfather was a builder and decorator. My father came out as what would now be called a hospital administrator, but was then called just a clerk. My mother – unheard of in a small Oxfordshire village – went to the grammar school and became a teacher eventually and probably had the ability to do more. But that step was big enough, from a carpenter's daughter, in a small village. She was the same generation as Laurie Lee, you know, coming out of what was really a Victorian village effectively, to being a school-teacher, it's quite a long way to jump. But the thrust was on, definitely from my mother. That, you know, the profession and the qualifications and the upward climb was the way to go on and this was the route to success and I think perhaps that if I'd come from a family that had already made that success, perhaps not so much score would have been put on it. I don't know. I would have been more allowed to float. And I think perhaps the people who allow themselves to float a little bit more are more comfortable in life. I'm a victim of upward social mobility. I don't quite know what my children will do – if any. They'll probably go back to being builders and decorators and be very, very happy.'

He described how sometimes he thought 'My God, I'm not practising medicine, I'm not being a decent husband, I'm not happy. I want to leave.'

'You meet different people in medicine. You meet a lot of people like me. Probably more people like me than of the old school whose fathers and grandfathers had been doctors, but those of us in my position are probably a slightly restless bunch, where the satisfaction is a little bit tenuous and the escape route is non-existent. We wonder if we haven't put our heads into a very nicely velvet-lined trap.'

I only saw three GPs who weren't happy in their work. To conform to the national – or Cartwright – average, I should have seen half a GP more. She found 7 per cent didn't enjoy their work; 7 per cent of fifty is three and a half. She found 55 per cent enjoyed it a lot and 36 per cent moderately – this compared with 52 per cent, 37 per cent and 9 per cent respectively in 1964.

Cartwright noted that considering the many improvements – more money, better premises, more help and so on – these figures showed little change. Dr Axmouth, I felt, wasn't totally suited to being a GP. He was rather authoritarian and impatient. He said, 'It's probably a revealing statement, but I haven't actually *got* a lot of friends.' There was something not so much lonely as isolated about him. 'Most of my friends are medical.' But it was clearly the nature of his work that didn't suit him – the host of what he saw as trivial complaints and demands, the non-medical element of it all – 'I'm not practising medicine.' This was true of both the other GPs (both of whom could have been brilliant doctors of another sort). I suspect this is true of most of Cartwright's 7 per cent. The 'improvements', the 'conditions' are irrelevant to them. Indeed, the 'velvet lining' makes it all the more irksome, shaming almost.

This leads us into the whole field of what GPs treat and how, their attitudes towards and feelings about their patients, all the things related to what I described as the heart of GP life – the consultation.

18
THE CONSULTATION

Women consult more than men, particularly (and probably for this reason) when reproductive (aged eighteen to forty-four); the average for women is 4.6 consultations a year, for men, 2.7. But those who consult least are also women, those between the ages of forty-five and fifty-four. They were thought to be racked by menopausal difficulty, but Cartwright found this not to be so. Among men, the lower socio-economic classes consult more than the upper, partly because their jobs are physically more demanding, and at the time of the survey they still needed short-term sick notes. Finally, old people are the least likely to worry about wasting GPs' time; this probably is because by then something chronic has set in, which is recognized, serious, and requires regular attention.

What else goes wrong? We've seen how all the fevers and decimating infections went; what remains? Here is the main pattern in a practice numbering 2,500 – figures in brackets are the number of cases this GP could expect in a year:

1) NEOPLASMS (growths), 1 per cent (twenty-five patients). This is higher than the actual number found, because there is a high fear rate.

2) GENITO-URINARY DISEASES, 5.4 per cent (135 patients).

3) INFECTIVE AND PARASITIC (like measles, glandular fever, mumps etc.), 8 per cent (140 patients).

4) MENTAL DISORDERS (clear-cut psychiatric disease, like schizophrenia), 8 per cent (125 patients).

But if you add in the whole psychosomatic 'mental' group, that is another 25 per cent (550 patients).

5) RESPIRATORY (including colds), 26 per cent (650 patients). This, therefore, is the most common. But many of these will also have partial or total psychosomatic elements, and in fact this is probably the largest component of the GP's sick list. *The Future General Practitioner*, from which these figures come, later puts it at 50 per cent. No one knows how large it is, except everyone agrees it's large. Another study, *Doctors Talking to Patients*, says it could be as high as 80 per cent. One doctor I spoke to said that 95 per cent of the patients really had mental problems of one sort or another (but I think she had slightly gone over the top on aspects of this).

The GP's prime task, the reason he is trained, the reason he exists, is to pick out disease as early as possible, and then to see it gets the best treatment. The most important part of his life, therefore, is the diagnosis.

The Diagnosis

DR JOHN MARTHAN: 'My father said to me, "In a busy surgery, amongst all the moans and groans and trivialities you have to pick out the ones who need urgent attention." Your chap comes in, and goes home and says "I'm all right." Then it happens again and he say, "I'm not going back. The doctor said I was all right." That's when it happens. You've always got to be careful of the patient who only comes once in four years. He says he might have a bit of a cough. That's the one who's going to have a carcinoma of the lung.

'But it's not just slog, nor knowledge and experience gone in and forgotten. There's a bit of intuition. I had a patient, an old girl, who was a spiritualist. She gripped my hand and there was a funny movement in my arm. She said, "You've got the healing movement very strongly, doctor." '

DR CHATHILL: 'The fear is missing something that you ought to find and therefore killing somebody. If not immediately killing, not finding quick enough. All our training is picking up illness *early*.

'It's a combination of tiny points – the severity of the pain, the way it presents, how ill the patient looks. Sometimes something seems to go off in your mind, alerts you, before you've even looked at them. And that's what goes, if you start getting flu. Something like a virus infection and the perceptive faculty goes and that's a dangerous time to examine patients.'

DR THRIPLOW: 'If there's a diagnosis, you've usually made it within a few minutes of talking to them, and then everything else just confirms your opinion. Some, you're pretty sure there's nothing the matter with, and then there are others that you feel are not well, but you can't put your finger on it and yet you feel you've got to go on looking and these are perhaps the worrying ones.

'But the great thing about general practice is that time is on your side as it were. Whereas a hospital doctor or a clinic has one look at them and doesn't know any more than that. *We* know what sort of home background they have, and if we're not very happy we can perhaps pop in when we're passing, or say, "Look in again next week." And time will usually reveal whether there is anything.'

DR ABNEY: 'The triumphs – oh yes, can be lovely. There's Harry – I knew him. I drink out away from here to be out of sight of patients, and Harry and his father had often popped in there for a beer. Harry came to see me one afternoon here and said "I've got a terrible headache. A really frightful one and *nobody* is taking it seriously at all." He'd been the rounds. He'd been to

casualty departments. And he said, "Nobody takes this headache seriously."
I said, "OK, right, let's give you a good going over." He'd got a cerebral
tumour anyway. No doubt about it. I rang up. The brain pressure was
obviously acute. He was a different man. He changed mood. He'd got
absolutely *classical* . . . Well, I mean, OK, one's always suspicious of things.
I'm perhaps over-suspicious. But anyway the next day he was in hospital and
they did an operation to relieve the pressure first. It suddenly started
enlarging rather quickly and they decompressed him and put a shunt in, and
then it was obvious the thing was still romping away. And then about a
month later they went in and removed it. Yes, it was operable. He lost the
sight of one eye but then, slowly, the sight came back. He's back at work
now; back to his normal work. And yet he hawked himself round GPs and
God knows where, trying to get someone to take him seriously.'

DR MARY TRIMDON: 'One of my partners looked at this patient's eyes
yesterday and when he did that there's a thing moved up and down like a
bubble. And he got another doctor to look at it and in *both* eyes this thing
moved up and down like a bubble. Never seen anything like this before. The
patient was suffering from severe headaches. And he had a look but couldn't
see her discs, thought they might be a little bit cloudy. So he sent her up to the
eye pavilion and the patient came in today. I saw the letter saying there was
nothing wrong with the patient – the handwritten letter which had come
back. He said to me, "Would you like to have a look at the patient?" And
when I did that I said, "You know what it is? It's contact lenses." Now I've
never seen contact lenses before, but it was so obvious. And he'd sent them
up to the hospital!'

Psychotherapy
Patients, particularly poorer ones, have always come to the doctor with
problems – 'life' problems like their jobs, family problems, personal
problems like depression.
  It is not really possible to be certain if patients do this more or less than they
used to – though most GPs think more. It is likely to be more, since it is part of
a much greater movement. As the great army of historical disease was
destroyed, it sometimes seems that all that was left were the psycho-
somatic/social/life-caused/stress-caused diseases. And this is not just a
relatively larger proportion (as we saw, anything from 30 per cent to 80 per
cent). It is absolutely larger. This for several reasons. In the twenty-five years
from 1950 the *average* wealth in the country, right down through the classes,
quadrupled. This has never happened before at any time in the history of the
world. It was an astounding economic explosion, and gave rise to extraordinary expectations in the most diverse fields. People began to come to
their GP with anxieties, fears, complaints which they would not have dreamt

of coming with before; and which a good many GPs think they should not come with now.

Second, there is the enormous and pervasive influence of what can loosely be called the psychoanalytic movement over the last fifty years. This, and studies which ultimately derive from it, have shown the astonishing extent to which the mind is involved with and influences the body – its ills expressed there, distressing, distorting, destroying.

It is not difficult to conceive how mental illness can have a physical cause. Mental depression and anxiety were recognized as physical illnesses in the fourteenth century. It is harder for people to realize that mental distress can create actual physical, sometimes fatal, illnesses.

Yet this, too, was understood in the past. Hippocrates was aware of it; so were the great Arab doctors of the Moslem Empire. There is a fascinating passage in a treatise by William Harvey*, early in the seventeenth century:

> I was acquainted with another strong man, who having received an injury, and affront from one more powerful than himself, and upon whom he could not have his revenge, was so overcome with hatred and spite and passion, which he yet communicated to no one, that at last he fell into a strange distemper, suffering from extreme oppression and pain of the heart and breast and in the course of a few years died. His friends thought him poisoned by some maleficent influence, or possessed with an evil spirit . . . in the dead body I found the heart and aorta so much gorged and distended with blood, that the cavities of the ventricles equalled those of a bullock's heart in size. Such is the force of the blood pent up, and such are the effects of its impulse.

And then suddenly Harvey seems to glimpse for a moment, in a flash, the extraordinary possibilities of his observation:

> And indeed, such a flood of light and truth breaks in upon me here; occasion offers of explaining so many problems, of resolving so many doubts, of discovering the causes of so many slighter and more serious diseases, and of suggesting remedies for their cure, that the subject seems almost to demand a separate treatise . . .

For an instant one thinks – suppose he had pursued this line? But he didn't. Two and a half centuries were to pass before, after Freud, medicine was to become aware of this truth again. But it is an extraordinary moment.

As well as affecting the heart, prolonged stress or anxiety can lead to tissue change in intestine, lungs and skin. There is suggestive, but not conclusive, evidence linking cancer with states of mind.

More general evidence shows the same thing. After extensive flooding in Bristol, Glin Bennet notes in *Patients and Their Doctors*, in 1968, attendance at surgeries increased by 58 per cent and hospital attendance more than doubled (this was random illness, not directly caused attendance due to exposure or whatever). An American study he quotes found a 'cluster' effect. It had been noted that a quarter of the population had half the illness. When studied, this revealed the cluster effect; illness occurred when several aspects of the life

*Quoted in Brian Inglis' *A History of Medicine*.

situation went wrong – job, money, marriage – and the patient couldn't solve them or see a way out.

The second way mental stress manifests itself is in the now familiar concept of 'presenting'. The patient turns up with boils or a sore throat because they can't quite admit to the real reason – their boss or rows with their husband. The real reason might not emerge, or emerges at the end of the consultation in those words which make every GP's heart sink – 'Oh, while I'm here,' 'By the way,' etc.

But if the real reason does *not* emerge, then the patient will return again. Every GP has a patient who seems to have nothing wrong, but comes back again and again, with more and more bizarre symptoms. It may take time to get to their root, but not, in the end, nearly as much time as *not* getting there. The point is, since personal conflicts, stress and problems are a common cause of physical illness and disease, the cure of these diseases lies in 'curing' or alleviating the conflicts. The furious young champion of the seventeenth century with the heart of a bullock could have been saved. And often the 'presenting' and the illness are one, as the anxiety manifests itself in a physical form – Balint quotes the case of a woman, aged thirty-two, who had an appendicectomy, hysterectomy and cholecystectomy over three years, and was still vomiting when seen. Her husband was out of work and she had been supporting the family for three years. She was presenting the symptoms of someone overstretched. When this was pointed out the symptoms disappeared. She was very upset, but could now concentrate on solving the real problems.

So much importance do many doctors attach to this 'holistic' approach – that illness can be, and often is, an interaction between the purely clinical, the inner psychology of the patient, and his social and familial environment – that the Royal College of General Practitioners now requires diagnoses to be made at all three levels. And the main tool, both for diagnoses and also often for treatment, lies in the technique of consultation.

Techniques of Consultation

Since anything from 30 per cent to 80 per cent of GPs' work has an emotional/mental content, and since the way into this content is largely dependent on how they consult, you would suppose it was an important part of student training. It is not. It is virtually not taught at all. GPs now have to do a year training to be GPs after they have qualified as doctors, and here of course they can learn to consult. But since their trainer has himself never learnt to consult and may be no good at it this is of somewhat random value.

However, both to remedy this situation and also as a consequence of the importance now attached to it, a great many books and studies have been published over the last fifteen years or so going deeply into the subject. And, before very briefly indicating some of the things they suggest, it is interesting to look at some of the things their analyses of untrained GP consultations have thrown up.

Patterns have emerged. GPs are more friendly to old patients and to women patients (one GP studied by Byrne and Long in *Doctors Talking to Patients* actually had a special accent for women).

Doctors will go to surprising lengths when faced with disorders they don't like or want. Seven doctors in the Byrne study became very aggressive faced with this situation. One went so far as to say, 'I shall tell you what your symptoms are.' Many doctors prefer to withhold information.

PATIENT: 'Did the specialist say I was all right?'

DOCTOR: 'Nothing there at all. False alarms. Now – I want you back in a month.'

The fact that he also prescribed showed that something was wrong. He simply didn't want to share the information.

Doctors will avoid emotional content; in fact difficulties in consultations nearly always arise because the doctor wishes to treat an organic illness, the patient wants counselling.

PATIENT: 'What on earth am I going to do about him, doctor?'

DOCTOR: 'Let's concentrate on your rash, shall we, and leave that to another time.'

Or, another example:

PATIENT: 'I do feel badly about the whole thing, doctor.'

DOCTOR: 'Well, take your tablets.'

Patients play on the GP's feelings. If they can arouse his sympathy, they will obtain more attention. Doctors feel they are being used and learn to suppress sympathy, almost automatically. Again, for a GP's skills to be fully alerted his anxiety must to some extent be aroused. Patients are aware of this and will exaggerate their symptoms. If false, the GP is naturally enough angry, and may miss whatever it was that was there. (Another anger-making situation is the unnecessary night call – this can sometimes be 'presenting' for something else.)

Quite often the patient 'presents' with some trivial symptom, meaning to somehow get into all sorts of other, far more important reasons for her visit ('her' – the examples are usually feminine). The doctor, who already suspects the worst, seizes the symptom and starts to treat it. Upon which, the patient, realizing what has happened, starts to offer the real causes for her attendance. In order to find out what is happening one of them has to stop. Chaos can result, as happened here, apparently bang in the middle of a consultation, to the immense surprise of the researchers listening to the tape. The doctor had examined the patient for chest pains, which she had already said started in the night.

DOCTOR: 'What time did the pains start?'

PATIENT: 'I saw him at three or four in the afternoon . . . but he didn't seem to notice me then . . .'

DOCTOR: 'Yes, but what time did it start?'

PATIENT: 'There was nothing to be said. Nothing at all [crying]. I wasn't there at first. It didn't seem real.'

DOCTOR: 'What?'

PATIENT: 'When I came home.'

DOCTOR: 'At what time did it . . .?'

PATIENT: 'It started at nine.'

DOCTOR: 'The pains started at nine?'

PATIENT: 'What pains?'

DOCTOR: 'The ones you said you had last night.'

PATIENT: 'I'm not talking about them.'

DOCTOR: 'Oh.'

Doctors also claim that they alter their styles with, say, immigrant patients or British patients with little verbal ability. In fact, it seems they just ask the same questions only more slowly and much louder.

These errors can be dangerous. There is a good deal of anecdotal evidence that the body 'organizes' itself for major illness. There is a feeling of general malaise. And it is at this point that the doctor can actually dictate the form it will take. An anxious patient, given a barium meal, may develop into an ulcer sufferer – a disease likely to be harder to cure than the original anxiety state, which will in any case return in some other form. It is this aspect of dealing with the whole complex *life* of a patient that requires the GPs' work to be so much more dextrous than the lifeless clinical skills of the hospital specialist – and, *if they have that bent*, so much more fascinating.

Finally, sometimes all these GP clumsinesses irritate, alarm or frustrate the patient and he gets better in order not to have to see the doctor again. Balint called this 'the retreat into health'. But – he will be back.

There are two root troubles. The first is that even simple therapy demands that the doctor should feel. He has to respond to the patient, sympathize, to an extent feel with him. For a whole complex of reasons, a great many GPs resent this.

Second, their entire early training is in the diagnosis and treatment of organic disease. Here is laid down the pattern of consultation. History taking, examination, diagnosis, treatment. The doctor is an authority figure, in charge of a goal-orientated process, his questions designed to elicit the truth, which he usually half knows (the patient has been sent to hospital, in any case, with suspected kidney trouble or spleen or whatever), and to block off irrelevancies. This process, one might note, is a great deal easier than anything more subtle. It is also perfectly adequate for such purely organic diseases the GP will meet. What one might term the 'new style consultation' attempts to turn all this on its head.

I say 'new', but in fact this has been going on since the fifties. The seminal figure here is Michael Balint.

DR RIARD: 'He was a tremendous man, extraordinary man. Big man in every sense of the word. He was a Hungarian who came over here to escape from Hitler in the late thirties. A mixture of an enormously powerful theoretical mind, and a great pragmatist, very down to earth. He could be very aggressive. He believed that doctors really would learn a lot if they could only listen to their patients, and he really taught them how to listen. I think that he showed the way forward for a kind of research – and this is my own personal view – which is not fully exploited yet. It's what's called narrative research as opposed to numerative research. It's looking for models and pictures of what's going on in people's lives and interpreting them. And in that I *guess* he drew upon his psychoanalytical background. Perhaps the most important thing he did was that he actually changed the morale of general practice more than anybody else did. He believed that what we did was fascinating, important, capable of scientific analysis, and his influence was I think out of all proportion to the number of groups that he held and so on.

'Michael was a great debunker and he was very gruffly honest. He doesn't come out well in his books because he wrote appallingly. I mean, he wrote and spoke like some steam train without rails running uphill through treacle. But put him in a group of doctors and the thing would come alive. He would with an absolute shaft suddenly open a case up for you and show you what was there under your eyes. And he would never say, "That is what is there," but "Maybe you should go back and see whether it's there or not," and that was a marvellous experience.'

And that is, in fact, quite simply the sum of it. The essence is, finding the right problem, not the one presented. The way is to let the patient explain it himself. And this involvement of the GP with the patient has two advantages. As a result the patient becomes 'real'; work therefore becomes more satisfying. Second, if the patient can cause his own illness he can also cure himself. This ability is best tapped if the patient is left free, not dictated to by the doctor.

The method of letting the patient in is by listening and observing, not blocking him off with direct questions – 'What's wrong?' or 'What's hurting today?' But asking open questions – 'What can I do for you?' Reassurance can block. Encouragement too. It is not therefore easy. Silence is a tool, but busy GPs don't like sitting in silence, Dr Blairhall's 'head of steam' building up in the waiting room. It is easy to slip into direct questions. 'What is your schedule? Do you have lunch?' The patient says yes, he has lunch, and the GP passes on.

The result of learning such techniques is to add one or two minutes to each consultation. Not, one might think, a great deal.

But lessons in consultation offer psychoanalytic insights also, and ones that can go beyond the frequent GP discovery that a patient who comes with 'a pain in the neck' is having difficulty with the boss, or a woman 'sick to the stomach' is in trouble with her husband.

One clue is feeling. A patient who cannot express a feeling verbally or does not know *what* he is really feeling, will act these feelings out: aggression, depression, sexual attraction or whatever it is. The doctor reacts appropriately, and this gives him the clue as to what is going on. His feelings are a tool. A patient who makes him feel sick or angry or frightened is telling him as much about his symptoms as if he had a temperature.

It was, to diverge for a moment, fascinating to find how relevant to the researching of this book all these particular observations were. I learned early that I must shut up when talking to GPs. If I talked too, although the results were often stimulating, they told me little or told me what they thought I wanted to hear. (Patients do the same to over-directing GPs.) But I often felt quite strong feelings talking to them. With Dr Anne Uplees, I began to feel overwhelming depression. It was not until near the end of our interview that she revealed that she was being analysed for depression. I felt this too with Dr Chathill and Dr Axmouth. With Dr Nyewood I was aware of quite strong feelings of antagonism and aggression and had to control my reactions. When we looked at his health centre he showed me the incoming mail. There was a vast pile for him, five letters for the next partner, no letters for the senior partner. 'There is no way of dealing with disparity of work. It can be a source of great friction in a practice.' But I think my feelings about both him and Dr Chathill were revealing something still more profound and distressing, as we'll see – in Dr Nyewood's case revealing it in quite an odd way.

Michael Balint, and after his death his wife and collaborators, wanted to find some way in which the insights and help possible in full psychotherapy, but which take an hour once or several times a week, could be applied to the situation of general practice – where the average consultation time is six or seven minutes, and GPs certainly don't want to see a patient more than once a week. They developed what they called the 'flash' technique. The idea of this is two-fold. The doctor doesn't concentrate on deep-seated psychological areas – childhood, relations with parents or siblings – but focuses on something more superficial. The focal point is chosen by the patient. The way of recognizing what it is is the 'flash'. This utilizes the GP's feelings, but it must be a flash of feeling between him and the patient, which both recognize as significant and which they can then follow. These doctors also found that so far from the shortness of time being a difficulty, it in fact had the effect of concentrating the mind of both doctor and patient. The book edited by Enid Balint – *Six Minutes for the Patient* – gives many case histories, some quite subtle. Here is one.

A woman of thirty-eight, with three children, came quite often with tension headaches, and was always anxious about her children. She refused to discuss her headaches with her GP. One session she was rather flirtatious and the GP felt he didn't really know her at all, and wondered therefore if her husband did. He said, 'Somehow I feel your husband and I are missing what you want.' She answered at once (so a mini-flash), 'It's funny you should say that. I've been working for some men who run a flower shop and one of them has been paying me attention lately.' Her husband had stopped her working there. Doctor: 'Would you like to come and discuss this later?' She said, 'No, I'll drop in and see you in two weeks' time perhaps.' Doctor: 'So it seems I must pay you enough attention but not too much.' She smiled and agreed. This was the true flash.

She came thereafter much more often. She talked of her husband in a rather derogatory way – 'Men are funny' etc. The doctor pointed out she enjoyed making her husband look small, though this didn't really help. Next time she said, 'I've been thinking it over and you're right, my husband and I have been having an argument without words.' She began to work on this, and on her unsureness about herself, on her feelings about other people.

All this came about because of the GP's sudden intuitions – one of which she shared – which broke down the tensions between them and started her working on her main problem – her relationship with her husband (and also made her become a 'real person' to the doctor). She had not allowed him to question her directly, nor would she have gone to a psychiatrist (she didn't need one). Her tension headaches went, she ceased to be so anxious about the children, but she was not a 'new' woman. She had gained a small improvement in understanding herself and her life and that was worthwhile, and more realistic than a total psychotherapeutic 'cure'.

And that is the fairly limited aim of all this – to prevent wrong diagnoses, to let a patient have greater understanding of a problem and to live with it. Also, one might add, to bring greater satisfaction to the doctor. 'How,' asked *The Future General Practitioner*, quoting J. Spence, 'are we to maintain in doctors the sympathetic understanding of so many individuals, without which their work becomes a weariness of spirit and flesh?'

I did not go more deeply into the 'flash' technique, which is fairly complex, because the suggestion in the book is that only a very small number of GPs are capable of practising it. (One only of the doctors I spoke to used the word flash, and then in the wrong sense — as a personal flash of insight, not as the instant and *mutual* moment of realization meant here.) Only a very small number of GPs *want* to practise it. We have already met a good many who, it will have been clear, would have had nothing to do with such airy embellishments of their hard-pressed lives. Many GPs are against the whole concept. In their view, their job is to detect and treat organic disease. 'You don't die of unhappiness, but you die of appendicitis.' They feel it's impertinent to probe in this way.

As far as Cartwright went, facts emerged on this from her indefatigable labours, as they do on most things. She found no difference between men and women GPs in the number of consultations they thought trivial and the appropriateness of patients consulting them on personal problems. In general, 92 per cent of GPs thought the tendency to ask for help was growing; and more thought this was inappropriate than had done so in 1964. Those who thought it was appropriate, and who also thought less of their work was trivial, were happier than doctors who thought the reverse (64 per cent enjoyed their work a lot, compared to only 39 per cent of the others). They also attended more courses, were more likely to be trainers and to become members of the Royal College of General Practitioners (conversely, the GPs who thought their consultations were often trivial found the Royal College irritating). It is hardly surprising to find that the Hesse Sachs bunch of hand-picked GPs maintained there was no such thing as a trivial presentation.

The point about doing even minor therapy is time. Time is of the essence. I said one or two minutes added to a consultation wasn't much. But if you are seeing thirty patients a surgery, which is quite possible, that could be an hour in the morning and an hour in the evening. Many GPs feel they are already pressed enough, that is they find it is already hard enough, if not impossible, to respond to 'concealed offers', look out for 'flashes' and the like.

Yet there are odd facts about this pressure of work. GPs thought they were busier in 1977 than in 1964, but in fact there had been no change in numbers seen or lengths of consultation time, and the number of visits had dropped dramatically. They may have simply been spending less time on the job, and felt pressured in the shorter time they had left for the patient. This is borne out by fewer complaining they have too little leisure time.

In a survey done of fifteen countries, *Pulse* reported in July 1982 that British GPs spent less time than any other doctor consulting patients – less than European doctors, than American, Scandinavian, Israeli, Canadian or other Commonwealth doctors. They spent an average of four hours a day consulting patients in their surgeries. Canadians spend seven hours a day doing it.

And Hesse Sachs discovered something interesting in her sample. She found that the doctor who spent the least time on average with his patients was the one whose patients consistently said he always gave them enough time. He never hurried over a consultation and was always relaxed. The researchers asked him how he achieved this apparently paradoxical result and he said that he did it by focusing *entirely* on the patient. He gave them his full attention. It seems that a good concentrated dose of attention is more valuable than longer attention which is distracted and dissipated. (The same has been found with children, incidentally.)

But the problems of consultation only come alive, the perspectives alter, when we hear what GPs themselves feel about the subject.

DR CHATHILL: 'Yes. It takes a lot out of you, actually. I think that people don't appreciate that is why you should retire early – the fact that you're giving the whole time. Somebody comes into you, they plonk their problem into your lap, they then sit back, leaving the responsibility for caring entirely with you. And one has to give them total attention and interest and then they walk out feeling better and you've given something and by the time you've given that forty times a day, you get tired. One gets very tired, actually, and maybe one gets more tired the older one gets.'

DR JOHN MARTHAN: 'When you're doing a surgery session of two or three hours you don't get much break. One patient goes out and the next one comes in and you're dealing with him, and it's constant strain, diagnosing. When you're visiting you get a break between patients. Just a few minutes perhaps, but your mind is taken off medical matters. Either you're concentrating on driving or thinking, but it gives you a chance to freshen up.'

DR NYEWOOD: 'I think this business is sort of encapsulated in the idea that a patient comes to you with a nasty carbuncle, or severe athlete's foot, or tonsillitis, or a Potts fracture or something, and you say, "Ah yes, very interesting, but what have you *really* come for?" This is the sort of thing and I think there is an awful lot of crap about it really. I mean, of *course*, when you have a busy surgery and someone has spent a lot of time talking about their ankle or whatever, and when they get up and you are writing up the notes, and very pleased it is all over, they say "And by the way", and you have got to know that this is what they have really come for, and up to what has happened now you can forget about. This is very important, and is maddening of course, but at the same time you are in a way a plumber, and if somebody comes to you with athlete's foot or a sore throat, you must treat their athlete's foot or sore throat and stop buggering about.'

DR CULROY: 'Sometimes at the end of surgery I feel I've done no *good* at all. A wart, a cold, a sore throat, catarrh. What am I *here* for? I've saved no one.'

DR JANE EDSTONE: 'We are the only people that anyone can approach without labelling themselves. I think the churches should be far more involved. It's a complete waste of our training, but on the other hand I think we have quite a useful function in society.'

DR TELSCOMBE: 'I think 80 per cent is mostly reassurance. One talks about the patients who come in with nothing wrong with them. I don't think I've ever had a patient who's come in with *nothing* wrong. You get a lot coming in with very little wrong but that's all they want to be told: "You have very little wrong with you", but they thought it was something worse. And this didn't dawn on me until many years after I'd been in general practice.'

DR ANNE UPLEES: 'I find it strange that people go to a doctor if they've had a sore throat for a day or whatever. One could probably wait a few days to see if it goes. An awful lot of trivia really. On the other hand it doesn't take me long to deal with and I'm really quite pleased they haven't got something dreadful.'

DR CERNEY: 'I do make a claim to be becoming more expert on helping people to see that anxiety and worry cause pain and aches and bodily symptoms. And that's actually something that's very, very difficult for people to accept. It never ceases to amaze me how difficult it is to accept, that patients have some huge life event of tremendous significance to them, and they come with a pain, it's extremely difficult for them to see the link between the two. Perhaps I'm making an unfair judgement inasmuch as it's something that I'm experiencing – at least by proxy – through a patient, many times a day. Yet for each individual patient it may seldom happen.

'But of course it's true of doctors too. And the absolutely classic case is a clinical/pathological conference which is written up in the *British Medical Journal* in 1968, and consists of contributions from all the learned professors and doctors who looked after this chap during his long, long stay in Hammersmith Hospital in London. It was a patient, just "A Man", and he had a terrible disease of his guts and all these clever doctors, professors of this and that and the other, took him to pieces, literally. They examined single enzyme systems in the lining of his gut. They almost took molecules of the poor man, and they got nowhere near finding out what was wrong with him. And after about fifteen years he died. And at the post-mortem conference when they looked at all the material, and all the medical contributors came, they also had his family doctor there and half-way through the Professor of Medicine turned to the family doctor and said, "Dr Hatfield, can you tell us something about the home life of this patient, as you may feel it has a bearing on it?" And the doctor said, "Yes, I think this man's illness started when his father died. Then it got much worse when his adopted daughter made what he regarded as an unsatisfactory marrage, and the final relapse, followed by his death, occurred when he was sacked from his job into which he'd put many, many years of hard work and he was sacked without having any kind of adequate recompense made to him." And the Professor of Medicine said "Yes, thank you very much, but I don't think really we can take psychological facts into account here. Professor Somebody, could you tell us about the something or other?" And they took absolutely no notice of that man, because doctors don't have a framework of reference to enable them to translate things like anger or sadness into diseases.'

DR JANE EDSTONE: 'You see the extreme in Mrs Grey. She has changed from being a most difficult patient to a very co-operative one. When I first came here, not knowing her history, she was on my doorstep complaining the whole time. Finally, one gets out of her the problem of her daughter and her son. She's obsessive about them. First of all it takes a bit of time for people to admit, or to relax and talk to you about their problems, so first of all they've got to meet you as a person and perhaps cook up some minor complaint to make the introduction. Perhaps "cook up" is unkind – everyone has aches and pains – and when they relax on the second or third, or even tenth time, they start to say what's really upsetting them. It's obviously her daughter at the moment, plus a son. But I haven't quite come to the son. I can't quite remember what he does at the moment, but I know she gets very upset about him from time to time, and I'm not sure what the situation is but it will clarify itself.'

DR VERYAN: 'Yes, we can teach them. For instance, do you, as a GP, want to find out how to cope with yourself? How do you cope with an angry patient, an upset patient, a bereaved patient, and how do you cope with your own emotions? If a man starts crying in the surgery, how do you cope with him? Do you fend him off and say, "Look, I'm sorry, I can't cope with you crying, will you please stop," or do you allow him to cry because you are comfortable yourself with somebody crying in the surgery? We try and get them to become more sensitive to this sort of thing.

   'But it can be quite simple. We had one girl who was on the point of giving up general practice. Her surgeries took three times as long as anybody else's. She was there five or six hours sometimes. So what we did was a mock consultation and it became very obvious on the video screen that what she just couldn't wrap up was the conversation. She'd take twenty minutes even with a sore throat. And this she learnt very fast. It was just a matter of teaching her how to stop.'

DR BLAIRHALL: 'I find that if I introduce the word "love" into a discussion with a patient about problems, it's an absolutely key word. Because it's not a word they expect to hear from many people, and certainly not from a doctor. But if you discuss whether they love somebody, or whether they feel love, or what love means to them, you get into that person and it's very helpful in solving stressful situations. Another interesting question is to say to them,

"What's the worst thing?" – I'm doing vocational training here, you've got me teaching – "What's the worst thing that could happen to you?" and if it's a married person and they pause and think before they answer, my flash is, "What's wrong with the marriage?" because if you were to say to me, "What's the worst thing that could happen to you?" I would say "If June died." So if they pause, or say, "If I were to die" I would say, "Well, that's not the worst thing that could happen to you. That's the worst thing that could happen to your wife.""Oh yes." '

Mistakes

All doctors make mistakes, and there is no need to dwell on them. One might note that as medicine becomes more effective, so what you miss or don't do becomes more critical. It didn't matter so much when you could do little anyway.

The mistakes they have made, those they will make in the future, are a potent part of doctors' cohesion, the protectiveness they show each other.

As Dr Warfield said, easiest are hearts, coronaries which the GP mistakes as wind or acid.

Worst are children, because of the speed, because they are heartrending.

DR SUGNAL: 'I had the unfortunate experience of a child that I'd seen dying earlier this year, a baby who had meningitis. Not usually one of my patients, but one I'd had on the rota, I saw it early in the morning and it certainly wasn't very well, worse than having a cold and it certainly went off in a big way. In the afternoon he was rushed into hospital and he died that night but it's the sort of thing that happens to everybody once or twice and it set me back a bit, you know. I might have noticed sooner. I think I probably would. Or perhaps enough to worry me. It's bad luck. It's the sort of thing that does happen; it's happened to other people and it'll happen again. But I think I did all the right things but perhaps I wasn't quite inspired enough. At least I visited it when they asked me to.'

DR CHATHILL: 'I missed one diabetic child I didn't diagnose. I was too tired. I'd said I'd do somebody else's surgery and the child was terribly constipated and I didn't realize that constipation was due to dehydration from his diabetes and the mother didn't tell me that he was getting up about eight times in the night to pass water which as he was a five-year-old, she might have done. And I didn't realize why he looked so thin – he was about the fiftieth person I'd seen that day in somebody else's surgery. He nearly went into a coma about six hours later and one of my other partners was called out and by that stage it was very obvious he needed a hospital and they gave him insulin and he recovered. But it's always stuck in my mind ever since and I've never failed to examine another child's urine over the last twenty years. I've never seen

another case like it either. But I think that's really the only serious mistake
. . . I think that's why it stuck in my mind.'

DR MARY IFFORD: 'My partner made the most appalling mistakes. Often.
And you try and handle that as tactfully as you can. Those were the sorts of
things I found very difficult to cope with. And probably why I like working
on my own.'

DR THRIPLOW: 'Must I admit them? No. Well, one or two that really stick in
my mind are a couple of people I saw at branch surgeries; ladies that came in
complaining of swelling of the feet. I gave them a diuretic to try and clear the
fluid away; came back a few weeks later, still complaining, and one of them
went on for about three months and then I thought, "Well, I must examine
this woman, I can't just go on treating her like this." So I said, "Well, go back
home and I'll come round after the surgery and examine you." She had a big,
palpable ovarian tumour, and this turned out to be the root and she died and I
still feel a little bit guilty when I see the husband. Probably by the time she
presented it would have been too late anyway. But that's the sort of thing that
can happen, particularly at a branch surgery where you've few facilities. This
is one of the nice things about having four or five doctors in a practice.
Perhaps, if you're not happy, you can arrange for your partner to see them
next time. They see them with a new eye and between us we usually manage
to find something.'

GPs' Discoveries

GPs have always done original research. You may remember Andrew's paper
in *The Citadel*. Now they do so more than ever. In one of the large group
practices I visited in the South all five partners were engaged in research and,
with the aid of drug company funds, they were building up quite an extensive
reference library in the health centre.

There is no need to go into this, though it is one of the most fruitful ways
they keep up to date. But all sorts of GPs, like people in all professions,
make small, accidental, experimental discoveries as they go through their
lives.

DR WARFIELD: 'I say to my trainees, "If you're not sure whether they've got
sinusitis, ask them whether it hurts when they bend over. If you've got a
sinusitis that really is a sinusitis it hurts like hell." My little diagnostic find
that isn't necessarily in the books. Another one, which very often trainees
don't know, is if they get a patient with swollen ankles, they say, "God, is it
cardiac failure?" or is it just that when they stand up for long enough they get
swollen ankles, which has no great significance but is a thundering nuisance? I
say that they've only got to ask them one question – what are their ankles like

in the morning? If they're down in the morning, it just means they fill up during the day and it doesn't matter. It's not a sign of heart failure. But if they've got swollen ankles when they get out of bed in the morning, then they've got heart failure for certain. There are exceptions to the rule, in fact. So I certainly have some aphorisms which I pass on to my trainees.'

DR YETTS: 'I've found that touch is very important. With old people and children. In the majority of cases, with an old person, touch happens somewhere. As a contact. On the way out. "Bye." Something like that. And more subtly, if you've a more equal relationship with someone your own age. They may be expecting an examination and they don't get it, then a touch replaces it and soothes them. They feel cheated if they've not had the touch.'

DR COLKIRK: 'I've recently got this new sphygmomanometer – Japanese, it takes blood pressure and lets you know by sound. I discovered that women have far more volatile blood pressure readings than men. Does anyone else know this? I've never read it. I announced it at this huge meeting at Dundee. Were they interested? Were they heck. "What does that prove?" asked the chairman aggressively. "All it proves," shouted a voice from the back, "is that you're not a nancy boy." The sphygmomanometer itself isn't really known about in Britain.'

MARIUS, A STUDENT: 'This GP told us ill people seem to live longer. They've got chronic diseases and they've always been ill, they seem to cope much better. Whereas if you get someone like you who's been healthy all their life, suddenly gets something like lung cancer, they just die. Whereas if you've had, say, TB all your life and you suddenly develop cancer, those sort seem to last longer, they hang on and cope. Training for ill health is ill health.'

19
KEEPING UP TO DATE

In the 1920s and thirties it was fairly easy to keep up to date since new discoveries were quite rare. The reverse is true today. Most GPs use some or all of these different sources: post-graduate courses, drug reps, journals and talks with consultants and colleagues, with varying degrees of intensity. My GPs seemed remarkably conscientious, though I daresay they laid it on a bit for me. A number skated through the subject fairly lightly; one or two hardly skated at all. Most groups of three or four GPs took six weeks' holiday. This often used to be five weeks' holiday and one week on a course, which, becoming optional, has turned into six weeks' holiday.

Whether this is typical or not, I don't know, since Cartwright doesn't go into it. She notes that 43 per cent of GPs also have hospital appointments, and this is certainly another way they become stimulated and learn. It used to be compulsory to have five sessions on refresher courses a year to obtain seniority payments, but this has been stopped, which seems a pity. (A 'session' was a morning or afternoon, so you could get away with a long weekend.)

Dr Chathill said he thought single-handed GPs lacked colleague stimulus to keep up to date. I didn't find any patterns. Of the four who were distinctly vague, two were single-handed, two in groups. It depended on inclination. Dr Velling enjoyed his surgery, his invented operation and the like, very much; he enjoyed the practical, clinical side of medicine. This made him rather impatient with the psychotherapy side of GP work, but it gave him a sort of medical restlessness. (I think he also liked getting away from his home.) He darted off weekly, sometimes twice weekly, often at weekends as well, on every sort of course. He was tremendously up to date. He much appreciated that the NHS paid overnight expenses and mileage.

The most powerful rejuvenating influence on GPs today is the trainee system. The effects of this are going to be so profound that I shall leave it till we deal fully with the whole training, student area.

DR TRIMDON: 'Oh yes, you have to keep up to date. You're lost in two years. I mean, advances are so phenomenal. I think the primary way is reading research done in hospital – that's where you get the first of the new stuff. Parallel with that you've got your drug reps, all your mailings. There's too many journals to really digest them, *I* think. But you might read a snippet of this, a snippet of that, and I think just discussion with your colleagues, you know, over your drug dos, or coffee time. It's not so difficult as *you'd* think, as a layman. I'll take your broad point that in the run-of-the-mill things, you know, the same old cough medicines and the same old penicillins will do, but of course, with the media, patients are very much on to the new things so you've got to know them.'

DR THRIPLOW: 'If there are particularly good meetings, like the one in Aberystwyth on acupuncture or something interesting, or we had a lecture there on Cicely Saunders, the doctor who started the hospice idea, and that was very well attended; I go to those. And once a quarter I have to chair one of the vocational training meetings. So on the whole you get involved in a little bit of medical education. And all the journals – we're practically bombarded with journals; all very good, very well done. And just by skimming through you can pick up all the latest things that are happening.'

DR NYEWOOD: 'But the great thing about general practice is that you have your little obsessions and you can decide that your interest is chronic bronchitis, emphysema and asthma, cardiovascular disease and hypertension or psychiatry or family pathology, or psychosexual problems, you can run a particular horse whenever you feel that you've got to, and you can become famous for it in the district and a frightful bore to your friends. And you can do this and after a few years you can change and become interested in skin and go on a course and do that.'

DR BLAIRHALL: 'I am very keen on going and *working* for a week in a hospital in a particular department. Rather than going and being lectured at solidly for a week, to go and actually do the work is absolutely first class. That week I spent at Nottingham, I had to interpret as many X-rays as I normally would take about ten years to be offered, working at our local casualty department. The same with obstetrics. It was a *marvellous* week. I got to do forceps and breaches and whatever was going, whatever it was it was for me to do. And talking to the junior staff you learned as much as talking to consultants. In the medical unit, having to do the resuscitation of patients with the defibrillator, which was a new machine for me; absolutely fine. I can't think there's a better method. In fact, I'm going up to London next month to two hospitals on a course of psychiatry. But I've got an ulterior motive for this, which is partly associated with what I've just mentioned about our psychiatric service.' [How bad it was. His six-man group practice in the Home Counties was 'at present running on a locum who worked as a registrar at Broadmoor'.]

'I'm going up nominally to refresh, but the hidden agenda is to try and identify one or two psychiatrists who will help my practice; who will help my patients.'

DR YETTS: 'We have occasional meetings where the college group of GPs in the town invite new consultants to come and sit round the table. To give a talk if they want, but more to sit in a circle and talk about problems, and so they're very much equal with us, and we've done this with a gynaecologist, a physician, and a surgeon.

'We only have visiting speakers occasionally. We try and do things ourselves. So either one of us gives a talk or we bring cases along. You bring a rheumatology case or you bring a chest case, or you bring a death or something like this, and everybody brings the same sort of thing and we have a round robin. And one discusses his case and gets quizzed on it, and so you learn and it goes round.'

20
PREVENTATIVE MEDICINE

DR AXMOUTH: 'I would certainly like to be doing routine cervical smears, blood pressures, and to some extent I do these already, and I screen and see small babies and children – see they're developing all right. But I think it's become a bit of a parrot cry.'

DR NYEWOOD: 'The only real one is routine blood pressure testing. You see, you may have a very high blood pressure and be on the verge of a stroke and feel perfectly well. In fact you feel very well sometimes. The only way to spot it is to check it. And you do. Of course, you should not also base the decision to put somebody on some kind of treatment on a single reading. That is why it should be taken when quite young, so you have a series of readings. If you can look at someone's records, you can say "Well look, five years ago it was this, two years ago this, a year ago this, and now this. We have a progressive gradient. We know you have a problem." This give us reasonable grounds for saying – "We must take this seriously." A chest X-ray, an ECG, urine test, and repeat these so it's quite clear. These days it is possible to control it with, say, a single pill each morning. Some modifications in life style – reduction of salt, loss of weight, that sort of thing. The heavy death rate from cardiovascular diseases is one we can do something about.'

DR WARFIELD: 'We do very little. Obviously we do immunization. But for one thing there's the cost. It would be nice, perhaps, to do a mammogram on every woman aged forty-five and pick up a few cancers of the breast at a very early stage, which is *alleged* to improve the prognosis, but it might cost you £20 – £50 a patient and whether the NHS could stand that is another thing. Are you with me?

'But the pick-up rate is abysmally small – you'd hardly ever find anything of note that hadn't been found already.

'And do you really influence the course of the disease by picking it up early? You pick up something, a synovitis of the joint, there's nothing you can do about it. It's thought that you don't really influence the course of diabetes by catching it. If they are reasonably thin and eat sensibly it probably makes no difference. Even picking up a carcinoma of the breast very early probably doesn't influence the prognosis. In fact, the prognosis of carcinoma of the breast has not changed for fifty years. A lot of docotors think that by the time cancer shows up on an X-ray the patient is dying of it. So therefore one has to take a fairly gloomy view of preventative medicine. I think the only thing I know of where you do influence the outcome is picking up early hypertension.'

DR TELSCOMBE: 'I've got a couple of plasticine big toes in my cupboard there on which I show them how to cut their toenails. I've found my practice is now much more explaining to people what to do.'

DR TRIMDON: 'We do baby jabs. We do cervical smears. Far more than we're paid for. We're only paid for one every five years for women between the ages of thirty-five and sixty-five, who are not at high risk. We're paid for doing smears on the wrong people. We should be doing the young, sexually extremely active female, between sixteen and twenty-six. I think it's terrible the way GPs have shown that if you start giving them money, they'll do things and if you don't, they'll just say, "Oh, to heck." And we have an obesity clinic – sixteen people. But nobody here does much else, I don't think.'

Dr Thriplow was using his age-sex register to do smears on women between the ages of thirty-five and sixty-five – he would take blood pressures and urine at the same time. Dr Abney did get young girls in – but neither practice did much else. The Lincolnshire practice got diabetic families to test their own urine – because diabetes is statistically high in East Anglia, but they did nothing else rigorous. Dr Cerney, on the other hand, did a good deal. Among much else, all the over-seventy-fives were visited once a year with a questionnaire designed to measure physical health and social contacts, to discover which ones needed regular visits and from whom. Dr Telscombe did smears if people asked, blood pressures somewhat at random, immunizations.

GPs, that is to say, are extremely variable in the amount they do, and the amount they believe it is worth doing. Over the country as a whole, there is little doubt they could do a lot more. Where high blood pressure is concerned, for instance, which they all agree could be treated, it was found in 1981 that out of thirty-eight British practices studied, 53 per cent of men in their forties had had no blood pressure taken over the past ten years. Another study showed that 27 per cent out of a large group of patients had not had their condition recognized, 20 per cent had been recognized but not treated, 51 per cent treated but not controlled, and only 2 per cent were recognized, treated and controlled.

The same is true of immunization, about which GPs in general agree, and which on the whole they carry out. Yet there are gaps here too. By October

1982 America had virtually eliminated measles as a disease. Yet in Britain there are still 125,000 cases a year, twenty-five children die, many more suffer permanent damage. A new German measles epidemic rages as I write, and will bring in its wake maimed babies and abortions in hundreds.

There are really three issues here. The first is the amount of work involved. Studies over the last twenty years show this would be enormous. In any regional screening only sixty-seven in 1,000 would be found to be fit. Half would be referred to a doctor, one sixth would be found to be suffering from one to nine serious illnesses. For every case of diabetes, rheumatism or epilepsy known to a GP there is another case undiscovered. For every psychiatric case, bronchitis, hypertension, glaucoma or urinary tract infection, there are five cases undisclosed. There is eight times more untreated anaemia than treated.*

This is often called the 'iceberg of sickness' in our society. Two arguments flow from it. One, that in the current set-up, GPs couldn't possibly cope with it. Two, some sort of ill health seems almost normal. The greater the medical provision the less people can cope with this 'normal' situation. I don't really see the validity of the last argument. It could have been said at any point in the last 200 years and about any advance. We could still be in the eighteenth century as regards, say, our teeth, all falling out with huge holes when we were thirty.

Second, what good can you do preventatively? There is, as Dr Warfield rightly pointed out, controversy here, and certainly areas where at the moment there doesn't seem to be much you can do. But it is also clear from the preceding three paragraphs that there are areas where you *can* do a great deal.

Finally, and crucially, there is the attitude of the doctor himself. For centuries he has been a shop, responding to demand. People arrived *with symptoms*. A great many of the GPs I spoke to took blood pressures, smears, did urine tests, breast examinations etc., 'if the patient asked'. This is a stage ahead of the shop mentality; or at least it is the shop used for a different purpose. However, it throws the preventative onus on to the patient. It is still a long way from a far wider vision of preventative medicine which those who advocate it call 'anticipatory care'. We will come to this, and in doing so return to and resolve these questions, when we look at some of the possible futures for general practice.

Two last, slightly random points: an age-sex register, which about ten of the practices had, is a list of all the members of the practice arranged in groups showing their age and sex. It is essential for research. It makes selecting 'at risk' groups much quicker – men over fifty for blood pressure, those over eighty who live alone, etc. On it immunization, those on the pill, and other relevant information can be noted and this information used – the old who

* Figures from *Limits to Medecine*, Ivan Illich, London 1976; citing *The Changing National Health Service*, R. G. S. Brown, London 1973; I. S. Israel, G. Teeling-Smith, 'The Submerged Iceberg of Sickness in Society', *Social and Economic Administration* Vol. I, No 1 (1967).

haven't had flu jabs, for instance, when an epidemic starts up.

All doctors tell their patients not to smoke, and though they all said it achieved very little, in fact cumulatively something like a million smokers a year – 5 per cent of people told by their GPs to give up smoking, do so.

The pressure to give up smoking among the GPs themselves has been almost irresistible. So strong is the disapproval that while seeing the doctors, although I only smoke about five a day, I gave up altogether.

But there are still a very few smoking doctors, who gave me a good deal of pleasure. Dr Locking simply started his pipe without comment after supper and gradually vanished like something in a convoy. Dr Abney grew increasingly restive after he'd started to talk, drumming his fingers and hurrumphing, and finally said, did I mind old man, as a matter of fact, an occasional puff – lit up with vast relief and then had ten pipes in quick succession until he too more or less disappeared from view. Worst were the Trimdons, husband and wife, who simply chain-smoked cigarettes. They smoked wildly, guiltily, in front of patients, out on visits. But they were too frightened to smoke at medical meetings – which had become hell. Dr Henry Trimdon described going to a party of GPs and their wives and families, up the road. A special 'smoking room' had been set aside, and into this he had had to quietly creep – alone.

21

FRINGE MEDICINE

DR BLAIRHALL: 'I think it helps patients sometimes; I'm not opposed to it. Again my views have changed in thirty years. We were taught at university that 'covering' was a sin – that's the technical name for co-operating with someone who's gone to a bone setter or a charlatan of any kind. So we were taught that was a sin. But over the years so many people with these bad backs and various muscle pains have been helped by these bone-setters, or masseurs or what else, that I'm sure they help. I'm not saying that if I didn't have a bad back I wouldn't go and see one myself. And certainly as far as acupuncture – a fellow GP has started doing acupuncture now. And I mean, he's a good GP, he's an excellent doctor, and if he knows what he's doing, then that's fair enough for me. I don't think I'd refer anyone, or be awfully keen on someone going to an acupuncturist that wasn't medically qualified.'

DR ABNEY: 'Well, acupuncture, there's a Chinese girl – she's quite dishy actually. They like her. She's bloody awful. The smokers are great on her – I'm terrible, I smoke a pipe myself. [A comment that was quite unnecessary. It was now, as I've noted, difficult to see Dr Abney.] But she shoves needles here, there and everywhere and they still go on smoking. She's just 300 or 400 yards up the road. If it keeps the patients out of my hair, I don't mind who the hell they see. But some people get terribly uptight. If somebody gives their patient a tetanus jab at the factory – we've got one doctor round here who *takes off*, absolutely. Actually, that's because he loses a fee for doing it – that's the trouble.'

DR WARFIELD: 'I play about with hypnosis occasionally, more for fun than anything else. I send the occasional patient for acupuncture. I send the occasional patient to a back manipulator who is in fact medically qualified. I don't refer patients to osteopaths at all. That's really about the limit of my views on fringe medicine.'

DR TELSCOMBE: 'Certainly personally I'm not enormously keen on getting into that side of it. Probably something in it, but I think medicine has enough to offer.'

DR AXMOUTH: 'It's not something I have strong feelings about. I think people should try if they want to. I'm not going to get uppity if it's someone else who does the curing of them. In fact, I've found that a number of people with chronic problems have been to acupuncturists and appear to have had no benefit, and then to osteopaths and so forth. It does give me a certain amount of quiet satisfaction, because although I don't wish them ill, it's quite nice to know that they're actually not magicians.'

DR CHATHILL: 'I'm sure things like meditation help. I don't have formal sessions, but one teaches people how to relax a lot, if they get in a state or for asthma.

'I've been to a couple of courses on acupuncture and my impression is it works for pain relief very well, and also some cases of drug dependence. I don't think it cures a lot of the diseases they say it cures. But pain is reasonable actually because it produces a form of morphia in the brain, a naturally occurring morphia derivative, encephalin, after one of these jabs. I don't think there's anything in the positions, or these elaborate charts. Nowadays, you put an electric current into the needle instead of manipulating it. In fact, they've gone further, and just stimulate the skin with an electric current for pain relief. Electrodes in the neck and then perhaps a very small pulse vibration. The Marie Curie Institute is using that as pain relief for terminal cancer and it works like a charm. But I don't see a use in general practice because it only works while you're doing it. You can give total relief for half an hour but they can't go on being switched to their machines indefinitely.'

22
THE PATIENTS

The relationship of a GP to his patient is complex. It is for one thing legal, contractual. Based, according to Dr Yetts, on the signing of the medical card. 'If you phone up your doctor and say "I've a terrible pain in my chest", and he says "Go away", he's broken his contract and he will be penalized legally by the FPC.'

But it is also a personal relationship, and this mitigates the legal one. 'If you make a mistake,' went on Dr Yetts, 'they'll say, "You are human. We'll forgive you." And this has happened in our practice. A mistake was made, and they came to see the doctor about whether or not to make a formal complaint, and he said, "You've every right to make a complaint. I agree with you." They said, "Oh no, I wouldn't do that. It might get you into trouble." ' Dr Yetts thought that this was what saved us from the US-style litigation, which is no doubt true, though I suspect the fact that the NHS is free has a good deal to do with it as well. (In fact, litigation is rising. Ten years ago GPs paid £12 p.a. for anti-litigation insurance; today – £264. Only about 60% is inflation. More GPs are sued; judges award more; there are more delayed claims.)

Yet it is in this personal side that the complexity enters. There is a vast variety of patients and a great variety of response – a GP will be fond of some patients, amused by others, indifferent, disgusted, enraged and so on. Dr Telscombe felt that as a GP he didn't respond differently to each patient – how could he with forty or fifty different patients a day? But the knowledge that he wasn't but should be doing so was one of the things that tired him.

We have just seen that there are moves to bring GPs closer to their patients in consultation – to be more sympathetic, to listen, be less authoritarian; and benefits to be gained from this. Yet the relationship can be too primitive for that to be possible. When ill we regress to childhood. We become dependent on those around us and they all to some extent become parental, but none more so than the doctor. People, often GPs themselves, attack doctors for being too 'authoritative', but it is a role which is to a considerable extent thrust on them, or which arises naturally out of a patient's sickness. (Childhood is also a time when intimate physical handling goes on without a sexual basis, as John Berger observes in *A Fortunate Man*. At the same time, childhood is charged with sexual feeling. He thinks this is why people are so outraged by sex between doctor and patient. It is not just a betrayal of trust, paramount in childhood. It also raises buried feelings about incest.)

Another facet of the relationship is that doctors prefer it not to be too intimate – some distance must be kept. This too is criticized. Glin Bennet, for instance, in an interesting book called *Patients and Their Doctors*, makes a fairly familiar charge. Doctors are trained as students not to feel. Patients are referred to as 'the spleen in bed four'. Later on, this makes doctors cold and distant, unable to 'relate' (the ubiquitous and hideous modern word Bennet uses three times a page) to their patients.

But this, too, is complex. Once again, society imposes some distance. Doctors are always slightly isolated and special. Berger's Dr Sassall felt himself an equal, a real part of his society, because he could say anything to his patients, and they to him. But this was the precise indication that he was *not* part of society. You can't say *anything* to your equals. You learn quickly the limits of their tolerance. Doctors complain that people come up to them and talk about medicine at parties (you will recall Dr Locking's 'sod off'). Dr Nyewood once asked someone about this. 'She said, "I thought it was all you could talk about".' This difference society assigns doctors – which one would expect – even shows up in odd patterns in the research. Cartwright found that the older the doctor the less likely patients were to consult him. This had nothing to do with older doctors having less time or being less interested (on the contrary, they were more interested). It seems to be a 'ritual of courtship, extending over several years, during which, as patients get to know their GP better, they feel able to see him less'.

Feeling and emotion are not really susceptible to steering, but GPs have to try and steer a line between distance and involvement. Too close, and they become anxious, their performance impaired. That is why few GPs like treating their families. Also, how much strong and painful involvement should we expect of them? Doctors do feel for their patients, as we'll see more fully when we come to the sections on stress and death. Berger, when Sassall (a real GP – the book is in essence a biographical portrait) was unaware he was being watched, saw him weep as he crossed the field away from a house where a young boy was dying. There are limits to the amount of reality people can stand, and GPs see a great deal of it.

One or two doctors didn't seem to see this as a problem. Dr Thriplow – 'Oh yes, I have close friends as patients. And the family as patients. It doesn't seem to interfere.' But Hesse Sachs found, and so did I, overwhelmingly, that some distance was felt to be necessary. Quotations to this effect could be repeated indefinitely.

DR BILSBY: 'That is one thing I don't like, somebody I know personally coming to see me as a patient. You're looking at your watch beforehand, wondering how long they're going to be kept waiting, and then you are slightly anxious. It is far better to be seeing patients as sort of anonymous. And family too. Not family.'

JANET BILSBY: 'To say that David is tense with his mother is an understatement.'

There is one final attitude in a GP's relationship with his patients – and one which they by no means all shared – and that is an attitude of total, absorbed, fascinated interest. This will, I think, in the end turn out to be completely fundamental.

DR JOHN WHEATACRE (Thinning hair, a long face lined with smile lines, twinkling eyes, spectacles on loops. It was late at night, in front of the fire.): 'What I'm really saying is that this is the real interest for a GP. And however you look at it, it's more interesting for people of my temperament and your temperament to see the way people accept things than it is to say, "Ah, this is another case of multiple sclerosis taking an extremely long time."

'Mr Parker, for instance, he's a statistic in the neurologists' case books but he was a man who at the age of twenty-four – and I only know this from his notes; he was a patient of my uncle's – who got the first symptoms of multiple sclerosis, and it was confirmed by the then Professor of Neurology. I knew nothing of this. He became my patient when he was in his fifties, I suppose. He had a slight limp and I said "What happened?" and he said, "Oh well, I had something wrong", and I looked up the notes and there was a letter confirming the diagnosis of multiple sclerosis. But he then went on and his job was kicking with his good leg, kicking tyres on and off at a big motor works – a firm that dealt with lorries. He retired from that and died of cancer of the colon.

'But what would have happened to this man if I'd been his doctor and his wife had also been my patient, which she was of my uncle's? When he got this multiple sclerosis, I would have said to him, "I think you should tell your wife you've got multiple sclerosis and ask her to come and see me"; and I might then have said to the wife, "He may do very well, but there are certain things you should know; one of which is impotence and the other, of course, is that he may become completely bed-ridden." A third die within ten years; a third live like this fellow finally did – doing their job until old age; and the other third are midway between. I might have interfered and she might have said, "Well, I'm very keen on having children if this is possible, and I really couldn't stand nursing a man . . ." and the whole course of that life might have been changed. And this was just an ordinary labourer; they had two daughters so he clearly wasn't always impotent – whether he was at the end I don't know. One daughter became a teacher and one became a ward sister and when I think back – if I'd been interfering and officious, knowing this married couple, I feel I might very well have actually said something to her which might have put her off. My uncle didn't. And he didn't, I think, because in those days he wouldn't have regarded it as within his sphere to do it. He may well have been right.

'You see, my whole attitude to these things was formed by a particular man – a school-teacher – who came here when he was already badly crippled with multiple sclerosis. He was in an electric wheelchair: he could scarcely do anything. And his *wife* impressed me by the enormous care she put into him. It was a sort of cold but efficient care. There was something about her that I couldn't quite make out. She was absolutely devoted to his welfare to the extent, on one occasion, when there was some strike on, the various incontinence pads were not available, and the district nurse very properly said, "Well, we're sorry, there's a shortage of supplies. We'll have to cut your supply by half or even more." The wife then went down to find out where the district supplies of these things were, went down, talked to the caretaker, persuaded her – the caretaker – that she had permission, and took enough to serve her husband's needs for the next month or so. The district nurse was absolutely *incensed* about it and, you know, said, "This is disgraceful. We've got poor Mr Bottomley who's in just as bad a state as this man." They were absolutely incensed and I said, "You know, I appreciate your feelings, but you shouldn't have taken so many." And she said, "To hell with everybody else. I'm going to look after my husband." Well, that confirmed her determination. But one of my partners got closer to her than me – the young one – and she said to him – he must have said something that started her off. And she said, "You know, when we were engaged the diagnosis of multiple sclerosis was made and my mother-in-law and father-in-law" – who had deliberately come to move nearer to help a *bit* with looking after her husband – "they didn't tell me. They didn't tell me at all, and it was only after we'd been married a year that I realized that the next symptoms were multiple sclerosis." And she expressed, not in words but in emotions to him, her *bitterness* towards the mother-in-law particularly, and it was quite obvious that she was going to show the mother-in-law. The mother-in-law let her into a situation which was almost intolerable, but *by God* she was going to look after him. She would plunder all the supplies and get all the help she could.

'And perhaps I was wrong to be so affected by this woman whose whole life was undoubtedly ruined, I think. He's dead now. She was then about forty-five. She never had any children. And she has left the district and I don't know what's happened to her. I'll find out because she had neighbours. But her reaction, her bitterness, at finding out after a year that her mother-in-law knew and deliberately withheld it to bring about the marriage.

'And the mother – the mother's not a bad woman. I can see myself – well no, I can't. But you can sympathize with the mother thinking, "Well, if he marries when I die, or even now, this is the one way to look after him." But the wife's life was really ruined. She taught. You know, she would get up early; she would set him up in his chair; she would have neighbours there. She taught full-time because that brought in the money to pay off the mortgage of the house. Yet when she'd married him he was a young teacher who might have expected to be quite rich.

'And *that* is the interest. All that's far more interesting, it seems to me and I think it would seem to many people, but not to enough doctors. Because they are taught as scientists, you see.'

Dr Wheatacre raises issues beyond simply how GPs feel about their patients (to which we will return, as we will to Dr Wheatacre himself). One of these issues is class, and even superficially there are some curious aspects to GPs and class and to class differences themselves.

Class

Different classes have different diseases. Classes one and two have coronary diseases, leukaemia, alcoholism, cancer, psychoneuroses and the men over sixty-five get ulcers. Classes four and five get infectious diseases, bronchitis, pneumonia, TB, ulcers, cancer of the stomach and rheumatic heart disease. Schizophrenia rises sharply from class one to class five. No one knows why. Some people think social factors are a cause. Others that schizophrenia is so incapacitating that people with it tend to drift downward into the unrewarding but undemanding occupations of that class – labourers, kitchen hands, tramps. In the 1930s circumcision and tonsillectomies were much commoner among the middle than the working classes; today the reverse is true.

GPs have to be sensitive to differences in class occupations. Backache which an office worker can support is intolerable to a docker; if a manual worker is absent for a month his work is done by others; a manager's work piles up on his desk. The article from which these facts come, in *The Future General Practitioner*, is an educative article, and I was glad to see it told GPs that 'poverty occurs in middle class homes' – something about which they now need reminding.

Class is not a factor in what you might call patient efficiency (except perhaps in Glasgow, where Glin Bennet noted that only one fifth of patients asked knew where the stomach was). Nor is intelligence. The stupid remember as much as the intelligent. Out of six statements, both will forget two. Both remember best if only told two. The old remember as much as the young. Half the medicines prescribed are not taken.

Some GPs don't mind which class they see.

DR ABBERLEY: 'I can switch from one to the other without any alteration of gear. I can talk to anyone that comes in and I've known so many of them for such a long time. There's no difficulty in the transition.'

Some prefer classes one and two.

DR NYEWOOD: 'It is easier to deal with educated people who have the same attitudes to life as myself. I'm not saying they are always easy people to deal with – very often they are very demanding. They have very high expectations and they want the best, sort of thing. They are not the sort who say, "I know my rights", but they do. But it is easier because they speak the same language.'

But most of the GPs I saw (and this is borne out by research) preferred classes four and five. We have in fact already seen this several times. The main and obvious reason is given in this answer:

DR AXMOUTH: 'I find the older working classes and generally the lower middle classes of all ages easier to deal with than my own sort. My own sort ask complicated questions and are often dissatisfied with the answers. And want long discussions in the middle of a busy surgery. The others simply listen and do what you ask.'

A number of GPs had ideological reasons (or in some cases middle-class guilt creating an ideological drive) which led to their preference. But to most it was because classes four and five were, quite simply, easier. But questions of power arise here. Where the dependence and deference are greater, the power is greater, and the GPs' feelings of doing good are greater.

And they are objectively right. It is, apparently, well documented* that doctors do not perform so efficiently with patients from the same or higher socio-economic groups. This is supposedly because patients can ignore instructions, or persuade the doctor to give them what they want more easily with this additional class clout.

It may be GPs prefer their class four and five patients because they are more grateful. Certainly, more of them think their GP does a good job. And the class structure itself would enhance this: even if all the patient gets is sympathy, it has added value coming from someone in authority, like the Queen visiting wounded soldiers in a ward.

The Gratitude of Patients

DR THRIPLOW: 'They say "glad to see you" and the odd half-dozen eggs are very welcome, and the odd bottle of milk, which we usually boil before drinking, even though we are now brucellosis free.

'Then you get chickens and turkeys at Christmas. A bottle of whisky now and again. And it doesn't bear any relation to the actual work you've done for people. Somebody you've seen once in the year may drop you in a turkey at Christmas, and someone you've seen twenty times may not even say "Hello"

*The Myth of Mental Illness by T.Szasz, Paladin, 1972

if you see them.'

DR JANE EDSTONE: 'It feeds your soul, or whatever. I think we get far more undeserved thanks than blame. People are terribly grateful 99 per cent of the time. And very sweet. When I had Simon, the number of people who sent me cards. I put them all round the waiting room; they were knitting me matinée coats and one woman – pathetic, she was dying of cancer and she was knitting me a matinée jacket – awful things that I'd never put on a child – but she was knitting that and she couldn't finish the last bit and she asked one of the ward sisters to finish it for her. I've still got that.'

DR TRIMDON: 'You never have any problem getting help in the house. And I've a bloke who's had a heart attack, he comes and works on my car – washes it every Sunday morning and shammies it dry. That's the sort of luxury I have, in addition to my shoe cleaning.

'And then you get a salmon or a couple of pheasant or a bottle of whisky. And one old lady, she's actually English but she lived in Canada and I was sorry for her and I used to go and see her quite a lot. She loved it when you went in the evening. She's an awful boozer. And when I was so busy I had to go in the evenings because she was sort of half an hour's time. And there was nothing she'd enjoy more than pouring out two doubles of whatever – if it was before dinner it was gin, after, it was whisky. And every Christmas she would give me 30 quids' worth of something. You know, a litre of Glen Morangie, a litre of gin, and I had to tell her nicely we'd quite enough apricot brandy one year. A carton of cigarettes, and an RSPB tie, and she gave me 500 quid once. She's never done it again. I keep thinking she might.

'But that's not the most of it. We had a doctor in this area was left a house and its contents some years ago. We reckoned some £16,000's worth of house and £16,000 of antiques. An old patient of his father's.'

DR LUCY VERYAN: 'We've got another partner – the younger chap – who we found quite frightening to start with. But we are just beginning to see that he has exactly the same frailties as we have, and we find that we have to prop him up now and then. Just tell him that he is good and that that was the right thing to do and that was the best way to handle someone. I'm sure as a breed we need an awful lot of pats on the back to keep us going and I think this business of reward and anguish is a balanced thing and according to one's personality one swings more or less. But I'm sure the pats on the back, the gratitude, presents at Christmas and Easter, but gratefulness throughout the year, keeps one going.'

Difficult Patients, Dreaded Cases

DR ULLEY: 'There are some people who annoy me so much that I really cannot stand to examine them any further because they're making me so cross. And they're not really getting their full medical due because the man, or personality, has made me so cross that I'm anxious to get them out of the room because it's such an effort to keep on seeing them.'

DR ANNE UPLEES: 'She was a funny, white, pale lady who sat polishing her nails and seemed to do very little else at all all day. Her husband was a very strange West Indian who said he knew all sorts of West Indian authors. I never found out whether he did or not, but he reckoned he was an important sort of person, and he wasn't my patient but he used to come and chat sometimes about his wife. I can't remember having very much of a relationship with him. But he was quite threatening to the wife, because she came one day, sat down and said, "Do you know that my husband is going round telling people that you're paying him to have sex with him?" So I said, "No, I didn't know that", and I said I thought she'd better get off my list.'

MRS NYEWOOD: 'But you get some real bloodsuckers, some emotional bloodsuckers, don't you? People who want to go round and round and round, totally self-centred people who never seem to tire of their own problems. We have got one particular one I think, Janet, who pounds in regularly once a week, usually drunk. She always causes a sensation in the waiting room because she comes in sort of screaming how much she loves Dr Nyewood, all this sop you see and she scares me actually, she scares quite a lot of people because she has got very dark hair and wild eyes, and she foams at the mouth. And she can hit out. There was a terrible day when she came up here, do you remember? I was all by myself in the house one afternoon and there was this pounding on the door. I opened the door and to my horror there was this woman, absolutely drunk, and so I said, "I am sorry, Janet, you can't come in here. Dr Nyewood is not here. I'll ring the surgery." And I of course shut the door and she kept trying to get in and I thought she was going to go round the house and break the windows. She is quite frightening – so finally I rang the police and they came up, by which time she had passed out in the drive, so then they rang the ambulance, so this is the minus side of being a doctor's wife.'

DR MARY IFFORD: 'The worst is the one that comes in day after day, with niggling complaints. You know they're rather inadequate, they've got no back-up. The family is breaking up, the marriage is breaking up, the housing's awful. And there's very little you can do or say or do that . . . it's being impotent really. They need proper housing, reasonable food, a lot more money, and a little support from the family. The other thing is alcoholics. Unless they want something done, agree to have something done, there's nothing you can do.'

DR AXMOUTH: 'I think that probably hysteria is the most difficult thing to deal with. The patient who's making a lot of noise, particularly a noisy hysteric who is actually enjoying making a lot of noise and is likely to make more noise the more attention you pay to them and who none the less the relatives – who have already been caught – would like you to do something about. That is an impossible situation, in fact, and is well worth avoiding almost at any cost, if you can. That's sort of psychological. I think that on the physical side of things, the chronic bad back in a man of working age is very depressing, particularly when you're not absolutely plum certain that there isn't some underlying – some psychological – reason why his back is so bad. He is depressed, angry, a bit defensive, you haven't cured his back, he goes on and on, he's lost his job and he's been on the waiting list for so long; you can't get him in to see a specialist though you try very hard. That, I think, is the physical problem that is most difficult.'

DR THRIPLOW: 'If you look at somebody's notes as they come in through the door, you think, "Oh God, not again!" There is obviously a failure of something there, whether it's medical care or understanding or what, these poor people move backwards and forwards to clinics and surgeries and specialists of one sort and another. Nobody ever gets to the bottom of their problem and their notes get thicker and thicker and thicker. But it's the one with the nagging fear at the back of your mind that there is something there. And it's surprising how many of these – it may be ten years later – develop some fairly major pathology, and looking back over the notes you think, "Could I have spotted it perhaps five years ago?"; and these are the ones where my heart sinks when I see their names on the visiting lists, or I see their notes coming in to me.'

DR TELSCOMBE: 'So then they change doctors. I know a lot of doctors feel hurt when this happens. I used to feel terribly hurt if someone left me. I'd done something wrong. But now I feel, well, I change my garage every so often. Somebody charges too much or they're not doing a good job on the car. They're perfectly entitled to change. They've only come for a professional opinion. They don't come for a statement of fact.'

Critical Patients

DR RIARD: 'Anne [Cartwright] takes a very left-wing view of things, but the lovely thing about Anne is, she's very critical about doctors, and she's a super woman, you'd like her. She's very amazing and very, very knowledgeable. But although she denies it, Anne at heart is very critical of doctors. And yet in all her surveys, to her astonishment, she shows that general practitioners are not diligent enough, not caring enough, fail at so many different things, *but* somehow persistently, even though her populations that she administers questionnaires to are very disapproving of *doctors*, they take a very different view of *their* doctor. *Their* doctor is all right. He's special. Of course there are critics. I'm giving you a very rosy view. But the majority have very strong, warm, positive feelings about their doctors. And I think Anne says sometimes that "I think people are just too complacent. They're not critical enough", and then she'll whoop with joy if there's a trend to be more critical in one particular survey.'

Anne Cartwright would have given a whoop while compiling her last survey, but it would have been a small whoop. Her doctors thought patients were more critical and knew more than ten years before, but these effects were not quantified – except that 58 per cent of patients too thought they knew more. But patients changing doctors due to dissatisfaction had declined from 8 per cent to 4 per cent (though she thought this was because in a lot of partnerships you can choose who you see).

A number of the GPs I saw agreed patients knew more. 'Oh yes, they'll come and say, didn't I know, such and such is the new thing for rheumatism; or they want to come off something. "Jimmy Young said you shouldn't take this" [Dr Telscombe].' And some agreed patients, middle-class patients especially, were more critical.

I saw three or four mildly critical patients. The only really critical ones were medical students.

SUE, A STUDENT: 'I mean, sometimes I've gone in and asked for a prescription for something, and he says "What's that? I haven't used that yet." And he has to look it up. And I'm always watching to see what he's going to ask and if he doesn't ask that he could have missed a brain tumour. But I expect medics make terrible patients.'

But as Riard says and as we noted already, the vast majority in Cartwright's survey were 'highly satisfied'. Other surveys agree. When the readers of the magazine *Choice* were polled, 90 per cent could only think of nice things to say about their GP.

Why is this? One answer, the one preferred by GPs, is that they are, quite simply, satisfactory. But I think there are other factors involved. With single-handed GPs, still numerically quite a large number, there is no standard of comparison. But the same is true of groups and partnerships. Few people have belonged to more than one. In each case the GP or the group is the standard, and people prefer to think that what they have is good. That is the clue. Hesse Sachs puts it with admirable clarity.

HESSE SACHS: 'I think if there is a principle operating it is that you don't like to be dissatisfied with what you've got. We found in housing that people were very seldom critical of where they lived. The moment they decided to move, *then* they were critical.

You can't take the dissonance, you can't tolerate the idea of disliking what you've got. How can you cope with it if you dislike it that much? I think that is why people don't complain. Most people say, "Yes, he's OK, I'm satisfied" – otherwise, "why the hell am I with him?" '

23
AN INNER-CITY PRACTICE:
DR TIM CERNEY

After leaving Dr Locking, I had planned to drive at once to the north of Scotland. But for a variety of reasons it became clear that it would be simpler to take in my first inner-city practice just below the border, cross Scotland for my second and then head north.

When I'd first come up from the South, I'd been sharply aware of the major physical differences – the massed cities turning into great uprising slabs of moor and dale and fell, the hedges into dry-stone walls. But now, as I recrossed the vast industrial heart of England, I saw that it was stopping, the body sprawled decaying, falling to bits. Half, no three quarters, of the tall chimneys stood smokeless, pointless. The factories had a derelict look, tiles falling in on their huge silent structures with their thousand windows, abandoned bits of equipment, broken gates, debris – muck without brass.

The Cerneys had a pleasant house, with nice furniture. Only their daughter was there when I arrived, about fifteen, with long, shimmering, palest gold hair. She had a slight, attractive northern accent, compared to their ordinary middle-class one. She gave me tea, put on the radio and went up to do homework.

Tim Cerney was about forty-six, but looked younger (rare for a GP). He had a strong, handsome face, like D.H.Lawrence only better-looking – a film star Lawrence. A number of younger doctors have beards, I suppose for speed in the mornings; for the same reason they often have electric razors. He had an engaging manner, something not quite naïve, but boyish about him. One wanted to help him (but left-wing GPs are on the whole more sympathetic than right-wing ones). A certain inner tension, more or less understood and, perhaps, under control. He was open, honest, dedicated – tempted to work too hard. Very strong; strong arms and hands. The day after our first talk, which itself went on late into the night, he was up working until 3 o'clock, and had to get up early for an emergency call (I heard the phone go at 6), and that afternoon was off to London. Despite his openness, a sense of reserve.

DR CERNEY: 'Unfortunately I didn't get on with the partners in my first practice and had to take another practice rather quickly. So I moved on to this enormous housing estate. The whole housing estate is about two miles square, and it's council houses bar a handful of houses, as far as the eye can see in every direction. We're about in the middle of it and it was built in the twenty years between the early thirties and the early fifties and it's various different parts. Some of the parts are, as it were, *good* parts; some of the parts are not-so-good parts and are well known as areas of great social deprivation, and that means an awful lot of unemployed, single mothers, chronic handicapped, elderly people, and those sort of people just do get sick a tremendous amount. The rate of somatic illness is very, very high. The rate of cancer, for instance, is very high. I remember one weekend I was on duty about two years ago, three of my patients, all with terminal cancer of the lung, died, all in one weekend. That has never happened before or since. But that's the kind of thing that happens in a small practice – you know, just over only 5,000 patients it was then.

'You do know that social class is inversely linked to cancer? In other words, the lower your social class the more likely you are to get cancer. You need to know that. And it is, of course, another fact that any cancer will somewhere in the world be very rare, which argues that there must be environmental factors that come into it. And doubtless one, of course, is cancer of the lungs – smoking. But I think that people – the sort of people who live on the estate where I work – are very often eating a poor diet, are very often exposed to external hazards, chemicals, gaseous fumes, pollution of one sort or another in their work, and always have been, and hence have a very high rate of cancer. And we have many, many cases. The sort of cancer which in the textbooks they say you'll see one case every twenty years, and we've had five in the past six. I'm thinking of cancer of the pancreas, for instance. It's supposed to be a very rare cancer. Brain tumours – you're supposed to see one every ten years; we've had four in the last two.

'The other thing we have is unemployment. I think for all the people who come in wanting a quick week off because they don't like their job, there are now the people who know very well that if you fall sick for a bit then you'll be chucked out of your job. Working people know very well that the boundary between sickness absence and sort of unlicensed absence, if you like, is now very narrow and employers are only too willing to get you out if you have too much time off work, for whatever reason.

'I'm quite sure that there are people who are desperately worried about their job and desperately worried about their situation in general. Whether one could say that they would not have got ill if it had not been for that is, of course, impossible. And I don't give any global figures for the whole practice on the rates for this or that. But certainly people come and say "I'm desperately worried about my job", or whatever, when they, of course, didn't before. I think that, in a sense, may be passing. I don't seem to have heard it so much lately. I think people may be, on our estate, settling down to just sort of putting their head down or waiting until better times come as people of that sort always have done. They know by direct observation or experience or by hearsay what the Depression of the thirties was like and they know that things picked up. And I think they just – there's a sort of fatalism amongst a lot of my patients, waiting for things to pick up; hoping they will.

'Another factor in this practice is that people have very low expectations. In my first practice I would get called out at two in the morning for a child with earache. I can't remember when that last happened, but it's not uncommon, even now, for a parent to bring a child and say, "His ear's been running for the last two or three days." And this is an earache which was bad four days ago maybe, the eardrum perforated three days ago and now the child is brought in because the mother or father's tumbled to the fact that this isn't quite right. So expectations of what you can get out of your doctor are very low. And we are constantly trying to raise them.

'It is a problem. Everybody has this. "My doctor says I've got to let him know if I think anything is wrong and I went along and they said it was nothing", which is the most putting-down feeling to get. I think what I'm aiming at is not to make people feel put down when I say "There isn't anything wrong."

'But if we are here, as GPs, to detect the earliest possible departure from abnormality, we are going to get a lot of false positives. People with a cough who think it's cancer of the lung; a headache is a brain tumour; who have a pain in the chest because of muscle strain and think it's a heart attack. By the nature of one's invitations to come early, they'll come with unserious symptoms. That's our business.

'And this also enables people to go when they know deep down that their worrying pains are due to anxiety or something more profound. Because they do know that.

'I can illustrate this best with my own example. Over the years I found that my practising of medicine was distancing me from my family and that it was very easy to get caught by the intellectual fascination of my work and the sort of extras that people put in on me. I became a teacher of general practice, I became a part-time university lecturer in general practice and I sat on 1,001 committees. The result was that I separated from my wife and needed an enormous amount of help from counsellors for a period of about eighteen months and during that time came to accept within myself the nature of my emotions and their power over me – not power over me but the power of them, and came to see that in patients at the same time. And as soon as it became known, and it became known it seems within the first millisecond of my telling anyone just about, that I was having trouble with my marriage, people flooded in to see me with troubles with their marriages almost straight away. And having, during that time, been able to gain some insight into the nature of my own difficulties, I was able to help some people a great deal. In the same way that my young women partners who are pregnant have lots and lots of pregnant women coming to see them. There's nothing surprising about that although it always hurts one's feelings as the older male GP when the women who become pregnant desert one and go and see one's partners. But this is just identification with the doctor – it's a pretty frightening concept actually. I didn't think of that before and maybe it's very threatening that patients actually identify themselves and their problems or illnesses with their doctor. It's as though the doctor may actually have those, the doctor by his understanding of the nature of them may himself be a personal sufferer from them. I've never thought of that. But how much does one actually take on of one's patients' suffering? I think one takes a great deal actually.

'Anyway, it was during the period of, if you like, self-analysis and emotional regression that I came to understand and accept my own emotions and accept and understand those of our patients a great deal more. So coming back to what I was saying, this was the time I realized that the emotional life of my patients, even though they were verbally unexpressive, they were emotionally suffering in exactly the same way. And another thing, I've come to rate intelligence very much lower as a predictor of sensible behaviour. The common sense that a great many of my patients evince when dealing with their children or simple symptoms or difficulties in general, is not necessarily immensely related to intelligence.

'Of course, to share people's emotions is in a sense hard. But if one is putting up a defence against someone else's emotions, that's actually very hard work in itself. Whereas acceptance of emotion carries with it a sense of achievement and means that one doesn't spend a lot of energy pushing away emotion.

'Is that true? Actually, now I think, I don't think so. Of course, it's not *all* at an emotional level. You know that Katherine Whitehorn thing when she was castigating the Balint doctors – "Forget about the sex life, doctor, just bung across the throat pills." Well, there are times when, obviously, probing into people's emotional lives is a grotesque intrusion and totally inappropriate. But there are lots of times when it is appropriate and then to do it on a succession of patients, on a quick-firing time scale, is extremely exhausting.

'And the other thing is, if people know you won't accept their emotional symptoms they stop offering them. They offer something extremely trivial. "Can I have some more throat pills, doctor?" and you bung across the throat pills and you don't do anything. You're acting at some very, very low level as a doctor. If people know you're willing to accept their emotional difficulties then they will throw very difficult, exhausting things at you and in they come, bang, bang, bang. "Battered by the commonplace" is what John Stevens used to call it.

'I found it very difficult to throw John off. He was an enormously powerful character who impressed one as soon as one met him. But the thing was, he took over his patients – he controlled them pure and simple. Now, it's not necessary to control your patients. I've come to realize over the last ten years that in fact doctors are very fringe to people's lives. OK, there are certain moments – birth, death, serious illness, trauma, or something, where doctors are vital and they will actually save lives sometimes, but for most of the day-to-day running of our patients' lives, doctors are extremely fringe. They're extremely fringe to their state of health. OK, I give them antibiotics, I give them tranquillizers, or anti-depressants, or whatever it might be. I treat this or that, but to the general state of health of most of our patients I make very little difference and so this calls a bluff on control by the doctor. It isn't necessary.

'And another thing about our practice is the old. I've never done a calculation as to what proportion of our work is done with the elderly, but it feels like about half sometimes, and certainly most of our home visits are to the elderly. I do like the old. I had a very happy example of four grandparents, all born in 1886, all who lived to a ripe old age and all who I knew well as a child and as a teenager. And I had the example of a happy, adapting, successful old age from these four people and it's made me have quite a close link with elderly people. And it's not an unselfish thing either. It is actually very super to give good care to the elderly because they seem to get specially poor care most of the time, and it's so easy to find elderly people who've been badly looked after by a previous doctor, you can suddenly make them feel better. You give them the proper pills for their arthritis or you get their heart failure under control and they feel so much better. Or you can get them a hearing aid or you can get their cataracts done, or just be nice to them. And this seems to make an enormous difference. You can take on board their fears about their dying and you can say "Yes, it's OK to feel frightened of being old." I don't find that in the least bit hard to do, not least because it's, you know, selfishly, it's very rewarding. Their gratitude, yes.

'Also, intellectually, the medicine of old age is very difficult. Well, inasmuch as you've very often got a number of problems intermingled. Somebody will have a bit of heart failure, a bit of arthritis, a bit of high blood pressure, a bit of that, perhaps a little bit of thyroid failure, and which of all these is causing their dizziness? you'll say to yourself. Jolly difficult. And you need a lot of energy and enthusiasm to look after elderly people because it's so easy to say "It's old age" and so you don't take another blood test to see whether, in fact, their chemicals have become out of order due to your treatment, for instance. Maybe you've run them out of potassium through over-enthusiastic treatment of their heart failure and unless you take a blood test you won't know. And it needs energy to have a syringe in your bag and to take the blood and bottles in your car, and get it into the laboratory, and go back a week later, rather than a month later, in order to tell them about the results.

'It was a conscious decision to come here. It was early to be one of a training scheme twelve, thirteen years ago. We could have had the pick of the practices anywhere in the country. But I decided I would come to a place where they were a bit short of doctors and where doing good was more likely than if one went to Shepton Mallet or Sherbourne or somewhere nice.

'The other reason I came here was political. It's had a Labour council for years, it's got a total comprehensive system and it looked a good place for one's kids to go to school.

'And I suppose personal reasons. There was a strong tradition of service in our family. My parents were idealists – political idealists. My mother, in particular, was always sort of doing good. She was a JP, she was always helping the more unfortunate members of the community. At Christmas, I can remember, we always used to have to go and take down to our charwoman in the village where we lived presents for her and her four children – her four illegitimate children.

'I had a lot of psychosomatic illnesses as a child. I had a fairly traumatic childhood inasmuch as I was evacuated to Canada when I was two for the duration of the war. From 1940 to 45, I lived apart from my parents. I think it was a very traumatic thing to do and for most of my life I lived in the denial of that trauma. My parents did their best to make up for it when we came back, but it was a very traumatic thing and it was only again during my own – I only grew up emotionally I think – during the period of being separated from my wife.'

'Battered by the Commonplace'

The next morning we set out at 8 o'clock for the surgery. We drove through acre after acre of factory lots 'for sale' or 'to let', the names – Regent Works, Samuel Osborn – inscribed on confident Victorian cast-iron plaques.

'So Japan could make them cheaper, so they were out of date – there must have been a better way,' said Dr Cerney.

His surgery was set plum in the middle of the huge 60,000-strong Claywood Council Estate (his practice had about 6,000 – him and two other partners). It was in one of the detached houses. Small, neat, efficient. In his surgery he had the patients sit beside him. There were a lot of toys about for children.

All the patients were class four and five with soft northern accents.

MRS THOMAS: Fifty-five, greying, stick, trousers. Comes in, sits down, 'I've still got this nasty peppy cough.' He puts her on the couch and, behind curtains, she undresses. Doctor listens. 'Still sounds a bit ruckly. Get dressed while I have another think what to do.'

Lots of puffing while she dresses. Returns, with sticks (when she came in she'd laid the sticks on the couch – 'You have a rest').

Doctor has read notes. He says he thinks she'll find she gets better soon. Patient: 'I felt better today for the first time.' Doctor: 'That's it. That's the antibiotics still working. The rest you'll cure yourself.'

Her real worry was about her husband, whom she now spoke of. He was dying. 'I try and cheer him up. He won't take those vitamins. He'll be in tomorrow.' Doctor listening, noises of encouragement.

MRS WATSON: Rather plump, forty-five with a brown, lined, round face, discontented expression. Doctor: 'Feeling any better?' 'Better than I did last week, but still far from better.' Doctor: 'I don't know what we can do.' She agrees. This is clearly part of a long dialogue. Feeling of gloom. Doctor says she's been worse than this, but she climbs out of it. Mrs Watson: 'I haven't been out for a month.' They gain comfort from the fact that some recent tests have shown there *was* a real infection (urinary I think). The dose of antibiotics is changed.

She goes out. Doctor says he doesn't have the faintest idea what's wrong – she's had anti-depressants, every conceivable test, psychotherapy and psychiatric referral. No one knows what it is. She still feels down. Life?

MRS RIVEN, MRS HILL: Two large women with short, plentiful hair like big fair sponges round their heads. One thirty-five (Mrs Riven), one about fifty-five (Mrs Hill). Both spectacles.

Mrs Riven has been given the wrong prescription and has also come for an injection (of iron it turns out). She bares her plump arm and grips it with plump fingers. The moment of bravery, then *looks* while needle is pushed in. He wipes with cotton wool, she holds. Chat.

Mrs Hill is the mother of the first. Has catarrh. Doctor: 'Colour?' Mrs Hill: 'Not green. A sort of greyish.' Doctor: 'Isn't this just cigarettes again?' Mrs Hill: 'I think antibiotics would help. I feel tired all the time. Me arms and legs hurt.' Doctor says her diabetes is under control. How many is she smoking? 'Twenty a day.' Her daughter volunteers that she managed to give up once for six weeks. Doctor ignores this feat. 'It's too much, bad with lungs like hers. I think the catarrh is just the end of an old cold. I'll give you some paracetamol for your arms and legs. You must try not to smoke so much.'

They go. 'Both diabetics,' says the doctor. 'A whole three generations of obesity. Now the granddaughter weighs nineteen stone. She's dieting. If she doesn't come well down, she'll have diabetes sure as eggs is eggs. She'll wear out the pancreas's ability to deal with all that carbohydrate.'

MRS JAMES: A little, fairly old lady. (They're coming in about every seven to nine minutes, no sense of hurry.) She has a woolly green skull cap, grey curls coming out. She thought (croaky voice) she might have an X-ray to see if her 'croaks' could be cured. Had this 'flu', a flu-like illness a month ago; 'I haven't got over it.'

Examination behind curtains so I wasn't able to see. He listens. 'Breathe deeply.' Mrs James: 'Do I open my mouth to breathe?' Doctor: 'Yes, open your mouth.' Loud breathing and listening behind the curtain.

Doctor says there are some patches of infection. He'll give antibiotics. It becomes clear that her daughter had made her come – Mrs James talks of pain in the chest (cancer?). She's going to Malta on Wednesday. 'That'll make you better,' says Doctor, giving her prescription.

I wonder if she's apprehensive about going abroad, wants to lay in a store of good British antibiotics in case. But Doctor says no. Oddly enough she has money ('very rare here, she may have cashed in her husband's insurance'). She goes abroad five or six times a year, always off season – Malta, Marbella, Majorca.

MR MOOTHAM: Big, sixty, balding, fluent. Doctor: 'I've got a colleague here . . . writing a book . . .' Mr Mootham: 'I thought you said you'd got a *comic* here.'

Trouble with the right testicle. Fairly lengthy 'history'. 'Intermittent pain . . . on and off . . . didn't want to bother you, but the wife said "Let Dr Cerney 'ave a look." '

On to couch. Doctor examines. I discreetly look away, listening: 'No hernia – tough as boots down here. The cord here is absolutely fine.' Clearly in splendid condition.

'I gave it a fortnight before troubling you – it's erratic, see. Wife says "I'm sick of you. Go and see Dr Cerney." '

There is further trouble with an elbow which keeps giving him electric shocks. Dr Cerney says it must be striking a nerve. That can happen. 'I don't think we have anything untoward. Let me know if anything alters.'

When he goes, nodding good-bye to the comic, Dr Cerney says, 'He's one of nature's hypochondriacs. He's here the whole time. Always blames it on his wife.'

JOHN CHILDS: Young man, soft northern voice. He's had a sore throat for two weeks, 'I've had strepsils and all sorts, nowt shifts it.' Doctor immediately notices a vast, now healing wound in his lips, a black gash. Boy quite unconcerned. Dog got his lip two weeks ago.

Doctor tuts, looks at throat, feels glands, takes temperature. 'All the signs are I can't help you with antibiotics on this. I go by this – they'll help if there are two of these signs, white spots on the tonsils, glands swollen, a temperature. But you have none. I can't help. But that should be reassuring – nothing seems to be wrong. Sorry, I can't cure you – but nature will.'

I say it's odd how concerned they are with sore throats. Dr Cerney agrees. 'I wonder if it's a folk memory of diphtheria – could easily be that.'

SALLY DAVIS: Youngish, pretty, tough-faced girl, high cheekbones, broad hips, eyebrows just pencilled-in lines, high-heeled boots, long gold hair pulled back. Rapidly gets upset, twisting hands.

Dr Cerney gives a survey of her case, ending 'You've seen four specialists about not conceiving. It isn't going to work. Seven people out of 100 can't have children.'

'Can't I go to the test-tube baby people? Couldn't I – even if it means waiting a year? All I've wanted in life is a child.'

'I don't think you can go there. It's not possible. You'll have to face up to it – you're not going to get children with the help of a doctor.'

She pleads to be allowed to go. He says the trouble is she's had a very irregular existence, trouble with her husband, many attacks of VD. 'It's all telling against you. And you're not married now. They wouldn't touch you.'

'But I am going to get married.' Talk of results of tests. She says her womb is OK. Doctor: 'You can't be sure, with the tubes so damaged.' Sally Davis: 'But the right tube's OK.' Doctor: 'Yes, and that's another reason they won't take you. With one tube OK there's no *reason* you shouldn't conceive.'

This goes on and on. She's been on the fertility drug for some time, and is till March. He gradually becomes more gentle, continually says she can conceive, nothing's been found to say she can't.

Sally Davis: 'I'm twenty-eight next March.' Doctor: 'You're not on the shelf.' Sally Davis: 'At least I'm having some good news. My divorce is coming through.' He gives her a small prescription for Mogadon (she asks for a large one). He'll see her soon. Somehow, there is an air of hope. Sally Davis: 'What'll I tell Bob? He'll go mad if I tell him about the VD.'

'Why not tell him the truth? That the test-tube people won't see you with one sound tube, but that with that you may conceive.'

She agrees, but goes out clearly planning some tale to keep Bob expecting her to conceive as a result of future actions by the doctor. Face tense and sad.

Dr Cerney says she's been in and out of prison, is an alcoholic and an addict of Mogadon. Perhaps she will conceive. They vet test-tube mothers as *mothers*.

MRS ALTON: With her two kids: about four and five, a girl and a boy. 'Am I just fussing? Kelly's had a right bad cough. She's had penicillin but she's no better. I'm frightened it'll be *whooping cough*!'

Does she whoop? Dr Cerney describes what she should be doing and Kelly's mother gets vaguer and vaguer, but throws in a few not eatings and being sick at nights as a make-weight.

The doctor examines Kelly, feels her, deliberates, looks at his notes. 'I think this is really the tail end of an ordinary cold. Mrs Alton is reassured, but still keeping her end up. 'It keeps her awake at night.'

Doctor: 'I can't be *sure* it isn't or wasn't whooping cough, but it's not really dangerous at her age. Bring her in again on Monday. And *always* bring her in if you're worried.'

MRS SMITH AND MRS HUGHES: Two young women, sisters, come in with their children: a one-year-old baby and a toddler of two and a half. The first mother is Mrs Smith, aged eighteen (looked fifteen). She is a new patient, so the doctor takes various details – baby (boy), weight at birth (seven and a half pounds). He can walk, has been bottle fed, has had two immunizations and is now to have a third. The old GP's address had been in Cemetery Road. ('Not very appropriate' says Dr Cerney. No response.) She's also come to see about a coil, which her elder sister has. 'Not the pill?' asks doctor. 'Can't seem to swallow them,' says her sister (Mrs Hughes). Doctor doesn't comment on this rather odd bit of information. I don't think he noticed it. Baby is undressed for examination and then has the jab. The mother flinches and looks away as the needle goes in, as though it were her being jabbed. I am amazed at the doctor's speed and skill, which is lightning; baby hardly cries. As she is dressing him, a packet of ten cigarettes falls.

'Ah, the guilty evidence,' laughs doctor. The little girl is running about the surgery, playing with the toys. 'Did you ever try and stop?' Mrs Smith: 'Yes.' Doctor: 'What happened?' Mrs Smith: 'Temper.'

Her sister, Mrs Hughes, now comes up. Her little girl is hot, no appetite, quiet. (I thought she'd been toddling about fairly normally.) Doctor examines – she is *extremely* reluctant to open her mouth – but he does eventually get a glimpse down. He says they'll check her urine. 'Urinary infections are very common in children – it makes them poorly and listless so we do a lot of checking of that.' He says two spoonfuls of paracetamol liquid every four hours.

Mrs Hughes now says that she too is listless and only want to sit about. (I have the feeling that the daughter was an excuse to come herself.) Doctor: 'Had any more arguments with hubby?' She says that's OK now. 'Appetite?' 'I'm only eating out of boredom.' 'And cooking for him?' 'That's boring too.' Doctor: 'So you *do* argue about that?' Mrs Hughes: 'No, we've sorted that out.' 'Does he notice how you're feeling?' 'He says it's laziness.' Doctor reassures, says these things aren't laziness, they're in the mind. 'Have you discussed it with him?' 'He doesn't repond.' Does she mind this? She shrugs. 'How do you feel?' She doesn't feel miserable, just a lack of energy. Finally he gives up. 'Think about it. I think you'll find it cures itself. But come back in a week.' He wants to see the little girl again.

'Well, I failed there,' he says ruefully when they've gone. 'I think I gave her every opportunity. She came before and it was rows with the husband then.'

YOUNG MAN comes in and is extremely brisk with me. He'll see the doctor alone if I don't mind.

He's with him thirty-five minutes. I sit in the waiting area, two small square areas with waist-high divisions – about five people on the banquettes. I feel a vague loss of status, from near-GP back to patient. They sit, two mums talking, people come in for repeats, a new patient comes, a sitter goes along to a partner's surgery, children and toddlers wander about, picking up waste-paper baskets, magazines, lying bored on the banquettes. A large repro-duction of a Swiss lakeside, with Disney cuckoo-clock cottages is on one wall, all highly, almost luridly coloured. On the other, a severe grey reproduction, like a Piper design for the stage set of a castle. Framed photograph of the old senior partner.

Eventually the young man appears and goes out without looking at anyone.

Dr Cerney says, as I go in, 'That's my psychotherapy patient. He was feeling pretty desperate. He's articulate but not too intelligent.' He describes a long case. The young man concerned was a twin; at birth, his mother felt she couldn't cope with two children, so she kept the daughter and gave the son to his grandmother. When he was fourteen his grandmother started to die; she disintegrated over three years, nursed by the boy, and eventually died. He went back to the family he'd hardly seen. Subsequently he became set in a long history of disturbance and delinquency – psychiatrists, therapists, hospitals, etc. etc. He's now twenty-four and slowly on the mend.

We went out to the car and set off on the first visits. The case that seemed to preoccupy Dr Cerney was the young mother who'd had arguments with her husband. There was something there. I suggested the fact she'd come with her sister meant, if there was something, she was reluctant to spill it and had brought the sister to guard herself. My presence may have had an effect too. In which case it would eventually come out; Monday perhaps. He agreed.

But the case I thought the saddest was the delinquent woman who couldn't have children. Her anguish was patent, her anxiety, 'What shall I tell Bob?' But I suppose there was little or nothing he could do about her. She wouldn't be accepted for a test-tube implant; he could only hope she'd conceive, and comfort her. No point, therefore, in thinking about her. The other, he might be able to help.

The Visits

Dr Cerney's ratio of surgery to home visits was about 3 to 1, very high by modern standards. This was partly because, where 14 per cent is the national average, 20 per cent of his practice was geriatrics. ('Worn out often by the nature of their lives and work.') But also because he believed that was the role of the GP – both to seek out illness, and to *actively* assist. 'We won't bully people to get taxis or lifts or to get their children out of work to take them to the doctor.' Thus he did about thirteen visits a day – except during epidemics when the number soars.

It was now about mid November – getting colder as I went north. Intermittent to violent rain drifted or stormed in off the moors over the city. The estate was built in long, well made, endless, identical rows not at all the same to those who lived in them.

MRS ROCKWELL: Seventy-nine, in a ground floor, one-room flat, recovering from a stroke. Tight, grey hair, rather wide eyes, apprehensive. Started right in – 'pain in the head, when I lie down at night, it drives me crackers!' Doctor: 'In the head?' Mrs Rockwell: 'No – right up *here*,' rubbing head. Doctor examines head. 'You seem to have some permanent bruise.' 'It was last *year* I fell,' she says, while he looks in her ears, on both sides. She is leading up to the real worry, 'But have I *damaged* the brain, doctor?' (Laughing, but looking apprehensive.) Doctor rather briskly reassures her she hasn't, says it will pass. 'There's not much I can do in any case.' Prescribes paracetamol. Doctor: 'How's the dizziness?' Mrs Rockwell: 'A bit better.' The room is like them all, small, square, clean (daughter does it regular), a sofa, two chairs, telly, plastic flowers, gas fire. Hot. As we go out, she says 'Is "he" a doctor?' When she learns I'm not, 'Oh, pity – I was going to say, more the merrier.'

Outside Dr Cerney says, 'Most of our time is spent dealing with baffling, incomprehensible pain.'

MRS BRYAND: Ground floor flat, assisted by a warden and home help and several daughters-in-law, eighty-eight, been bed-bound for eight years. 'But,' Dr Cerney said, 'great spirit.' 'God is good to me', and she meant it. Rheumatoid arthritis had suddenly meant she'd lost the use of all her joints, no strength in them. Huge bed in room at side, facing gas fire and telly, by dresser at back with plastic flowers, pills, piles of things. A big strong woman, grown small, skin a bit yellow. A nurse there, who left as we arrived. Daughter, forty to fifty, smiling and attending and prompting.

Accent quite strong, 'I've had a stuffed-up nose, but right better today. I'm ashamed at asking doctor out.' Daughter prompts, 'You were coughing last night.' Mrs Bryand: 'You want me to be telling tales. I wasn't.' He listens to her chest on the front. Then, like lifting a limp sack they, as it were, drape her forward as he listens to her back. As they do this she murmurs, 'I'm useless.' Doctor: 'It's a bit sickly.' Mrs Bryand, dropping brave front: 'It's been worse, doctor. I've been terrible.' Doctor: 'But I reckon you're all right.' Mrs Bryand: 'I'm not *dying*.' Laughter. As he writes out new prescription they discuss when he should come again. Is it to be six weeks? 'I *want* you to come,' suddenly face strained, pleading. 'I'll come in a fortnight.' She relaxes. Looks stronger. 'You'll come – or you'll be out of a job.' Laughing. As we go she fills with energy, manages to pull herself about in the bed. 'We're having a party when I'm ninety.' 'Can I come?' 'Of course you can.'

We go. No visit lasts more than seven minutes or so – we started at 12 and the next surgery is at 3. In the car he says, 'The daughter's lost a lot of weight. There's *something* wrong. She's not my patient, though. But that's an example. The hospital wouldn't know – but the whole picture would have to include that.' He suspects it's cancer. He says, 'They hate that, when their children go before them. They feel cheated. That's a terrible thing.'

Old People's Home
Just outside the town and, immediately, we are in the country. A huge,

mock–Tudor rambling house. Private geriatric home, but fees very low. As we come in, bolting out of the rain, I'm hit by the smell – impossible to describe: hotness, fug, Vitamin B in the pee, urine smothered by washing, old bodies, a solid, fusty, thick smell. Through the kitchens, lots of cheerful cooks, etc. dishing up (*sloshing* up) apple pie, glimpse of nodding geriatrics and upstairs, following the young, attractive, flower-faced figure who, I learn, runs it.

Stairs, paper peeling from ceiling, wheelchairs parked in large, carpeted 'baronial' hall, in one wheelchair was a cat. A big aquarium. Corridor and then she knocks briskly at a door. A rather sprightly old man – eighty? ninety? – in his small bed-sitter watching telly. He fumbles with his programme-change gadget and after a while Sir Geoffrey Howe falls silent. Scabs and discolouration on his ankles. He has very thick glasses and a high voice, almost a yelp, but is alert and bright. As they look at his ankle you feel the *intensity* of his knowledge of it – this scab off yesterday, that the day before. Horny toenails. Dr Cerney changes his drug. He nods, takes in new instructions, pipes 'Thank you very much, thank you very much.' As we walk back downstairs, Dr Cerney says, 'I changed his drug because it can have side effects on his circulation and it was the circulation that had been affected.'

The room next to the kitchens is full of the rest of the inmates sitting about nodding, waving, wobbling in their seats, eating, some looking as mad as hatters. One of them gives vent to piercing whistles from time to time. 'Those *whistles*,' says Tim. He had to explain to one bald, tiny figure that her house was being sold to pay for her keep. She didn't really seem to follow but realized something was up and plucked at the tray on her lap.

Up different stairs. Mrs W, ninety-three, been in a week and not eating, 'She's on the way out.' She was in what seemed like the best room, two beds, big and chintzy, a wall electric fire. In the bed, a tiny, frail figure, the look of death on her bony face, eyes wide, one drooping. The doctor was incredibly gentle, felt her, found she wasn't in pain. As we left, the young girl stroked the dying woman's forehead.

They discussed her death certificate before we left, standing outside the kitchens, where there was now a pram with the young girl's baby in it. Another cat. An air of friendliness. The young girl asked for some more Largactil prescriptions. We said good-bye.

'They've no facilities – they charge very little. £50 a week. You can pay up to £200. She's very good, very competent. An SRN and genuinely likes old people. She learned that from one of the nurses who's been here twenty years, and who's *devoted* – gives up her Christmas, works all hours.'

But if they can't pay the council won't – as some do – pay for them. 'They're doctrinaire in some respects.'

I commented how, after three minutes, one ceased to notice the smell.

'Yes – luckily the sense of smell is easily fatigued.'

MRS THOMAS: I was slightly apprehensive as Dr Cerney described Mrs Thomas. She'd totally neglected a tumour on the breast until it was (gesture) fist-sized. It was suppurating, and could now only be dressed (she'd refused a mastectomy – but he was quite sure that by the time she came it wouldn't have made any difference). She now had secondaries – recently in the femur of her left leg so that it had snapped. Did it hurt? He thought it might be beginning to as the tumour was reaching into the ribs. She'd been on anti-cancer agents and these had seemed to slow things up – though as she was seventy-eight it was hard to tell.

In fact, she was a plump, lively, very healthy looking woman, in a clean single room, bed, fire, same pictures (like village rooms in Spain – only warm). Had she dressed for the doctor? I would have thought so. Her leg hurting (very large calves and ankles). Clearly cancer (the same leg). 'It's really painful in the morning. Like toothache.' Doctor: 'Do the tablets help?' (Vehement) 'No. No. I just have to wait till the pain goes.' (Which suggested they did help.)

He wrote out new prescriptions (nearly all the visits were routine, to see, to renew prescriptions). She described the new rail at the door which the council had fitted, which allows her to get to the door on her zimmer, swing down and into her wheelchair. ('My chariot!') Again, all described vividly and graphically and I had the sense of how intense small details became in this almost horrifyingly circumscribed world.

As we left, she described some financial anxiety. Dr Cerney pointed out angrily to me that when she went into hospital her pension was docked. 'They talk about charging for hospitals – but hospitals are *already* charging. But only pensioners. Then they come out and run into this sort of worry about back rent.'

MRS JUDD: Obese, arthritic joints and suffering from some fall resulting from this, hence visit to hospital. Single room as usual. As we opened the door an absolute blast of urine so one was rocked on one's feet, or I was. Dr Cerney walked through it. Hot little room, plastic flowers, sideboard, little plaster objects, a round alarm clock, bottle of Walsingham water. Very hot. Carpet with pattern of flaming lipstick-red geraniums on it. Mrs Judd, short, large, colossal ankles and legs, came vaguely sluttishly into the room, extremely slowly on a zimmer hung with bags holding whatever she might need, wearing a gaudy striped dress, but put on so lots of vest was revealed. Face like ET. While Dr Cerney looked at her damaged leg, the home help banged and clanged in the background. Smell of urine already unnoticeable.

She complained bitterly about the hospital and rudeness of the sister as the doctor wrote out diuretics and other prescriptions. Mrs Judd: 'I *dread* going into hospital!' Long account of sister saying she must help the ambulance men. 'I help them ambulance men all ways I can!' 'Yes, it's bad when they get impatient,' said doctor, a bit absently. 'I'll come again in six weeks.'

'Good-bye luv,' said Mrs Judd, giving her loose smile, leaning into her zimmer as though thinking of getting up. There was a photo of her when young, on the sideboard – a strong fine woman, imperious, but beginning to be a bit plump.

MRS KING: Opposite flat. Four steps away. Deaf, and dizziness from angina – eight-three. But a sweet, clean-smelling paradise after Mrs Judd. (That easily fatigued sense of smell not that fatigued it couldn't, with delight, recognize the change.) Brisk and gay, lined face, looked seventy-three. I see they do put on an effort, these old women, for their male doctor. (The men make no effort at all. Did they respond to a woman?) 'If I sit and cry I wouldn't get any better.' Her briskness brisked us out.

MRS GORDON: Living in sheltered accommodation; expensive but a good rent rebate. (The council's policy was that people should have what they wanted and needed as far as possible, not what they could afford. So if, say, someone had brought up four children in a big house and loved it, the council would let them keep it, with a rebate.) She'd moved in from her own home eighteen months before, but was still disturbed by the change and kept getting vague apprehensive pains and illnesses. Now flu – 'I can't seem able to pick up' – which had led to pains in the stomach. Doctor said, after quite a long examination, 'a temporary upset which will right itself'.

As we went out I asked him if he ever gave placebos to that sort of person. He said no. 'I prefer to stay very low key, not alarm them. I say, "You were like this last year, remember? And you got better." They agree.'

We drove to the surgery, picked up three buns with corned beef in them (it was now 2.15), and drove on, munching them.

MR HART: In his own bungalow. Circulation trouble, difficulty walking, had been to hospital. Seventy-four. Came in unsteadily, in trousers and vest, braces over. Sat down. Hospital had said he was OK, he was really worrying about the expense of Christmas presents (five grandchildren). Prescription for circulation written out, also an injunction to have some sherry before meals.

Finally, doctor said, 'How much are you smoking now?' 'Five or six a day,' said the man, without much conviction.

'His trouble is smoking,' said Dr Cerney, as we walked away. 'He comes from that generation who smoked a fantastic lot at work and in the war, really took on board an immense amount of nicotine. That's what's wrong with his legs, why the circulation is so bad. The drugs are to open it up, and I said exercise too.'

'Would it make any difference if he gave it up now?'

'Oh yes. Each cigarette pulls in the elastic arteries a little – alcohol widens them, which is why I advised that.'

Later, in the car, he observed, 'I went on and on at him. In the end we came to a mutual agreement about his lack of success in giving up smoking.'

I thought later of his thin, spindly frame which had taken on board so much nicotine and was now as a result cracking up, filling, sinking.

Mrs Pearson: Seventy-six. She had a violently over-active thyroid, but complained that the pills made her lethargic. Tim said she had a man living with her, younger than her. When he came the man hid at the back of the house.

They had a long, inconclusive discussion, Mrs Pearson wanting to stop the pills (she'd been cutting down) – 'I get tired even in the flat.' Doctor sympathetic, but saying she remembered how when she stopped them her thyroid always got out of control. 'My heart thumps now.' 'That's because you've cut down on the pills.' She had a rather sensual face, with sweet, defined lips, and I could see how she might well be attractive. Perhaps she still made love and didn't like to say she thought the slowing was reducing her sex life. She said it was her husband's death gave her the thyroid condition, she was over that. Trying to get him to say she could give up. He wouldn't.

He said later that he had tried several times to do what she wanted. The thyroid condition – rapid weight loss, dangerous heart rate, etc., fatal if let go – always ensued. He said the condition had probably been precipitated by her husband's death.

Mr Sanding: Seventy. He irritated Tim, who lost his way several times, so much so that we had to go late, at 6.15, when surgery was over, when he lost his way again.

It was a check-up visit after a recovery from a stroke. Mr Sanding was – his wife told me – an ex-RSM. He was tall, talking with slight impediment, commanding, drumming large fat fingers on the sofa. Complained for some time that they wouldn't transfer him from the geriatric ward, full of incontinent men, where he'd been rushed on admission, to a better ward – where there were six beds. Also very irritated the way the doctor had called the nursing staff by their Christian names.

Diabetic too. Prescription pad. Instructions. Congratulations on swift recovery of speech. He would do better if friends came in to talk to him. It turned out they had almost no friends. Army ones had died or dropped away. 'Upstairs, the woman hasn't been out for three years,' said his wife. 'I see her on the stairs about once a fortnight. The woman below is ninety-two and deaf. They're very lonely places these flats.' They were trying for a bungalow nearer the shops. She hurried to show me the letter acknowledging their request, asking me to agree it was hopeful.

We drove back. I thought of all that lay behind these houses, all these old people alone. I could smell their little rooms, their urine, in my clothes all evening.

24

INNER CITY PROBLEMS:
TWO SLUM PRACTICES

I drove up into Scotland the next day. It was sunny and they were ploughing in the Lowlands, the gulls swooped and flocked, diving instantly the tractor had passed so the worms wouldn't have time to burrow down. I thought it must be like the pheasant season or oyster months for them – only shorter.

After a while I turned west. The earth started to heave, became moor-like, sensing the Highlands still 200 miles away. There must have been a lot of rain because the burns were very full, fed from dozens of tiny, gushing streams pouring off the bare, cropped grass, between the bracken and heather, glistening in the distance like twisting strips of mirror. Dotted here and there on the slopes were sheep, like pale rocks grazing.

Dr Mary Trimdon

I reached the Trimdons in the late afternoon. Both were doctors. We have already heard Dr Henry Trimdon on a number of things, and will do so again. (I mentioned their chain-smoking.) He was the son of a fisherman and proud of his working-class background. Proud, too, that he looked younger than he was. Her father had been a pastor, but for some reason I forget she was 'really' working class too.

He was short and did look younger than his fifty-six years. I think it was because he dyed his hair. He had large, pale eyes, dark jowls, a pasty face and was rather irritable. He treated his twenty-year-old son as if he were fourteen, though he was clearly very fond of him. They were a close family and he was justly proud of his achievements. Dr Mary was spry, lined, and clever but allowed her husband to lead.

Henry Trimdon was the senior partner in a modern health centre in a well-to-do part of the city. Dr Mary Trimdon, on the other hand, suddenly said of her own practice, 'That place down there would drive you round the bend. If you saw the area, the boarded-up houses, you just would not credit. There's a burn goes under one housing estate and the houses are all damp, and now they don't know whether to knock all the houses down. It's to be seen to be believed.'

I asked to see it and we went there on the second day.

The surgery was a big, drab, granite house set at the edge of the Glen

Moraig Housing Estate. This was another enormous council estate, but far more desolate and desperate than Tim Cerney's.

The receptionist/practice manager was replacing a lavatory seat when we arrived. The other had been torn off. So that I could be shown round, a cupboard was unlocked and inside it was a small metal wall safe. Inside that, row upon row of keys. It was like visiting a gaol.

DR MARY TRIMDON: 'We have to lock everything up. Every room, every door. They break in, getting after the drugs and scrip pads. They'll soak the scrip pads in brake fluid. Did you not know that? Och aye – they soak away the scrip and the name and address and just leave your signature. They'll add what they want. Diconal mostly (a strong narcotic pain-killer) – it makes them feel good, produces some elevation.

'And you have to be very, very firm. You hear them, in the waiting room, "Duin gae to her – she'll nae gie ye a line, and duinna gae to him either, he'll nae gie ye a line. The other two, they'll gie ye lines . . ." I bawl them out sometimes.'

It was an old house, all the doors were toughened against fire and break-in. The glass in all the downstairs windows was unbreakable. 'You can't break it but you can heat it and bend it. We came one morning and the windows here were buckled – so. Another time they picked the putty out of the windows and the glass fell in.'

We looked out of one of these siege windows. 'That's where they bring their prams for the ante-natal. We have a bar to padlock them to. Aye, it's true. We've had two or three prams nicked. They used to bring their grans to keep an eye on them.'

Outside her surgery was a toilet. It was like one in a rough pub. Here too the seat was torn off; there was a broken wire basket, but no paper. It was dank, wet, sordid, and dark. 'It's flooded at least once a fortnight – they stuff things down the loo. So now no paper. If you send a patient to give a specimen of urine you just give them a couple of tissues and say, "Right, there you are." You see there's no plug in the sink? That's because they leave the tap running to flood it.'

Her surgery was rather a bare room, walls painted dull institutional red and green. It had a buzzer to call patients, and was heated by a two-bar electric fire.

She re-locked her surgery, unlocked the nurse's waiting room door – a bare dark room with two chairs – and then unlocked the door into the nurse's treatment room. The room was very small and damp, paper peeling in a large curl down the edge of one wall, dark green worn lino, a sink, small unbreakable glass window, pot plants.

Dr Mary Trimdon's memory had been sparked off by something in the room. 'I'd two cases yesterday where I've been worried about children under school age. One mother is a perpetual criminal. Since nine years ago she's been in prison a couple of times. She *always* has fraud charges pending. She's supposed to be working out 200 hours of community service and she's done six. She came up in a great panic two days ago and she got an appointment today to have a smear done, and then I had a social worker on the phone saying she was worried about the children and what was *I* going to do about it? I said, "Look, I have no reason to suspect, I've never seen these children bruised." "Oh well, we must do something." So I said, "But unless we've any evidence we can't do a thing." And somebody at the nursery had seen the mother punching the child so I said, "Well, that's the person you want to go and see, not me."

'That was one. The other was a widow who stuck her hand through a glass window about six weeks ago, took the plaster off herself, never went back. She's going to be permanently left with a hand like that [making a claw gesture]. She's got two children that are completely uncontrollable and the social worker's worried about them. She'd an appointment yesterday and didna come, but she came for her prescriptions. She'd an appointment today. The health visitor went to the house to collect her and her child and could get no reply. So either she was lying in bed not opening the door – it was a first-floor flat, you see, so you couldn't see in the window – and if she doesn't want to open the door and come to the surgery, well what can you do now? What *can* you do with those two situations? Potentially four children under five are at risk.

'You can see how it runs on and on in the families. You'll find father was a bed-wetter till he was fifteen as well, but often the mother doesn't know that father was a bed-wetter. It's only when you manage to grab hold of father in a quiet corner and say, "Here, how old were you before you were dry?" And sometimes they take a while to tell you. And I say, "Well, you can't give young Jimmy a beating for being wet if that was the same as you were, because this is a familial thing."'

We went upstairs. The windows here had metal grilles. Outside, at the back, the surgery looked across to a block of council houses. I saw many boarded windows. Below was the area for the prams. The whole of the back was encircled by a high stone wall, along the top of which were dense coils of barbed wire. A sizeable wedge of new masonry showed where there'd been a recent collapse – or a break-in. 'They drove a lorry at it. Partly after drugs, partly vandalism.' She looked sideways, where the end of the surgery jutted into view. 'We put that non-dry paint on the drain pipes so that when they put their hands on it, they get their hands all wet and slip. That kept them off for a while but it's needing doing again.'

She unlocked door after door, then at the centre, the drugs cupboard. This was six foot square, several shelves packed full. Everything was supplied free by the drug reps: Benylin, packs of the pill, dressings, an enema, 'starter' containers of antibiotics they took on their rounds. 'We give them away free. There was a GP down the way, when you still had to pay for the pill. He'd sell them. I thought it was disgraceful.'

We had coffee in 'the doctors' room', sitting round a big table with piles of unopened *Pulses* and *General Practitioners* in the middle. Opposite, outside, was the local Paki shop, a betting shop, and the office of 'James Davieson – Solicitor'. 'He'll get you off anything.' 'You see those big mud patches,' said Dr Mary Trimdon, 'it was all grass.' I saw a pack of seven-year-olds, very scruffy – what Dr Watson would have called street arabs – clambering over a wire fence and scampering away over a derelict area of rubbish and grass.

'We have a drug problem – but they're not static, if you see what I mean. They're more wandering addicts who arrive from the London scene, stay as long as they can get their drugs, and then move on. There's quite a lot of selling of Diconal, DF 118 and some of the barbiturate sleeping capsules. There's quite a lot of that and my partner knows, he was telling me, of old patients in the practice who are eking out their pension by selling their sleeping pills.'

As we left the gaol-like, fortress surgery she pointed at the double locks on the door. In the car, 'Did you see that girl in the surgery, the one with the child? She jumped out of a third floor window two years ago. Fractured her pelvis. It was after a row with her drunken husband. We have a lot of recurrent cases here. Visits to the poisons unit, you know, with overdoses.'

It was a clear, cold, windy, sunny day. I'd seen many council estates apart from Tim Cerney's, all over England, but none I'd seen – or was to see – were as dirty, as run down, as destroyed as this one. The cracked, deeply pitted concrete roads, the rubbish blowing, littered about, piled, the lines and blocks of grey council estate, the sordid weed-filled, rubbish-filled patches of 'garden', wrecked cars – all sparkled in the sun. And the odd thing was, it was very close to countryside; quite soon was a steep hill, a little mountain rising above a loch which was a bird sanctuary. Flocks of geese on the soccer pitch of a comprehensive. In the distance, the fields and hills of lowland Scotland.

We passed a flattened derelict area from which 'travellers' had recently been evicted, and to which they would return.

'That's a terrible source of trouble to us. Not all of them. Some of them are lovely – the circus people, the ones with shows. There's one caravan, a beautiful one, must be worth £12,000, water, telephone, electricity laid on. Two sisters and a brother live there. The last of the Pinder Circus family. He's a very well-read chap this Pinder, and he's been trying to trace his ancestry. But these are no problem. They've a better standard than the local patients – they spend the winter here, and during the summer they move to wherever there's a gala or a fête. They're super. Very Romany. All the little girls from this size have their ears pierced – beautiful. And beautiful rings, gold rings, all the wives have great broad gold bands easily as wide as my three put together, and thick.

'But the really bad lot, the majority, are this lot from Southern Ireland – talk about filth and squalor and degradation. From the minute they arrive they draw unemployment benefit. They've never contributed, they've no intention of working. They work on the side, on the sly. Not window cleaning – you have to be registered if you window clean. But tar working, or with the potatoes or the harvest. A lot repair cars. They're illiterate – a cross for their names.

'And in the summer they move on. To Perthshire. They cut willow, which is flexible, and make like an igloo or tent covered in rugs or what they find. And if you're called you crawl in among all the muck; I had to do a confinement in one of those stinking little igloo tents.'

We'd driven on, and were now passing through an area of smarter houses, privately owned. 'You should see the surgery on a wet day, when it's crowded. The smell! These people here freely own to me, they won't come.

'But it's hard for some of our own lot. I mean our health visitors for instance keep a supply of clothes and only this week somebody phoned up to say she couldn't come to the surgery because she had no shoes. Now, in fact, she'd been out for messages in her bare feet and it was quite true, when the health visitor went down with a selection of shoes to see if anything was suitable, the child was washing her feet, and this was a girlie who's eighteen, has one baby and she's pregnant again and she couldn't keep her appointment at the ante-natal clinic because she was too poor to buy any shoes. I mean, that is actual fact. You wouldn't believe in this day and age that there'd be somebody with no shoes but the health visitors keep a big supply of clothes here. In fact we're always chasing the mothers – the better off mothers or the ones that look after their children more adequately, that when they've finished with clothes, if they hand them into the clinic we'll find a use for them. There are those who'll only come to the clinic if you bribe them by saying, "Right, if you bring the child up, we'll give you some more clothes", or somebody will ring and say, "I can't come because I haven't got a buggy to bring the child up", and we'll say, "Oh well, we've got a buggy. If you bring the child up we'll give you a buggy". A second-hand one. It's amazing. With the second-hand clothes we get we bribe them to come to the surgery themselves or bring their babies for immunizations.

'And I think it's very telling when patients say to you – you say to them "What's your occupation?" – maybe filling in an out-patient appointment form and "What's your job?", or to a girl "What's your husband do?" "He's *just* a labourer." And I keep saying to them, "But look, we need labourers, we can't all be brickies, and slickers and stonemasons and all the rest. We need the labourers as well." And they look at me as much to say, "Do you really mean that?". Poor things, so low an estimation. What an existance.'

We turned back into the huge estate – a big, dirty island bounded by smarter areas, then countryside. 'Good tenants won't accept a house here. They'd rather wait two years for a better area.' More litter. More dogs. 'They hunt in packs.' The houses – basically sound, solid, good square rooms – were again very shabby. Many were boarded-up. First stage was wood, then metal, big bits of rusty metal. 'If it's not done, they break the windows. Like those there. That lot. The authorities went in and found they'd come in through the roof. The place was gutted – radiators ripped out,lavatories. The place is emptying. That's why our list is shrinking.' I asked if that mattered. 'We've plenty of work,' she said drily.

'You see over there – the house with the chimney, beyond the tree? Phillip lives there, the doctor I told you sold the pill before it was free. He's crippled. It's a shame, he lives by himself.'

More bookies. Shops were open, but still kept their grilles down. The litter-strewn streets were fairly deserted. 'It's quiet now. They're in their beds. They're none of them up.' It was 11.30.

'That window up there, that's the one that girl threw herself out of.

'That was a fire. There was a fire in that house. And the woman was burnt to death. She was a McBride, needless to say.'

The cars had N, L, F or G registrations. When we passed a van, with a nearby cannibalized Escort, 'You can tell that type – Smart Alick living off his wits. A German girl lives there. She's going back to Germany I'm glad to say. They throw stones at her in the streets.'

Puppies and filthy toddlers were playing in the sun amongst the rubbish. 'Here were two murders, No. 20 or 22, at different times. Actually it doesn't look so bad today, maybe because the sun is shining.'

On the edge, after winding through the wide, deserted, dirty streets, we passed a pub, The Cooper's Crown. 'That's a very wild hostelry. It's a very wild area here in fact. I wouldn't do night calls here if you paid me. Too many drunks and wild people.'

Yet she didn't hate it. On the contrary. 'I wouldna look for another place. I enjoy it. They're a feckless immoral lot but I like them. The other doctor didn't bother with ante-natal but I got it going. There's still a lot of the personal element. One day, this old lady's blind, she lives alone, she's eighty-six, really pathetic. And she was trying to put loose covers on those squab seats, you know, one of the tapes was off, she was trying to sew it on. She'd sewn it on to the wrong place, so I ended up sewing all the tapes on to all her cushions.

'And they like it too, you know. Och aye. We rehouse them, a better area, better house. And they want back! They miss the company.'

The Problems of the Inner Cities

A good deal is written about the inner cities. And Dr Cerney and Dr Mary Trimdon have both illustrated something of what it is like. We can deal with the other problems fairly briefly, therefore; but deal with them we must – they are so pressing and they affect so many.

Britain is not alone here. It's an international problem. The World Health Organization thinks it's their worst. You find the same things in New York, San Paolo, Bangladesh, Paris, Sydney. (see *Health Care in Big Cities,* ed. Leslie Paine.)

Nor is all of it entirely new. Inner London was at its most crowded in 1910. There are reports of out-patient hospital surgeries in the 1890s with 150-200 patients, each getting thirty second 'consultations'. But these, obvious casualties and the like aside, were the old fever infections we looked at first. That layer rolled away – all the socio-economic-psychological-familial problems have been revealed.

What it amounts to is this. All practices regard these problems as the most difficult and tough. (Research has been done by the Acheson Committee and is so far unpublished.) All practices have them – but the inner cities have far more of them, and they are far more intense.

The problems I mean are elderly people living alone, unemployment, single-parent families, rootless highly mobile populations who vanish as soon as seen, alcoholics, drug addicts, immigrant populations, poverty. Many of these, like the immigrant populations, bring totally new problems. So do drug addicts. Dr Stane could no longer wander with 'the lassies of the Salvation Army' through the Gorbals secure with his little black bag. Drug addicts beat GPs up and kill them. On some of the big London estates the young girl GPs are too frightened, like Dr Mary Trimdon, to visit at night. At Stockwell, in Brixton, the group practice has to escort the receptionists home to be safe at nights in winter.

Schizophrenics can be violent and where the rest of the country has 1 per cent of these, London has 5 per cent. (This is because there are more social class five in inner cities – which, as Dr Cerney pointed out, means more ordinary disease as well.) Where the rest of the country has a 5 to 10 per cent turnover of patients – Paddington has a 30 per cent turnover. That is – *about a third of their patients each year are just not seen again.*

But, of course, within this general picture, there are wide variations. One city will have immigrant riots, another, like the area where Dr Cerney practiced, will have 20 per cent chronic geriatrics. There are variations within the cities. Take London. Lambeth, South London has immigrants, single-parent families, a lot of elderly people. Earls Court has an excess of mobile young people between fifteen and twenty; the problems are therefore drug addiction, suicide, and mental illness. Soho has the problem of single-handed often ancient GPs with tiny NHS lists and private patients.

A situation sufficiently catastrophic is made still more so by the way a good many GPs react. I talked to an Edinburgh GP who restricted his NHS list to 1,000 patients. Why 1,000? 'Because you get the basic practice allowance [then £7,000 per annum], 70 per cent of two ancillary staff, the rent and rates of my surgery.' His 1,000 NHS patients were carefully selected – 'Healthy adult males and females, under fifty. If they have any children – out.' (Just as you can choose your GP, so he – an independent contractor – can choose or not choose you.) He spent most of his time at, and gained his money from, the lucrative hotel trade in Edinburgh.

This is quite common in inner London. A thousand NHS patients gain the full benefits; but below that you gain pro-rata. That is, one tenth less if you have 900 patients and so on, down to 100. So, you live off private patients, but you have enough NHS ones to pay most of your rent, your receptionist, £5,000 or so capitation and basic practice allowance – and your NHS list is carefully weeded of the old, children, the chronic, etc. One result is that it is often difficult to get a GP in inner London (and in inner Edinburgh and to an extent elsewhere). Family Practitioner Committees can only appoint so many GPs per head of population. The inner-city area has a great many GPs, but they are not taking any more NHS patients.

Another reason for this situation – aside from greed and the desire not to deal with the intractable problems of inner-city patients – is that the inner cities are expensive. Over much of inner London a reasonable family house costs £100,000–£150,000–£200,000.

The primary care team hardly seems to have developed over much of the inner cities – and this is because it costs the GP money, no matter that the NHS helps generously. The proportion of GPs over seventy and single-handed is far higher in the inner cities (you will remember Dr Quainton tottering into view).

A lot of the wives I spoke to said they simply wouldn't have let their husbands apply for practices in the inner cities. They didn't want to live there. They didn't want their children to live there. So the ageing GPs linger on, fresh blood unwilling to replace them. That this is so is shown by the fact that there are far more overseas GPs in the inner cities (12 per cent compared to 2 per cent) – unfortunately always a sign an area is considered undesirable.

A final effect of all this is that the big teaching hospitals, which are usually concentrated in the inner cities (London, Sheffield, Glasgow, Edinburgh, Bristol and so on), base their view of GPs – the consultants who teach in them base their views of GPs – on the experience they have of them locally. This is frequently not at all good. In London in 1967, for example, St Thomas's view of GPs was so low that the only facility they allowed them to specify was X-rays. They simply didn't think they were capable of asking for anything else. This is historical, and almost certainly partly accounted for the extremely low status of GPs in the hierarchy of doctors until the improvements of the last ten years. But it is still a factor.

Dr John Hury

Dr John Hury said he could give me ten minutes. He'd got a golfing lesson with his pro and he didn't want to be late.

The surgery looked as though it had been converted from an old shop (as turned out to be the case). It was the first of three on the busy road. Large white plastic letters had been irregularly stuck on the inside of the window – SURGERY.

Inside was a bare 15 foot by 15 foot waiting room. Institutional green, wooden banquettes round the walls, holed linoleum on the floor. Off this were two smaller rooms – the consulting room and the receptionist's office.

The consulting room was too small for an examination couch and had no basin. Files, a calendar, a small table on either side of which we sat; the golf clubs more or less filled it.

Shirley, the receptionist, sat in on the interview, doing her nails and occasionally joining in – or rather being invited in by Dr Hury. She was an extremely attractive girl of about twenty-six, with high piled hair, a slender neck, humorous, slightly impatiently pouting mouth and a small chin. She swung her legs, showing them off with her high, red, stiletto heels.

Dr Hury himself was tall and strong, and gave an air of considerable vigour, with a red face and a mass of white hair. He was Australian, his accent totally untouched by his years in this country. He lived a good way away, very much uptown. Every now and again he got up and practised his swing.

DR HURY: 'The trouble we get is from the drunks, you see. I get a hell of a load of drunks. Someone's got to attend to them. It's because of the area. We have the two houses that cater for them – for these people who are down and out, derelict. If they need medical attention they come here. I'm the nearest one as they can hit it.

'*Coping* with these people, especially on Friday nights, sometimes. Some of them work, strangely enough. Some of them make the attempt. But as soon as they get paid on Friday, that's a hell of a job. I suppose everyone has that problem. But my percentage of drunks is far higher than the average I'd think.

'I wish I knew a solution to this. You've got to do something. You can't just kick them out and say, "You're drunk", you see. We give them vitamins when they need it. A lot of them need withdrawal tablets like Valium or Heminevrin. But a lot just use the Valium as an extra boost so I've had to stop it for some. I find drying out quite hopeless. It gives a sort of couple of weeks rest from them, that's all. But as soon as they come out they're straight back on it, you see. They've rested. We can't do anything. I've got so much cirrhosis round here you wouldn't believe. Let me say this, though, you expect much worse looking at them. You don't expect to see them in a couple of years and they carry on and on – it's amazing. And the symptoms aren't as bad as you think, although their livers may be buggered to hell. I mean, if you have their liver function tests done, I mean they're haywire. They've got huge, knobbly livers if you examine them. You get a lot of neuropathy here too, alcoholic neuropathy – their legs go. And I've had one or two cerebellar degeneration where they can't even hold their balance completely. No balance left at all. That's much worse than neuropathy. When it hits the brain, well then they go, you see.

'I never refuse them. My list is full now, over 3,000. I just have to put them on as temporary residents. They can be bloody trouble because they upset the other patients. We have a surgery full of kids and old ladies, you just need two or three drunks and the whole bloody equilibrium goes. But the way I look at it, everyone's entitled to medical care. It's bad luck they're alcoholics. Probably we're lucky we're not. They've got no women, nobody else. It's always the same story. "They won't have anything to do with me. Haven't seen them for years." Some of them have distinguished sons. "One of my sons is a specialist in Liverpool, doctor." Yes, it's true. Oh, it's a great curse, drink. We love it, yet it's such a damn curse.

'We used to have 80 per cent white and 20 per cent coloured. Now it's just the opposite way round. I hardly ever see a cockney. They've gone. God knows what's happened to them.

'Now, I'm not being racialist in any sense, but the difficult ones are not the black, not the African, not the Caribbean, but the Asians. They will come with anything. I mean a temperature's nothing, if he *feels* hot he's coming. "Feel it doctor." The most bizarre symptoms – if he hasn't passed a motion for a day. For that amount of constipation they'll come over. So that's my problem there – three times the workload from the Asian population.

'I got this by just applying. They just paid me something the first year because it was so-called under-doctored – 1,200 quid if I remember correctly. This was a tobacconist's. It wasn't a surgery. I didn't get one thrown at me, I can tell you that. It was bloody hard. We used to have 200 applicants in those days for one job. And if you didn't have higher qualifications, you had no bloody chance. I'll never forget my first patient who came in. I've always held the Rowton House people in high esteem for that – they sent him along.

'Incidentally they're trying to destroy it now. I hope they never do it. It'll be disastrous for this area, not for me. I couldn't care less. But for the people here. These are people who have nobody left in the world. It could happen to a lot of us. There but for the grace of God . . . Anyhow, they've 500 and I should think I look after 450 of them.

'I shall go on as long . . . well, when are you going to kick me out? When they've had enough of me. No, honestly, when I can't do the job properly I'm going to pack it up. When I start missing things, I'll say, "I'm no bloody good now. The old brain's gone." No, seriously, I'm not sort of saying I'll flog myself to death. In two and a half years I'll be sixty-eight, well, sixty-nine.

'But I *enjoy* it, you see. This is a super practice. You can't run a better practice. Whoever takes this over, they're really stepping into a paradise, aren't they? Don't laugh, Shirley. It's not a bloody building you go on, it's the set-up. If they've got the staying power to deal with all types of people. If they say "I'm not going to have drunks in here. I'm not having children with colds," they're going to be no bloody good.'

SHIRLEY: 'You get more depression here.'

DR HURY: 'Depression? I talk to them, don't I? Who gives them my time round here?'

SHIRLEY: 'No one.'

DR HURY: 'No one. You ask them and they'll tell me. I can give ten minutes for a patient. There's loads waiting.'

SHIRLEY: 'How many come really sick? Yesterday – one.'

DR HURY: 'One. I can't really think of yesterday. They keep me in touch you see. I have to have young people around me [indicating Shirley, who's started on her other hand]. Otherwise I'm lost. To stimulate, you know. Honestly. [Swings club.] I hope that bloody swing works today, Shirley.'
    'No, but honestly, my problems are *minimal*.'

SHIRLEY: 'We get a lot of depression. If the housing was better they wouldn't come.'

DR HURY: 'That's not a problem.'

SHIRLEY: 'Yes it is, because we can't help them.'

DR HURY: [not listening to her] 'I spend loads of time writing letters. Some of them are successful because I get thanks, and that's very nice when somebody says "Thank you for getting my house or my nice new flat." I'll never refuse a letter for anyone who wants better housing.'

SHIRLEY: 'They might have to wait for a little while.'

DR HURY: 'No, but we've done it, Shirley, I know. Hundreds of people have got flats through us and good luck to them.'

SHIRLEY: 'A lot are frightened to live in this area, aren't they? Muggings . . .'

DR HURY: 'There's a lot of muggings round here, you know. Every drunk I've had has been mugged. I should think 300 out of my 400 drunks have been mugged.
    'In the winter, I must say, I have to keep a wary eye myself. It's no good

just being flippant about it. You've got to be vigilant about that. Because I don't know who's behind me. They're not going to say, "Oh, it's that nice doctor, we're not going to hit him over the head." And especially, they do a funny mugging around here. You see, they go for blokes who come out of pubs and if he's just walking a little drunk he's had it. And we get them next morning. This is not unusual. My old ladies are barricaded in. You'd think they were at Fort Knox or something. They're hiding the crown jewels. *Really*! I'm waiting five minutes for this old lady to open the door. "Sorry doctor, won't be long now. That's the third padlock gone; the fourth one's off now." It's a scream. So you see how frightened they are. I can't just call now like I did in the old days. Just pop in. There's no such thing as these monthly seeing old ladies or something like that. That's out of the question. That's a thing of the past. They've got to call you and expect you before you go down. Otherwise they will not open the door. Because anybody can say "I'm the doctor."

'Nights are fine. I use a deputizing service. Perfectly OK. No, I'm not going to pass judgement on them. How well they get seen to – sometimes brilliantly, sometimes not so good. But that would happen if I was on duty in any case.

'I was a bit annoyed with them this morning. I mean – well I can trust this woman. She's not an exaggerator is she, Shirley? – anyway, the child had an earache and she'd managed to get him temporarily asleep. The doctor said "I can't examine him. Earache now subsided, baby asleep. Where's the lavatory." So they had to come in here. It hadn't subsided. It was still inflamed. But I'm not here to knock the Southern Relief Service. I've been with them twenty years. I would think I was one of their first customers round here. But they have varied. The standards.

'They're manned by Pakistanis. Exclusively almost. Now, they're good doctors. But the *reports*. Honestly – this bit of paper means nothing to me. "Earache subsided." When we used to get the old English doctors, Christ, they must have been tired at the time, but they did it properly. Very rarely did I see a bad report. That's what built up the Southern Relief Service originally. A doctor who went there originally does my locums for me. He'll be a consultant within a year. He's one of the top boys in veins and anything in the world. Goes lecturing all over. I shan't mention names but he used to work for them. That's how I met him. So he does my locums, my holidays, or fixes up with his friends. So I know I'm getting first-class people. I'm lucky that way.'

Deputizing Services

Deputizing services only operate in and around the large cities. Nevertheless, these are quite extensive areas. The Southern Relief Service, for example, patrols a huge area – including London, Kent, Middlesex, Surrey and Essex.

It comes at night and weekends for some 1,000 GPS and 2,000,000 patients.

There are four questions one should ask: does this matter, how many doctors nationally use the service, what do the patients feel, and what is the situation with doctors who still do their own night calls – if there are any such left?

It would perhaps not matter crucially if the relief services were reliable. I cannot find evidence about the services nationally, but as far as Southern Relief goes, Dr Hury is not the only one to worry. In May and June 1983 the *Sunday Times* carried a series of reports revealing a highly unsatisfactory state of affairs. Two patients had recently died following attendance by Southern Relief doctors; most of the doctors are Asian and some work incredible hours – one, Dr Ruwanysura Amareskera only slept twenty-four hours a week, working the rest of the time. Deputizing services are supposed to be an occasional relief for GPS, but a good many of them use the services continually; the financial set-up is complex. Southern Relief, which also owns a video shop and various properties, charges fees ranging from £8 50p to £20 a call. (The GP gets £12 75p a night call, even if it is made for him by a relief service, on which he pays tax but he can charge what he pays the relief service against tax.)

I write close to these reports. An inquiry has just been set up on behalf of the Family Practitioner Committees concerned. There is a possibility of litigation, but patients, as usual, are fairly non-committal. One fifth approved of the Service. Hesse Sachs found that if it was an emergency they didn't mind who came, as long as someone did though one imagines they'd be more concerned if they discovered the doctor only slept three hours a night.

There is undoubtedly a trend towards doctors using deputizing services. Cartwright found 9 per cent used the service in 1964, 26 per cent did in 1977. The *Sunday Times* quoted a third of all doctors. (Women GPS are more likely to use it than men.)

DR YETTS: 'It worked very well. We allowed ourselves six sessions a year of the deputizing service. Which meant six afternoons and six evenings a year completely off. It may not sound very much over a year – but it was the wedge widening.'

DR VELLING: 'It costs me £87 a month, plus £5 a visit during the day, plus £10 a visit for a night visit. So the average cost is about £150–£200 a month. Officially, I'm only supposed to use them two nights a week and alternate weekends – ah, but that's *whole* nights, and *whole* weekends. So I'll switch off one half Saturday, then switch *back* at midnight when I want to go to bed. Switch *off* again for a while in the morning . . . (Dr Velling, demonstrating, here switched the switch violently to and fro ten or eleven times in a way which must have caused considerable confusion to the sleepless Asians of

Southern Relief, whose aid he invoked.)

'People who have never tasted the freedom of the deputizing services can't imagine what it's like and are also slightly jealous of those that do have them. But for those that have, there can be no going back. Patients pretended to mind at first and made a great hoo-ha. Now they often use it to get a second opinion.

'But it's legal fiction. The general public seem to think they've bought the doctors body and soul, which in fact they haven't. It would be a mass resignation issue if they really tried to police the deputizing services.'

PROFESSOR MORRELL: 'It's not much fun for a GP doing a night call in Brixton, really. The chances of being knocked down and robbed are quite high. A lot of the young doctors now are ladies – it's difficult. So I haven't any time for a consultant in a teaching hospital who sits and complains about these GPs using the emergency deputizing service out of hours. If those consultants are prepared to drive their car down to the Stockwell Park Estate and get out and carry a doctor's bag and walk across the estate at 2 in the morning then that would be fine. But they're not. They're sheltering behind a registrar and a houseman up there in the hospital.'

Night calls

If a third use deputizing services, two thirds still do their own night calls – the vast majority of GPs. (A 'night' call is one between 11 p.m. and 7 a.m.)

There is no research as to how onerous this is. My strong impression was that it was not a terrible burden, though clearly no one likes getting up in the middle of the night, and likes it less as they get older.

Many GPs kept records of their night calls: Dr Cerney had an average of six a month – high; Dr Nyewood one every two weeks; Dr Telscombe, one every three weeks; the Kibanes once a month. Dr Trimdon, though he would have liked a deputizing service, in fact was called out so seldom he voluntarily did police night calls – 'It's worth getting out of bed for £20.' Dr Colkirk couldn't remember when he'd had one last. He talked vaguely of October (I was with him early in December).

DR CERNEY (who was in a deputizing area): 'How can I do terminal care, for instance, if I leave my dying patients to have any old doctor turn up? I want to be able to say to my partner who is on call, "Look, Mr Jones may possibly die tonight. It's been like this, and I've done that, and I'm giving him this", and so on.

'And we reckon it's better for them not to have some unknown character turning up to what by definition is an emergency and may therefore be more serious actually than most. I still believe that although our patients may be stupid sometimes, they never call us unless they're worried and so we reckon they deserve a doctor they know when they're worried – more worried than usual. Now, obviously, that's very idealistic and there are an awful lot of people who are you know, just a bit bothered. But there are times when crises blow up over the weekend, for instance, and when I reckon it's vital to have your own doctor around. And this may be a luxury. I may not have the energy to do that in ten years' time and I'm not criticizing those doctors who by their mid fifties have decided they haven't got the energy, and I think that's OK. The people I criticize are those young ones who work in practices of four, five or six doctors where it would be just one night a week on call but they can't just be bloody bothered. I can think of practices in this town where it's like that. Yes, yes. And I just don't think that you need to do that, or should do that.'

DR NYEWOOD: 'The reasons vary, but they are not trivial. Some you would say – "You're a bit wet." But everyone feels they have got themselves into an awful state about something. But again, maybe because of the class, people on the whole have a high level capacity to cope on their own and have pride in doing so. I mean, sometimes I have been amazed that people have telephoned me at 8 o'clock in the morning who have been in ferocious pain since 2 or 3 o'clock and have actually needed an injection or a drug or something. But they have felt "You can't call the doctor at this time of day."'

DR THRIPLOW: 'I must say that if a call comes in the night, and somebody phones up for advice about midnight, I'd really much rather go out and see them because I then find it very difficult to settle back to sleep, wondering if they're going to phone back again, or whether perhaps I should have gone out in the first place. Those I find to be the worrying sort of queries. If somebody phones up at 3 o'clock in the morning and says, "I don't want you to come out, but could you give me some advice?" and really it would be almost easier to go out and see them. I find it very hard to get off to sleep again after that.'

Solutions

The problems of the inner cities are complicated and often entangled with those that are far wider and deeper. But it is clear that private, profit-making deputizing services have got totally out of hand and should be taken under firm control by the BMA and Family Practitioner Committees.

Deputizing came in at first to relieve single-handed practitioners. But it could hardly have expanded as it has, unless there was spare capacity among GPs, in particular among Asian and other overseas GPs. (Since it is not really possible to both practise and deputize, though it is being done.) But this relates to unemployment generally and immigrant communities which are both inner-city and much wider national problems.

Again, medical problems have always been social and economic ones. Good drainage, better food, better water supplies, better housing did more to eradicate typhus, diphtheria and the rest than all the immunizations and vaccines. As Dr Hury's Shirley was aware, depression and a whole mass of psychosomatic presentations arise from poor housing, poverty, unemployment.

And there are those transmissions of learnt patterns that persist for hundreds of years and are not susceptible to surface tinkering.

PROFESSOR MORRELL: 'But I think in London the problems are a bit daunting. For your home visits, you've got a lot of steps to climb. And you've got these youngsters with their illegitimate children. It's very difficult for the older doctors to understand their behaviour and get to grips with them in such a way that one might be able to prevent this dreadful cycle of deprivation which you can forecast when these kids are about three years old: you know they're going to be the illegitimate mothers of another twelve years' time. They *are*. I've been here sixteen years and some of them I could have picked out ten years ago; they're coming for abortions now. Their homes are unhappy, desperately unhappy. There's no communication in the home. They want, as soon as they can, to get out and get away. All through their latter schooldays, all they can think of is getting away from home, and one of the ways of getting away from home is getting pregnant, having a baby and getting a council flat, yes. And then, you see, the next generation grow up exactly the same. The boy they get, he's maybe seventeen, eighteen, nineteen – they don't know what they want. In a year they're fighting and scrapping and in another year they've separated. Very few of those marriages really grow to anything, and the whole thing is perpetuated.'

Professor Donald Acheson chaired a committee and presented a report in May 1981. They considered making only one 'revolutionary' suggestion, and then rejected it. The solution was 'salaried doctors'. By paying a fixed high salary – say £30,000 per annum – in return for an undertaking to do NHS work alone, and rigorous selection, FPCs could have replaced the present gang of inner-city GPs with dedicated, highly trained practitioners. They rejected it because they thought the objections would be too strong.

I can't for the life of me see why. The principle has long been accepted and works perfectly well. Inducement practices are in essence salaried practices. It works perfectly well elsewhere, with Dr Axmouth and his 'velvet-lined trap' in a new town for instance, or with university GPs. Wherever I've seen it, none of the things GPs fear happen – there is no loss of independence; the GP doesn't suddenly work 'salaried' hours – 9 to 5; he can still charge just as much to tax (a secret but unadmitted fear). But I do see there would have been the most frightful fuss, and this is not the place to rehearse the arguments, in my view decisive, I had with GPs on this subject they find so sensitive.

Instead, Acheson made 115 recommendations. There should be a retirement age for GPs. (The DHSS pursues this. The age they suggest is seventy-five!) Group practice, primary health teams, ways of improving premises should all be financially and practically introduced. Money should be paid to compensate for the expenses of inner-city life. Selection – now made on the basis of whether applicants have five years GP experience – should be much more rigorous. GPs should be paid each time someone signs on, to compensate for high mobility. And so on.

Acheson's solution will cost money. So far the Government has decided to allocate £3 million to improve practice premises and to provide 'incentives' for GPs to retire (thus backing away from compulsory retirement). That is all. The rest is accepted 'in principle', but no one knows how long it will be before it is implemented.

We should now look briefly at the three more general problems of the inner cities; overseas GPs, unemployment, the old. Each brings us closer to, and with the old we are back in, the mainstream, once again at the centre of the major preoccupations of our lives and those of our GPs.

25

OVERSEAS GPs

DR THRIPLOW: 'At that time training wasn't mandatory – ten years ago – and the only response we got was from an Indian. He completed his year with us and he was very good. He went down very well with the local people. But he was very lonely here. There was nobody locally for him. He had to travel miles to meet any friends.'

DR SIMON KIBANE: 'When we advertised last year we had ninety-five applications. When we boiled it down by excluding the black population, we had about fifteen left. I don't know why I feel guilty about it, but I do. The written letters and curriculum vitae seemed much better from those who had graduated from an English university. But there's too much bias involved. I don't think I'm free of bias, I suspect.'

DR JANET KIBANE: 'The senior partner wouldn't have countenanced a Pakistani in the practice or an Indian, which were predominant. Yet we have 8 per cent Pakistani patients so it wouldn't have been to our disadvantage to have employed one.'

DR AXMOUTH: 'It's a hidden thing in general practice, you'll find quite a lot of white doctors, to my embarrassment, will be extremely rude about Indian, Pakistani and other foreign graduates in a blanket way. "Oh yes, our esteemed colleagues – ho ho ho," you know. I've seen a lot of curriculum vitaes in the applications who in various ways have been propping up this rotten health service of ours for years and years and years and are now finally trying to get out of their very tangled hospital careers and into general practice, and having a hell of a time and one feels very much for them.' (But Dr Axmouth was not going to pick an overseas doctor as the next partner.)

DR YETTS: 'He had such good references, and he was engaged to a white nurse from Oldham – she was a very, very nice girl and we thought, "Well, we'll just show that we are broad-minded, etc. etc. We'll take him." And it was a complete disaster. He didn't integrate with the rest of the practice at all. He spent as much time as he could sitting on his own in his room reading medical books and journals and things. He got on fairly well with a few middle-class patients. Most of the patients disliked him intensely. He wasn't doing his share of work in the practice and the time came when the rest of us were all agitating, agitating, agitating at the senior partner and saying, "Look, what are you doing about this?" He went to the senior partner and said, "Look, I'm going to Nottingham." It was a disaster, and he was a good one.'

DR SUGNAL: 'You can just be a doctor, do your job and clear off. Big lists, crash through, don't talk to your patients, just get through them and have a lot on your list. You can make a lot of money in a 9 to 5 job. A lot of Indians do very well financially.'

PROFESSOR MORRELL: 'We've got Indian and Pakistani doctors who are a great help. But variable, very variable. Two from Ceylon who are very good. But the whole Indian way of thinking is very different from the British way of thinking in terms of medicine. They don't solve problems in the same way as we do – they tend to learn things and try and apply them in a stereotyped way and it doesn't work like that in general practice because general practice isn't like that. There are too many variables you have to take in.'

DR RIARD: 'They have problems, to start off with, with their education system. Right from school onwards, it seems to me from everything I've heard from them, it militates against problem-solving, but towards remembering things. So they have enormous problems with, for example, our examination system here. Then, obviously, it's enormously difficult to come from a completely alien culture and then practise our particular kind of medicine. Open heart surgery would be a doddle. Or they're responding to immigrant roots themselves and there one has to remember two things. Here the immigrant root may be a very different root from their own. We tend to see immigrant doctors as a kind of amorphous mass but the difference of culture and country and race are as enormous between them as certainly any group of Europeans. And goodness knows how I would survive in France as a doctor, even if I could speak the language more fluently than I do. As I said, we can make judgements. I think they do represent a different sort of problem from home-bred doctors. And it is an education thing, a cultural thing. Nothing to do with intelligence, or ability, or even commitment, because if you have the sons of those overseas doctors, or overseas immigrants, going to our medical schools, who've had an English education, then they are among the brightest and the best doctors that we've got. It's entirely a question of the wrong preparation, I think, for the kind of doctors we need. It is, therefore, simply a question of time.'

Hard evidence of the complete picture is difficult to come by. *Pulse* is regularly filled with reports of overseas doctors almost automatically being turned down. One applicant sent off 300 applications and received only eight interviews. A GP who sits on a committee vetting applications in the Highlands said that out of fourteen who tried for a practice in a corner of Mull in 1980, six were Indians; for another remote island, seven out of fifteen were Indians. He conjured up a desperate picture of dozens of Indians wildly applying for the most distant, strange and unsuitable practices.

Cartwright offers no evidence as to whether the evident and widespread prejudice is justified in terms of skills or not. She notes only that overseas GPs are more common in health centres than elsewhere, that they are less likely than other GPs to see family matters as their province (29 per cent as compared to 69 per cent) but regarded it as more important that each family had the same GP (50 per cent compared to 24 per cent).

My efforts to find out for myself were frustrated, as I explained in the Introduction.

The one overseas GP I did manage to see was not totally reassuring.

Dr Rushdi

Dr Rushdi was a single-handed practitioner on a large inner city council estate in the north. Naturalized, married to an Englishwoman, he had been there twelve years. He was round, smooth, courteous, gentle and kind; he insisted on sending out for fish-and-chips which I ate out of a surgical bowl on a stand. We talked in his large warm surgery which had an efficient gas fire and was lined with medical books, also some Islamic tomes on his religion. He spoke excellent English.

He had qualified in Pakistan in 1963. It was a new school but 'the traditions were well set, even in a medical school which started in 1950. Very very up to date. The staff really lovingly taught us, and brought the moral fibre on.'

He came to England, did neurosurgery house jobs, was eventually asked to join the Irishman who had this practice and took it over when the doctor retired in 1970.

He seemed quite perfect. He had an age-sex register. He had the new A4 record forms in a large file, instead of the tatty, bulging little envelopes, like some administrative remnant of the war, which many GPs are sentimental about. He had a full list, and devoted two hours to each surgery, two surgeries a day. He felt most problems were social problems and were learnt from the families. 'We also learn alcoholism similarly from families. The wife wouldn't come and say "My husband is drinking" but you can always tell the tension is overflowing.' He felt his 'oriental sympathy' helped here. He also gave a lot more time. But he enjoyed this side. 'They really demand an equally investigating mind to find those challenges, a rewarding job.' He didn't think they were trivial.

He did about twelve visits a day, and never refused one. 'I never really say no to anybody.'

But it was in preventative medicine that he reached his peak. He gave a picture of successive and intense waves of attack. Three years before it had been hypertension. Within a year there had been a marked reduction of strokes and heart attacks. He felt he'd cracked hypertension. Then it was children with asthma, which had lasted two years. Now he was concentrating on diabetes.

He had three Pakistani families in the practice and they were maddening. These were easily the worst patients in his practice. One was the priest's family. 'They will not communicate. The women will always tell their husbands "I need my pill", and he will leave it to the last minute and at 8 p.m. he will ring me, "Can I have the pill?". I say, "You can have the pill, but how short are you?" and he says, "We ran out last night." Such a thing. It happened again and again and again.'

Another equally maddening family 'is just not conforming to anything. We told them, "This is the surgery time" – they'll come half an hour after, and you see half a dozen family load of people walking into the surgery, expecting to have a cup of tea as well, and two hours' chat as well and then be driven to their house as well. This is true.'

And so Dr Rushdi smoothly flowed on. The one temptation to doctors he felt was, 'They should not want to get rich, because if they want to get rich all the time they cloud the whole situation.' He thought GPs should retire at sixty-five. He kept up to date, courses and so on, he'd just been on an 'intensive refresher for a week'.

Yet I could somehow get no grip on amiable, kindly Dr Rushdi. Also I happened to know that he was losing a good many patients to the next door practice. His ex-patients complained bitterly he frequently refused to visit, and not just at night. I also suspected, and later confirmed, that his hypertension achievements were, to put it bluntly, pure crap. It would take ten to fifteen years before the sort of marked differences he claimed might start to show up. Finally, he said he telephoned his numerous relatives in Pakistan a great deal, but it did 'cost me a lot'. I wondered why, like other GPs, he didn't charge the customary 90 per cent of his telephone bill to tax. Perhaps he was fighting that temptation to become rich – the only GP who mentioned it to me as being a temptation.

26

UNEMPLOYMENT

DR KINSHAM: 'People don't tend to say much when they're unemployed usually. They tend to be a bit passive. They become passive after a year or so, and they don't complain much.'

HEALTH VISITOR (Dr Bilsby's practice): 'We see more dads. They sit watching the telly.'

DR ABNEY: 'Out of jobs; out of job teenagers; parents absolutely desperate. *Desperate*. They've got them at home all day long. There aren't that number of the sort of Youth Opportunity Scheme jobs round here. No, that's the most devastating thing I think, you know, and we may well have it ourselves. Our son, I can't see is frightfully jobworthy at the moment and I don't think that he stands out for employment. I mean, supposing we had all his 6 foot 3 inches, seventeen, around the whole time – he'd drive us both bonkers. I adore him – he's a super chap. All he thinks of is crumpet and money and if he's not getting both . . . Well, the money comes from us at the moment but he likes work. He works on the land in the holidays to get money to buy things – to buy stereos and cars and if he can't get a job – nightmare. His philosophy is that the job gets in money to enjoy himself. Well, OK, that's fair enough. On the other hand, if he *doesn't* get that job and he *doesn't* get the money, and he's round our shoulders all day long, what the hell are we to do? I mean, you can see it. You see, youth unemployment round here is high. And it's not the youth that comes in, but the parents – *desperate*.'

DR KERRIS: 'How it actually shows up in people is that some people come more often to the surgery and some people stay away. I think I've observed that a lot of people stay away really. They just lead boring tedious unhealthy lives, but they're not *so* ill that they have to come to the doctor and that sort of strain often comes out, not in the unemployed person himself, but it comes out in the rest of the family. The fact that he's around all the time and the fact that the *mood* – it's as much a mood thing as an illness thing. No self-esteem, and it just devastates families. Or the wife might get a little job, or what they call a "little job" which means a big job for little money, which upsets him again because he then feels resentful that she's having to go out to work.

'I think these surveys which show that people get desperately ill as soon as they're unemployed, I don't think it's quite as simple as that. There's a lot of work from Harvey Brenner and all that stuff. All sorts of multiple factors – poverty, changes in relationships and stress and things like that. Very, very complicated, and it is going to be a major thing because it is going to change people – the old family structure is just completely different now.

'The other thing that happens is that the other people who *are* still in work are terribly fearful about unemployment. They take risks and break legs and things like that because, say, there's one guy, in his fifties, who *was* able to cope at work – a slinger, which means when they have to lift big bits of steel, fitting ropes or fitting things round for the crane driver to take away. There's a lot of heavy lifting as well – the chains and manoeuvring these big bits of red-hot steel. I don't know exactly what he does, but it is a heavy job which he was able to cope with. But now, there have been redundancies. Two things have happened: one, that he is dead scared that he'll be redundant, and that makes him sort of take risks in the job, be seen to be active and put himself in a good light, and everything like that, whereas before he was able to pace himself. And the other thing is that a few of his mates have been made unemployed. Out of a gang of eight, there are now three or four or whatever it is. So he has to physically do a different job, twice as much, so it puts a lot of strain on people.

'It's something like 18 per cent unemployment around here. I'm not quite sure of the latest figures because there's a lot more mobility amongst the people who are unemployed; that's my observation. And people come at a very late stage for getting off sick, because if you're off sick a lot then you'll be the first person on the dole, and so they come very late, whether it's a bad chest or with a sprained ankle, or something like that, or infected finger. You've got to really beg people to take time off. And now there's almost no ill certification at all. I know the rules have just changed, but even allowing for that, people just don't come and ask for time off work, hardly at all. They're absolutely petrified by the current situation. So it's not as simple as just people who have been unemployed suddenly getting illnesses, although that does happen as well.'

27

THE OLD

We are not really designed by nature for old age. During the millenia during which we evolved, two or three million years, the fossil evidence shows that Homo sapiens died fairly young – twenty to thirty was old. (This is the reason, incidentally, why we are sexually at our most active and most fertile when young.) There was, that is to say, no particular reason during this long period for organs to be efficient into the seventies and eighties. The urino-genital system in the ageing male is almost ridiculously inefficient.

Not only did man not evolve to live into extreme old age, the pressure to pass on any evolutionary move which would have facilitated this was extremely mild. To breed such a development in and reinforce it really required the breeding of *two* old people; but women became infertile between forty and fifty, while men became less active and less fertile. Of course, a few old men will mate with younger women and pass on their own age-efficient genes (that is why longevity tends to run in families). Also those who have age-efficient genes will mate when young and may choose, by chance, a partner who also has age-efficient genes. It is also possible that age-efficient means that, by living longer, someone amasses wealth, and will give (or would have done in primitive societies) a better chance of mating to children and grandchildren. But there is no clear evidence of this. All we can say is that there is mild evolutionary pressure to live longer (a strong heart and good lungs are of use when young too); but that there is not the full-scale pressure that breeds in intelligence, for example, or breeds out infertility.

It is not surprising, therefore, if as we get older we begin to suffer from an increasing amount of major and minor illnesses, diseases and inconveniences. Over sixty-five, 25 per cent of us will have major disorders – chronic conditions of the respiratory, circulatory and urino-genital systems; 25 per cent will have minor disorders. All will be experiencing unpleasant developmental changes.

There are problem areas I had no idea existed. Feet, for example, are a major problem area. Few people over seventy-five can cut their own toenails, and many who are younger can't. It is here that Dr Telscombe's plasticine big toes, which made a brief, giant and slightly bizarre appearance earlier, slot into place. Yet there is a chronic shortage of chiropodists – and the lack is a major reason old people go off their feet. 'And chiropodists,' said Tim

Cerney, 'do far more than just cut toenails. They are often dealing with feet which are very distorted, which have a lot of callouses, which need padding and cutting and shaping. There are a lot of conditions chiropodists can diagnose and report – verrucas, for instance, or circulatory problems we might miss.'

These conditions require regular visits rather than crisis calls, and this raises an interesting, if slightly divergent, question about the future patterns of medical practice. One of the things that may have struck you, comparing the patterns before the war with those that have been unfolding as we progress, is that there has been some decline in personal doctoring. The feeling that they are being distanced from their patients worries a number of GPs. We must return to this, but the most convincing evidence that this is so comes from home visits. These have declined steadily and significantly – from being 22 per cent of a GPs work in 1971 to 16 per cent in 1977. Infrequent visits have dropped by a quarter. Cartwright thinks it possible we may reach the state of America, where there aren't any home visits at all.

But as the number of old people increases, so will the necessity for regular home visits. The pattern of general practice could well change back to what it was before. Certainly, I found evidence of this. In practices where the proportion of old people was high this certainly could happen – as with Dr Cerney's. Dr Thriplow, with 25 per cent over sixty-five and 10 per cent over seventy did 'look-in visits, things like that, putting your face round the door. Probably makes our prescribing rate rather higher than the rest of the country because old people, you tend to treat chest infections more vigorously, prescribe antibiotics quicker.'

This isn't an inevitable development. Some doctors don't see it as a doctoring problem. Professor Morrell says: 'We need a team approach. *We* can't help them. The nurses *can*. And home helps and people to bathe them – that's what they need. The doctor needs to be a good organizer of resources, but really he can't do much with his bare hands.'

My own view, to complete this, is that it will lead to more personal doctoring – at least as it is perceived by the patient. Some GPs will respond, like Thriplow and Cerney. Others will utilize their team. But Cartwright also shows that patients see the team, especially the nurse, as evidence of the GPs wider scope – that is to say, the nurse emanates from the GP and is part of his care. The net result will be an increase in personal care.

One thing is not in doubt. At this moment 13 per cent of the population is over sixty–five, by 2005 it is likely to be 19 per cent. (Along the South Coast – the Costa Geriatrica – it is already 33 per cent.) Does this mean a flood of steadily ageing figures gradually losing their powers and wits and requiring, fairly urgently, the building of giant near-mausoleums packed with beds? No one really seems to know about this. Some GPs think that all that is happening is that far more people are living to the age the old always did.

*   *   *

DR YETTS: 'The theory's been put forward that we needn't worry too much about people getting older and older because there seems to be a failure rate at about eighty. You know, that's a mean, so between seventy-five and eighty-five most people are gone just through natural senescence. We're programmed to live that long. This is a theory I've heard put forward recently and it makes sense. All our antibiotics, all that stuff, aren't going to make that much difference. More people may live to be sixty or seventy but not many more people are going to live to ninety, than did before.'

Dr Yett's confidence may be misplaced. Certainly this is not happening in America. According to the US Census Bureau, America is aging at a great rate. By July 1983 there were more Americans over sixty-five than in their teens. In forty years there will be twice as many pensioners as teenagers. And the faster-growing section of that elderly population is that known as the 'old old' or 'frail old' – the over eighty-fives. They are *not* just conveniently dying.

The likelihood is that we will follow the same pattern. We do so in other and similar social and medical fields, and have so far done so in this one. It is significant that energetic moves are now being made to improve our diet on lines common in the States for the last seven years.

Our cost pattern will be the same too. At the moment 28 per cent of the US medical budget is spent on those over sixty-five. The cost of dealing with each over-sixty-five rises 7 per cent faster than that of dealing with the rest of the population.

No doubt the old will be dealt with somehow or other, but to do so adequately will require billions of pounds. Can we afford this? Again, no one really knows. But there are convincing forecasts that by 1990-95 one tenth of the workforce will be able to produce all that we need. That is, thanks to technology, the country will be able to support a 25 per cent 65-100 population. If we will it. You could argue that if 25 per cent of the population is over sixty-five then we *will* will it. This is not certain. In Britain, the elderly vote less than other people.

The cost becomes clear if we look at what the NHS provisions are for the old in the GP community set-up. Quite apart from their drugs and medicines and operations, their zimmers and chairs and sticks and crutches, their in-continence pads, belts, loops, ladles, cradles, hoists, bars, belts, mats and other such movable equipment – all free – there is the vastly expensive accommodation structure.

There are usually three or four stages. First, comes a warden-assisted bungalow: half a dozen or a dozen little bungalows, looked after by a warden where you can either entirely cook for yourself or partly rely on council-provided meals. Next can come the same sort of thing, only a small flat, one of sixty or so under the same roof, with wardens, and the possibility of communal meals. Then comes part three accommodation, which is essentially an old people's home. Some are specially designed and built with comfortable bed-sitting rooms; far more are adapted old houses and fairly grim. Finally, there is the long-term geriatric hospital which is just a bed.

The variation across the country upon this is too great to make giving examples helpful, though as with other GP facilities the southern counties seem particularly well-equipped.

There were areas where long-term geriatric beds were in good supply, but they were rare. Endless battles rage – the GPs that have them trying to keep their own ten or twelve beds free for all the many uses they have for them; the consultants and area hospitals trying to get rid of the elderly who had come in with something acute and were now ready to be returned.

'The houseman will ring up,' said Dr Veryan, standing in his little GP ward and staring gloomily at what seemed little better than a corpse, 'and say, "Please can you take this patient. He's mobile and we're getting him up and about." We try and get more details but they're very devious, because this chap in fact wasn't mobile at all. He was paralysed in a stroke and he's incontinent and inarticulate and unable to do anything and he's been here nine months and he should really be in a geriatric bed where they're geared to cope with him.' He described how a woman consultant in his last practice had always kept one geriatric permanently in an ambulance waiting to be rushed into the first vacant bed in a long-term geriatric ward. 'Some of them must have driven thousands of miles, round and round and round.'

DR JANE EDSTONE: 'Over sixty-five we have, I think, an abysmal consultant who is absolutely useless. He just absolves himself from any unpleasant situations. He's always on holiday as far as I can make out. I've had two or three old people who were completely berserk. You can't cope with a really demented old lady who – well there is one just round the corner who literally had to be held down. From Friday to Sunday I was waiting for this wretched man to come back from his holiday. On Sunday when you let go she was rushing around, out the door, up the stairs and into the street, screaming and yelling.

'One uses everything one can. I know when I was in the west I had an old woman of eighty-two. She was formidable. She was built like an ox and was looked after by a very harassed daughter and son-in-law – or daughter-in-law, I think. And she kept falling out of bed. It was when there were no beds. But I rang up and said, "Please. I can't stand it any longer. The relatives can't." And he said, "I'm sorry, there just aren't any." I burst into tears and put the phone down and he rang me back and said, "Were you crying?", and I said "Yes", and he said, "All right, send her in." I wasn't putting it one, but I suppose a man wouldn't have burst into tears. I think it's the only time I've used being a woman, incidentally, and then I didn't mean to.'

A lot of people are looked after by relatives with jobs. As they become infirm, they either go into hospitals or the relative gives up their job. Yet they don't really need to go and rot in a hospital. A recent solution is day-care centres. I saw several of these, some so elaborate they were called day-care hospitals.

The Day-Care Hospital

The sister was Sister May Brown, plump, with a soft, serious, oval face like a nun, and wide, kind, brown eyes. She had a lilting Liverpudlian accent.

She'd left nursing and then come back. She'd gone into geriatrics with some trepidation. 'It's not a popular area for nurses. It's hard work, it's heavy. And before, when I'd trained, a geriatric ward smelled of incontinence, and they just lay in bed in white nighties and there was no *idea* of rehabilitation.'

Then by chance she'd been asked to relieve on a geriatric ward. And it had been a revelation. The consultant had been inspired. She'd suddenly realized you could help the old. They would respond. 'Because your expectations aren't too high, when you do have a success it's even more rewarding. It's amazing how much improvement can be made with so many of them.'

And she found she enjoyed it. 'I have a good rapport with elderly people; I love their company. If you've got time to listen to them they are fascinating.'

There was also something to do with her mother, who was dead, which gave her work an extra depth. This was too personal to tell me but I guessed, from a number of things she let slip, the general import.

The day-care hospital was more than a day-care centre. It cost as much as a hospital and for that reason they only came three days a week.

SISTER MAY BROWN: 'If you can stand getting up at 6 o'clock in the morning to be ready at 8 for the ambulance [old people require time to get ready] and then be bounced around while they pick other people up and not get back till 5.30 then, if you have the strength for that, you don't need four days a week. If you need more than three days a week, you've got severe problems and probably require hospital. But they love it. We've one old fellow wants to come every day.'

It costs as much as a hospital but was far better for them. It was run by the district authority but attached to Dr Chathill's cottage hospital, and they made full use of it.

The physiotherapy room was wide, bright, light and sunny; it was humming with activity, packed with equipment – two long, adjustably heighted parallel bars with a large mirror at the end to help the old recover the ability to walk; a small practice staircase like an Olympic podium with adjustable banisters and steps of different heights to practise climbing stairs; stationary bicycles for exercise. (Sister May noticed that the feet of one old man kept slipping forward, making his task harder.) There was a seat with pedals for those who'd topple off a stationary bicycle (the old lady on this had fallen asleep – 'They sleep in the day, then they don't sleep at night and get muddled about what time it is'). There were beds with pulleys and straps for getting old limbs to work again, ultra-sound for vibrating the tissues, facilities for wax baths for arthritis. The old people moved about on their zimmers heading for the next piece of equipment. There was none of the hopelessness I'd noticed before, or subdued irritation from the nurses.

Off the physio room were baths. They only bathed those who couldn't get in and out themselves, but it was a great time for confiding. Every morning there was a conference over coffee, the consultant, the physiotherapists, the social workers, nurses and the occupational therapists meeting to discuss each patient, plan for the day. In fact they had a project going at the moment, if I'd care to look at it.

This was next door in a large open plan area, divided up – I saw cookers in one, tables with bent figures weaving in another, chairs round a piano. The project was a whole series of photographs.

SISTER MAY BROWN: 'This lady, that was when she was seventeen, and she's now ninety-six. That gentleman isn't here today, there's his grandmother. He's eighty. It stimulates them no end. We're having a competition. They'll have a go guessing who everybody is. And they start talking, "Oh, I had a hat like that," "My mother used to do that." I've found it very enjoyable. You can visualize them as a young person, with the problems of a young person, the loves. They've lost sweethearts during the war, and children. It's part of their personality.

'There's a great thing about recall therapy. They don't remember things so well now because the input is faulty. But if you stimulate the past it makes them confident. We have one lady, she's very timid and frightened. We were looking at pictures of London and so on. It meant nothing. But then there was a picture of Liverpool, the pierhead plus the Liver Building, she became alive. I knew it too – but it was moving, her face suddenly got animated.'

She showed me the cookers, where they had baking sessions, and where people used to gas were retrained on electric for the warden flats. One old man was being retrained. Outside was a therapy garden with raised beds, and a greenhouse with doors wide enough for wheelchairs and benches of varying heights for the flowerpots. They had young nurses, and one of the physiotherapists had a young family who used to run in and out. 'But you don't want too many young. They feel comfortable with one another, they encourage each other, can go at their own pace.' On market day they went to market. A young hairdresser came once a week to do their hair.

SISTER MAY BROWN: 'We have two people who come in and play the piano and records and we have a sing-song. Older songs from the war years, music hall, all sorts. We had a session the other week went down very well. They were singing their heads off.'

The old are a problem to all GPs; the facilities, the response, the degree of care, the comments they made, differed with each doctor, each area, each team.

DR THRIPLOW: 'In the main old people are treated at home rather than in homes or hospitals. It isn't easy to get beds in these places and for most of them the family units still survive, so you get them caring for the patient. It's the odd one with no family that you really are sorry for but there is an incredible family, neighbourly spirit here. They keep an eye open, so if they are living next door to an old person they notice if they haven't taken their milk in, and that sort of thing, and they will go and see what is happening. And they will ring us if they are worried about them. There is very much more of the extended family: grandmothers, uncles, brothers, sisters, all living still in the area so there is much more support there.'

DR WARFIELD: 'Well – how do we cope? We've got all reasonable expertise in geriatrics – you've got to if you're going to stand up. The consultant geriatrician is damn good here. He'll come in and do a domiciliary within two days, or he'll take them in if the problem is such it cannot be dealt with at home.'

DR KIBANE (speaking of his post as clinical assistant at the local geriatric hospital): 'Yes I do. Do I enjoy anything? Insomuch as I enjoy anything, yes I enjoy it, yes. Because I enjoy the contact with people who are working as a team: physiotherapists, occupational therapists, the nurses. I enjoy taking them in and then reassessing them medically, and then putting them out with a different assessment to what they came in with. And I see the problems that other GPs have at the same time. It goes back to my own practice. You go to someone in their house and they're sat in – they got up that morning and it took them two hours to get dressed. They've got three corsets or roll-ons and several bras and eight petticoats and another dress, and nylons and shoes, and a cardigan, and they say, "I've got a pain in my stomach." If you want to examine them it's a major effort, virtually an operation. So, you know, to some extent I understand the problems when people come into hospital and the GP has sent them with pains in their stomach, and they've got a big tumour there, you can feel it easily, the size of a grapefruit – why the hell didn't the GP spot this? The poor GP, when they were in their armchair in front of their fire in their sixty-one petticoats, there was no way he could get *at* them.'

DR KERRIS: 'In a place like this there are fantastic services, really, amazing. Community work for the elderly – we've got a domiciliary physiotherapist for the elderly, we've got our own nurse for the elderly, we've got a team of social workers and community workers for the elderly people. We run a club for elderly mentally confused people. All sorts of church organizations.

'But how come it's the doctor's job to do something about that? It's to do with the aims of society at all sorts of levels – that people are left alone and all sorts of services and doctors have to pick up the pieces. It's political, really, that the people, in order to service the industries of the shape we've got, have had to be mobile, to have smaller families, to move away. Things like housing policy means that all the houses here are built in small units with two bedrooms and a teeny weeny box room, so there's no chance of the old mother staying. So it doesn't surprise me that the casualties are the people who are non-productive. We are really picking up the pieces that result from structural changes in society – sweeping families apart – which I believe actually effect the grannies you've been seeing. And the same things have actually often killed their husbands off anyway.'

Walking down the long, close-packed rows in local geriatric hospitals, going into yet another tiny warden-assisted bungalow or flat, whether in Newcastle or Glasgow, Bristol or Brighton or London, virtually the same, smelling the same thick smell, I often wondered – is it to produce this that the huge engine of modern medicine has worked and is still working? Was it for this that drains and houses and reservoirs were rebuilt, that all those antibiotics and the rest discovered? The end is often so long and difficult, happiness has to be fought for so hard.

Are they unhappy?

Few of the hospitals are like the day hospital of Sister Brown. Far more – 'Happy? No, why should they be? They are looked after well, they are kept bodily warm, fed. It's not a life, it's existing isn't it? For people who have had their own home, could do what they want, they have to go to bed at 8 o'clock because it suits the nurses. They have to rely on other people to carry out their bodily functions. Would you like it?'

And the others? The focus narrows and narrows, the wants become few. The old man reading a newspaper, hardly by word, almost letter by letter with a large magnifying glass – yet rapt. Dr Cerney said, 'I don't think they are unhappy if they are not lonely. Loneliness is worst. You could say, unhappiness *is* loneliness.' Yet, surely, many of them must be very lonely. They wouldn't brighten at the doctor's visit so much otherwise.

Telly has arrived in the nick of time, coinciding with the arrival of mass old age and able to make it tolerable, if soporific.

And then the old couples very close again, the basic drive now binding them together as strong or stronger than love or sex or children, the drive to preserve life itself. So, mutually dependent, the old RSM and his wife saw their future move, instinctively, in terms of the other. He said she'd get down to the shops easier; she that he'd be close to his one remaining friend. With them, she'd had three heart attacks and he'd been looking after her; now, with his stroke, there was a reversal. So old age does show, still, great achievements of the human spirit: courage and cheerfulness in adversity, the uses of love, above all stoicism in the face of death. Death becomes the great reality.

28
DEATH

DR ANNE UPLEES: 'I prefer not to be the one that tells them. Usually people have had things done to them in hospital and they get told in hospital, which I much prefer, or they don't get told, which means their relatives will. And then, if the relatives say they don't want him or her to know, then that's fine by me. I'm not quite sure, I haven't made up my mind whether people should know or not. But I guess that some people should and some people shouldn't. But how you tell those, I don't know. So I'm quite happy not to, unless pushed into it.'

DR JANE EDSTONE: 'I'm afraid I very rarely do. Usually people say, "I'm not going to die, am I?" and you say, "Well, we are all going to die sometime and I think we should be prepared for it." You'd always want to think there's a chink of hope. Don't you think so? They don't want to know. They always phrase it, "I'm not going to die, am I?" and not to go and say, "You are", but to say, "Well, you may. People don't always recover."

'I have told people. Once it was a success and twice it was a disaster. And it was so much a disaster that since then I have always left it as a rather indeterminate thing. With the disaster they were quite simply terrified. They said, "I can face it. I can take the truth. Am I going to die?" And after they'd said that so many times, I said, "Well, yes. You probably will," and then they were on the phone incessantly. Calling me out. Just panic. Not because they were ill – or any iller – but because they were frightened of dying. They thought if they shut their eyes and went to sleep, they wouldn't wake up.'

DR DOLWAR: 'I don't think you should tell people lies, frankly. People usually will accept the oblique remark and know more or less what's going on. Again, they don't always need to be told the bare bones and the absolute truth. And if they are, there's always a ring of optimism that they may be able to, it may be controllable. It may be possible to, if you can't completely eradicate your cancer, then you can keep it in check. You can live with it for a long, long time – that sort of thing. People will accept that sort of idea.'

DR WARFIELD: 'Consultants are not always good at handling patients. They are poor at managing people. One of the academic unit saw one of my partner's patients who'd got an inoperable carcinoma of the stomach. Instead of easing the blow for his family he said, "I'm afraid you've got a cancer of the stomach which is inoperable and the time limit is such and such." You just *don't* say things to a patient like that. Give them time. You go round the subject; you let it sink in gently and subtly, you inculcate the idea that things are not too good, but you don't come out with a blunt statement. And that's what happened to a patient, and the patient was absolutely shattered.'

DR YETTS: 'It's very unpleasant when you're met at the door by the wife who says, "You're not going to tell him. You mustn't tell him, will you?" and that means a problem in the relationship between the husband and the wife, which is a pity. The most comfortable thing is, "Well, you do what you think best, doctor." Or the most fascinating thing that I had once – this is another breast cancer – a youngish woman – and the husband was there and a grown-up daughter was there and she was working with some Christian mission, or something, somewhere, and had come to look after mum and I said to them, "Do you want me to tell your wife?" They said, "You shouldn't have to do that sort of thing, doctor. If anybody tells her, it should be us." They were horrified because they felt it was their responsibility and I thought that was marvellous, that they had taken that responsibility upon themselves. That's rare.'

DR THRIPLOW: 'I can think of many cases where we've visited two or three times a day. It's something I do quite happily. It's the *least* you can do, somehow. And another thing, we usually go and visit people after somebody's died. I think it's a help to the family to talk over why they died. Often they feel vaguely guilty or they wonder whether anything else could have been done and it often helps to air it at that stage. But we try and keep them at home as much as possible.

'The ones that do have to go in, I'm not very happy about because I don't think they get very good care. The local geriatric chronic sick ward where most of these terminally ill go is pretty grim. I don't think I'd like to send my mother there. I don't think I'd like to go there myself, certainly.

'Telling them is *very* difficult.

'I have one particular patient in my practice whose husband died of cancer of the lung and for a long time the family begged us not to say he had cancer. Anyway, one day he asked outright, "Have I got cancer?" and my partner said, "Yes, you have", and from that minute he perked up. His wife said later they were able to talk freely; they were able to make plans; he could plan out what was best for the future. There was no pretence that he was going to get better. And she said those last couple of months were the happiest of the lot whereas when everybody had been hiding it, everybody pretended that he was going to get better, there was a funny atmosphere. So I think at some time in the illness, the moment comes when you can break the news, and it doesn't seem to have any bad effects.'

DR ABNEY: 'I think the difficulty is with the younger people. You know, one gets some people who are absolutely coldly clinical. A chap up the road, only forty-two, about three years ago who'd got a really frightful kidney growth and it was one of those things that he was highly intelligent, a very gifted musician and his wife is a musician and they've got three children. Oh, it started so simply. He was well in January and desperately ill in July and then had a sort of remission and went on and on and on getting slightly worse and needing more and more attention. You know, the hospital were terribly good. They'd have him in for part of the day if it was difficult, and she could take him over there just for a bit of physio or a bit of something if he needed this, that or that done, they kept a bed open for him, which was marvellous. But he was terribly perceptive and wanted to know everything in the *minutest* detail; when he was going to die, how it was going to happen and everything. I found that a terrific strain. I really was absolutely done in. The hospital staff were absolutely whacked at the end of that. He would want to know the pathology; everything, absolutely in the minutest detail, and he questioned everybody whenever he went in.'

DR RUSHDI: 'My attitude to death – I'm a Moslem – is very, very open. We accept death, we're ready for it, any day, any minute. Never really shocked about it. There are no hang-ups about it – it happens to everyone. Many a time I say, "Find me a 200-year-old man or woman." It doesn't matter how many health precautions and how much money we can spend. We haven't got a 200-year-old in the world so we're all going some time.'

What can the books, the surveys, the studies tell us?

Not the least surprising thing about the training for medical students is that they are taught nothing at all about death – not how to break it, not how to deal psychologically with the dying, nor with the relatives afterwards.

Perhaps the thought is, death is something you can't teach. Yet it is one of the most sensitive and most difficult areas they will have to deal with. One would have thought the medical schools, however tentatively, might have given some thought to it. And the books, the studies, the surveys tell us very little.

Glin Bennet says it is the thing doctors are worst at. Thrust abruptly among the dying as students, they throw up defences, which are strengthened later as they become fearful of their own mortality. That is why they usually tell relatives, not patients – largely to spare themselves. He quotes, approvingly, Illich's maxim that in a cure-orientated profession, dying is 'The ultimate form of consumer resistance.'

Illich, incidentally, in a typically muddled and spurious passage in a typically muddled and spurious book, *Limits to Medicine*, is monumentally unhelpful. He compares the shallow, modern linking of death with 'causes', which can allow doctors or hospitals to be blamed, with a more primitive 'natural' view of death, where it was seen as an intrinsic part of life, and this gave death 'dignity'. (How do you give 'death' dignity? The person dying can have dignity; death itself is inhuman and has no human attributes.) The current view of death is equally 'intrinsic', it is simply that the mechanism of that 'intrinsicity' is better understood. Where doctors or hospitals get that mechanism wrong and allow someone to die who might have lived fruitfully for an appreciable time, why should they not be blamed? The present view of death may involve some people not facing up to it, but that has always been so. The Illich 'death is natural' view is romantic and sentimental claptrap, and invokes an invented, imagined tribal past. The remote past we know nothing about – hunter-gatherers very probably killed the aged in their tribes. In the past we do know, tribes and more lately Christians and other religions believed and believe in various forms of survival after death – i.e. that death doesn't exist.

But, to return, I don't think doctors are worst at death. It seemed to me that nearly all of them dealt with it courageously and compassionately, and that their experience was hard won – as I hope what they said bears out. Indeed, that experience is in essence all one can learn about death and how to deal with it. But I did read two or three other things, somewhat at random, which struck me.

In *Sociology in Medicine**, a book in fact written for nurses, R.J. and P.A. Jones suggested a view of death as a graded series of events: continent, forgetful, in a wheelchair, incontinent, occasionally incoherent, disorient-ated, etc. etc. ending finally, in coma and death. If the nurses, or the family, know this, acknowledge it and help *fight* each stage, and respect the patient's fight and value him during it, then it is possible to talk to the patient about it. The patient will accept death as the *eventual* and inevitable end, but it will be, in the sense that it is a battle, a positive process.

Bad news, death, is often broken in clichés. A cliché is a devalued and therefore weaker way of putting something.

The older people are the less they are affected by deaths. But being affected is also a process. Like the progress to death itself, grief has stages. The beginning, which can last hours, days or months, is characterized by numbness, punctuated by bursts of anger and acute distress.

The middle period is one of painful pining, with memories, continually gone over, of the events which led to the death. There are strong feelings that the dead person is present, and a desire to search for them as animals and children do. The sufferer may think these are signs of impending madness and is afraid to mention them. They get less in a week or two. People may be avoided as sympathy brings back the pain. A scapegoat is sought and is

Sociology in Medicine, by R.J. and P.A. Jones, English Universities Press Ltd., 1975

frequently the medical profession. This can be to relieve feelings of guilt which, if excessive, may need help.

The final stage, which lasts for about a year, brings depression, apathy, listlessness. By the end of the second year life will usually have been reorganized. Grief may never entirely go, but it should not affect or disorganize the bereaved person's life.

Many cultures have evolved rituals to help people through these stages. We have abandoned all but the funeral. The period of mourning is no longer practised.

Paul Ferris in his excellent book, *The Doctors*, quotes a study of patients in the last months of their lives; 'three quarters were well aware that they were dying'. But the range of reactions is large and often strange.

DR ABBERLEY: 'And it's a very strange thing, but nature is merciful. Among the things that might interest you is that I've been going to the gaol here for many years and in the early days I did a lot more – I was a locum there. Soon after I got there – this was many years ago – I'd seen the evening receptions, the chaps who'd come in, and the hospital officer said, "By the way, before you go home, I'd like you to see the CCs." So I asked what that was and he said, "That means capital charge. The men are under a sentence of death." This was in the days of the death penalty. So my knees shook a bit. So he took me around to the death cells and there were these two chaps in there. Two young men. They'd murdered a café proprietor in South London and they were due to die in about a fortnight. It gave me a most peculiar feeling. There were these two, fit young blokes playing a sort of silly game with their prison officers and there was a curtain and they knew at a definite time they were going to plunge into eternity. The curtain was at the end of the room covering a door leading to the gallows, you see.

'They were very nicely appointed cells, actually. But I couldn't sleep that night; but after I'd seen a few it didn't make any impression on me at all. It struck me then how I had always regarded myself as reasonably civilized, but how callous one can get. I remember one man and he was under sentence of death and the thing that really worried him was that he had an ulcer and he wanted a diet for his ulcer. It shows you that he could not accept the fact – fortunately that is where nature is kind. You can't accept the fact of your own extinction.'

DR NYEWOOD: 'Sometimes it is easier to cope with some major calamity, like the death of a parent, than it is to deal with a very nasty case of athlete's foot.'

DR YETTS: 'Sometimes the patient doesn't ask, but knows and very often they know that the doctors knows as well. They don't want to embarrass or upset the doctor by asking him, and you can not infrequently get a situation where the patient knows and knows that the doctor knows, and the doctor knows and knows the patient knows and both know each other knows as well, and you can be very comfortable in that relationship. I remember vividly one lady dying of breast cancer in the cottage hospital and she was only about in her forties or early fifties and she didn't ask or anything, but one day she just looked and put her hand on mine, and said, "You'll look after me, won't you?" and I said "Of course I will", and I'm quite sure that in that interchange it all happened. She was just an ordinary, simple, working-class mum. But I think this probably happens more than we realize.'

DR BLAIRHALL: 'I've noticed that religion is a positive comfort. The belief can be minimal. But, I mean, the majority of people in the country are nominal Christians, aren't they? They're not practising Christians. But when death comes up, the nomination produces a bit of practice with it.

'As for telling, by and large I will not tell the patient lies, but I will wait till I can assess whether the patient really wants to know or not. And my experience of patients, by and large, is that they don't want to discuss with *me* whether their illness is fatal, or terminal, or not. Either because they don't want to know – they don't want the doctor to say so, or I'm sure in quite a number of instances, to spare the doctor's feelings. And I've recognized a charade, and the charade that the patient plays is that he doesn't know. He does know, but he charades that he doesn't know. And he allots roles for his wife, and the nurse, and the doctor, and we play out the charade role that we appreciate from what he's told us. And I have experienced this charade with two relatives and they've confirmed afterwards that that's exactly what it was. That a wife will tell me, "You know, he *did* know, doctor, but he just . . . We talked about it together, but he couldn't bear his doctor or nursing attendants discussing it with him."

'Partly it's consideration for the doctor. But it is also because they think that's what's expected of them. By and large patients are very brave – and the expectation of bravery, of not making a fuss, extends to accepting death.'

DR CERNEY: 'Someone said to me, a month or two ago, that doctors are, almost by definition, afraid of death. They're almost self-selected to be afraid of death, and of their own dying. I've worked it out myself. This is one of the things I've been able to work out in the last two or three years, is to be able to come to terms with my own death – at least, I think I have. Certainly much, much more than I ever did before. But when I said this out loud to my partners, one of my partners said, "Yes, indeed, that very much rings a bell with me"; and he's in there, fighting off disease all around him, by proxy fighting off his own disease – his own death in other words. And I think this is again very often patients. Patients *know*, patients so often know, and doctors so seldom give them the credit for it. They will know that their doctor is hung up on the fear of death and they don't want to worry him too much with it.'

DR KERRIS: 'I wonder. It's really strange because I'm reading this book at the moment called *Short Lives* and it's all about people who have burnt themselves out very very young. And thence I'm doing all these sort of health freaky things myself. I mean I do lots of things to avoid my own death, like seat belts, and not smoking and not eating meat, and jamming down roughage, and I go for runs. And yet I sort of admire people who really *go* at things and all die at about – well, I think the age limit was about thirty-five or thirty-six. People like Janis Joplin, Marilyn Monroe, Albert Camus, and people like that. It's just a series of essays, about forty essays, and about people who really went at their life and the consequence was that they couldn't live for ever and didn't want to. Most of them were drug addicts or killed themselves doing silly stunts on motorways or something. So I admire that but I'm always doing things consciously to avoid my own death.'

29
EUTHANASIA

DR WARFIELD: 'I frequently give more. I don't mean that I give them massive doses, whack it in and they keel over and die. The answer is no, you give them largish doses of diamorph to keep them comfortable. It doesn't necessarily knock them off any quicker in actual fact, but it makes them a hell of a sight more comfortable. But I think that anything that hastens a terminally ill patient is justifiable short of actually murdering them. I think it's quite justifiable to give a massive dose of drugs to sedate them until they quietly slip away into unconsciousness, and I think this is absolutely reasonable and sound. What would be unreasonable would be to give them an intravenous injection of insulin, where they fell off the end of the needle and died. In other words, what some people would term euthanasia.'

DR EASTCOURT: 'I had one very tragic chap who lived just across the road, suffered from a terrible illness call motor-neurone disease – that's a progressive paralysis which creeps up from the limbs and eventually you choke to death, can't swallow, and he knew all this, and I said to him once, "Have you got a faith that helps you through all this?" We talked quite openly about the fact that he wasn't going to live too long. And he said, "No, no, I haven't got a faith at all. I know I'm not going to live long and when the time comes I will expect you just to put me to sleep quietly." And I said, "I will", and I did. Heroin and sodium amytal and when he wanted I saw him away to heaven in two days.

'You can't say that openly. You know, I couldn't write it in the local *Medical Journal*, but I take the patient's relatives into my confidence and I say, "Look, there's no bettering here; he's going to suffer a lot. My job's not to kill people, but my job's to relieve people of their suffering, and if I put him to sleep so that he'll never wake up again he'll just slip away, and I think that's what he would want and what you would want," and most of them say, "What a good idea." And the way I want to do it, in forty-eight hours, demands injections, eight-hourly, into the muscle. Barbiturate poisoning. It's not the morphia that does it. You can't kill people with morphine, you know.'

DR SALEBY: 'I think everyone's done it, if you admit it or not. It depends who you admit it to, really.'

DR YETTS: 'If it so happens that the treatment you give to somebody to relieve their symptoms shortens their life, which I think rarely happens, fair enough. I'm very orthodox on this. If somebody says to me "You know what to do now, doc," I say, "I'm sorry, it isn't my job to kill people." If you're talking in cold blood. I feel quite strongly that if a doctor comes to be known as a bringer of death, it's going to do untold harm to the relationship between doctors and patients. Just imagine a little old lady sitting at home waiting for the doctor to come. She can't *but* think, "Is he going to kill me this time or next time? When I'm so useless." OK, despite all the laws or safeguards and the signing or this sort of thing, people – just as now doctors abort – and if doctors become euthanasists, also I think if euthanasia ever comes in, it's got to be done by other than doctors because I think the harm that it will do to the profession will be fantastic. That's one thing I feel very strongly about – that one.'

DR MARY IFFORD: 'If I say I believe in euthanasia, it should never be legalized. But if someone was desperately ill and in a lot of pain I would certainly step up their drugs and I would leave them enough to enable them to end their lives. But I find it hard to go out and just kill somebody.

'I think my worst ever experience was having to kill a child of two. She had a tumour in her eye and at that time my daughter was two – my only child, incidentally. I think that added to it – and this little girl and my daughter had their birthdays within ten days of each other. They used to play together.

'They had a son and they wanted a little girl. They had had Susan and at the age of six months she had an operation to remove her eye – she had a false eye. She developed quite normally. She was trained, she learnt to talk, and then at twenty months her other eye looked funny.

'Anyway, she went up to the Royal Marsden and I went up to see her and there she was in this enormous great radio-therapy place and this little tot strapped down. No one with her, of course, and she cried and screamed for about half an hour – not because it was hurting her but because she was frightened. I went up to the wards and they had several children like her with the most terribly distorted faces being kept alive with drips.

'And she went home and I had to give her injections every day. And she got secondaries, and couldn't sit on her pot, and that upset her. She was a delightful child, and then she woke up one day and said "Switch the light on." The sunlight was absolutely streaming through the window. I thought, "My God, this is it."

'The mother couldn't have coped. She knew the situation. In fact I still see her. But to send that little girl into that hospital would have been awful. She coped as long as she could at home, but the child was obviously in pain. It sends cold shivers up my spine. I'd do the same thing again, and again, I hope. But it was like killing my own daughter, you know.'

30
STRESS

Dr Nyewood had been described to me as a socialist, a maverick. About sixty-five, 'tweedy', with thinning rather distrait hair, he had a habit of not looking at you and suddenly darting 'shrewd' glances. He had a sense of humour which consisted of saying the opposite of what he meant.

Like a number of GPs, he wanted to answer questions surrounded by his family. He wished to be protected. But as we talked I gradually detected a much deeper resistance than usual, which eventually led me to abandon my prepared questions. I also became aware, as I described earlier, of powerful, if controlled irritation – against the burdens of the three-man Berkshire practice and the unfair weight of them he carried.

He was, as usual, virtually tee-total. As we were going to bed he opened a cupboard and showed me some sloe gin he was making. 'Perhaps we could have a sip?' I suggested. 'No, it's not ready,' Dr Nyewood said. Then I heard him mutter, 'If I opened that I'd drink the lot.'

I was woken in the middle of the night by a sudden loud cry. I heard nothing else and thought I must have dreamt it. In fact, when I eventually fell asleep, I did have an extremely vivid and peculiar dream.

Dr Nyewood and his whole family had got up and were down in the drawing room. I went and joined them. Dr Nyewood was laid out on a table, like a corpse. Everyone sat about in silence and there was a feeling of great unease. After a while I retreated back to my room, wondering how I was going to get back to sleep.

It was so vivid, that I described it at breakfast to Mrs Nyewood. 'How funny,' she said. 'Trevor got up, unable to sleep, and came down to the drawing room at 3 o'clock. I joined him for a while.'

This was only the most peculiar and striking among the many ways GPs made me aware of the very considerable stress under which they laboured. It was this, ultimately, that lay behind the feelings of depression they occasionally engendered (even if they didn't seem particularly depressed characters).

And the tapes revealed signs I would have missed. On both Dr Chathill's and Dr Nyewood's tapes I became aware of an insistent, continuous nervous tapping, signet ring or watch or pen against a nail. Dr Jane Edstone was neatest. Early on I asked her how much holiday she took. Never more than two weeks a year, she said, and it was always ruined because after the fourth day she invariably got a cold. Much later on, I was asking her about stress, how she coped, what caused it. To my surprise this part of the tape, and this alone, was punctuated by the most enormous sneezes.

I do not, of course, mean by this that GPs were unaware they led stressful lives. They were perfectly aware of it. What did strike me was that very few of them realized just how profound the stress was.

With Dr Chathill, for example, who was quite clear how stressful his life was, I gradually sensed a good deal it is hard to put a finger on. Something was getting his wife down, although he was clearly extremely loving and 'supportive'. But there was something unemotional, or rather not un-emotional but repressed about him, a feeling that no one in the household ever lost control. I think that underneath he was under far greater pressure than he realized, and continuously having to control very strong reactions. And had been doing so for years.

The second thing I noticed about the GPs was that even fewer thought they could or should do anything about it.

Before embarking on a more wide-ranging discussion, I should perhaps say it can only be that. 'Stress' is a very inexact word and depends entirely on the person undergoing it. Dr Warfield said briskly that it was simply a question of decent office organization – being able to delegate, getting the receptionist to chase patients and consultants, routine, patients as an orderly sequence. A lot of people need some stress to function effectively. Stress under which one GP functions effectively would bring another to his knees. And in fact all the areas we are now entering – death, stress, the characters of GPs – are too vast to admit of generalization, the strands too diverse and contradictory to develop a single coherent argument. It is only possible to make, and let the GPs make, a number of separate and I hope illuminating observations, somewhat at random.

We have already seen the multitude of things which can cause stress (that they do will scarcely cause surprise) but it might be a good idea to put them all together under this one head.

1) There is the endless giving, endless dealing with people's problems – 'battered by the commonplace'. Some GPs think the sheer number of people with whom there is virtually no contact is tiring.

2) The work can be physically tiring – if night calls are frequent, if an epidemic requires a lot of visits, or partners fall ill or become alcoholic.

3) The nature of the work is anxious-making. It is composed of the unexpected – the unexpected event, the hidden disease. Life and death decisions are rare, but doubt and worry are not: did I make the right decision? The right diagnosis? Repeat visits to allay anxiety, especially to children, are common.

4) There is the endless effort and frustration of arranging things, getting patients into wards, getting them houses or flats.

5) A good deal of anger and conflict can arise from all this – from patients who want Valium to recalcitrant consultants. In a TV film on stress, it was an unfeeling consultant one of the GPs chose to attack.

6) There is the GP's emotional reaction to his patients. We have seen the difficult balance needed between sympathy and detachment. This is made more complicated because medical students were and to a considerable extent still are discouraged from having or displaying feelings towards patients. The implicit, or explicit, emphasis is to repress emotion.

This makes it much harder, especially for younger GPs, to deal with the powerful and complex emotions all these various situations produce – grief, affection, distate, anxiety, fear, anger. In particular, considerable aggression is involved, which has to be suppressed since the effect upon patients or consultants or social workers, though sometimes beneficial, is usually not productive.

7) All these stresses are cumulative. The strain begins to tell after about eight years.

There is also a wider aspect of the GP's life which should now be involved. On the one hand, it involves the acquisition and then application of a fairly considerable body of scientific knowledge. The deduction, testing and then acceptance or rejection of hypotheses, the subsequent use of that knowledge. On the other hand, since the problems are as much or more often social and psychological, with roots the patients cannot or will not express, strong intuitive gifts are needed which, if not precisely those of an artist or a novelist, are allied to them. These are what one might call feminine qualities, qualities of empathy, and are seen as – or seem to be – the direct opposite of the scientific mind. It is often the conflict posed when a GP has only one side of this dual armoury in abundance – nearly always the practical, scientific side – that imposes additional stress on his or her life.

This situation, long latent in what we have been observing, I would now like to make increasingly clear. It is, in my view, absolutely fundamental to the lives of the GPs, and therefore to this book.

We have seen GPs and those near them describe their stress, and will do so again. But the *level* of description was fairly superficial.

DR ABNEY: 'I was hoping, as I got older, that I'd get a little bit less to do but it's more. There's no doubt about it. More and more and more. Purely from the stress factors in life. The worries. But as I say, this is what I'm paid to do. I'm sure that a member of the cabinet feels the same, that they've got immense worries, and I do worry. I worry about children particularly.'

DR THRIPLOW'S WIFE, ALICE: 'When we're on holiday he gets no indigestion whatever. It doesn't matter what he eats, and yet if he has a really busy spell, he's complaining of his tummy. Even if he had the blandest milky diet. It's all the stress. Perhaps it would be better if he blew his top occasionally.'

DR JANET KIBANE: 'I would say one of the main strains is just hard work, because I think that if you are a good doctor you care for your patients but you try not to get too involved. The other major stress is what the patient wants and what you want, which can be two very different things. Dissonance. I had someone wanting a slimming pill, and I refused. Or a visit. That's when the stress comes; that's when the adrenalin rises – conflict. You've been asked to do something you don't want to do. You have to justify that and there's a lot of *anger* created, not necessarily from you, but directed at you! That is one of the main stresses. For me, anyway.'

RECEPTIONIST (DR TELSCOMBE'S PRACTICE): 'The doctors tend – I don't quite know how to put this – the doctors tend, I think, to turn on us when they're busy. They need, I suppose, somebody to kick then. Obviously days are going to happen when just too many patients want to be seen and the doctor is in a bad mood. The worst thing they do is tend to walk off and leave you with no answer, and that is difficult. You've got a patient on the phone or in reception and the doctor has walked off with nothing to say to them. Or they shout occasionally. Very different, all of them. Some of them are much much easier to deal with. Those are the ones you tend to shuffle work on to.'

Effects

John Berger called his biography/novel of Sassall *A Fortunate Man*. Sassall had become a GP because he'd identified with the heroes in Conrad – he was someone who had rejected the boredom and predictability of middle-class life ashore to pit himself against the unknown furies of the sea – but in his case a sea of disease and death. The pursuit was raised to nobleness, above normal self-seeking and advancement, by the ideal of service. As far as is possible in life, Sassall had realized the powerful inner dreams and ambitions of his youth.

Yet, long after the book was written, Sassall, this fortunate man, killed himself.

The facts are roughly known but must be repeated. An American study found that a quarter of all deaths in doctors aged twenty-five to thirty-nine were due to suicide, compared to 9 per cent in white collar workers of the same group. British figures show women doctors to be six times more likely, and male doctors three times more likely to kill themselves than other people over the complete age and occupation range, but ten times more likely than senior civil servants, six times more likely than university teachers. Their wives are also more likely to kill themselves than the wives of other professionals.*

*Report in the *Guardian*, 22 June 1983.

There is some argument about these figures. It is said they are high because doctors have easy access to drugs and the knowledge to use them. The same is true of chemists, whose suicide rate is much lower.

It is also said that the profession attracts to it people prone to suicide and other difficulties, and it is the factors causing this, and not the life itself, which are responsible. An American study quoted by Glin Bennet found that many doctors chose to care for patients because they had unloving and neglected childhoods – it was deprivation which led to their stress, and their stress reactions.

A third argument is that suicide is simply a straightforward reaction to unbearable stress – which the doctor cannot throw off by the usual methods, by behaving regressively, or by confession, because that is not how he is expected to behave.

I don't see there is a conflict here. No doubt both of the last two arguments are true. Certainly we shall find GPs whose drive comes from a neglected childhood or from childhood suffering. (And often the best GPs – just as homosexuals often make the best teachers or bravest war leaders.) This is no reason to somehow discount stress – it makes it all the more urgent and necessary to do something about it, since such people are more vulnerable.

And what is tragic is that the GPs themselves seem unaware how profound, how violent the feelings at work in them are, how suppressed, repressed, they can gather and gather until they burst out uncontrollably, overwhelmingly. The suicide comes instantly, unexpectedly – a sudden snap.

DR KIBANE: 'We're worried about one of our partners, aren't we? I mean Sally, that she's going to let it become too involving and too much of a strain. There are files everywhere; she's always behind. She doesn't write the records up. When somebody comes in, she'll leave it all because she's too involved.

'But that isn't too bad perhaps. It's obvious strain. You can see it by the look on her face, the time she finishes, the way her room is full of disarray. You can't always tell. We've a high suicide rate round here – two out of twenty in the last four years. It seems a lot anyway. But people didn't actually pick them out and say, "Look, he's going to commit suicide tonight." Like Henry Troutbeck did. Or like Jack Whilton did.

'With Jack Whilton, for instance, there were no clues at all. This was a chap in his, what, late fifties, committed suicide this year – one of the local GPs. A much-loved, conscientious doctor. No clues at all, he just went up into his attic and swallowed a bottle of barbiturates, or something, and some alcohol, and was found there by his wife, having left a tidy will and sorted everything out a few days before.'

One explanation of suicide is that it is aggression which, denied outlet, turns inward. But, of course, it is not just suicide. In the American study, 47 per cent of GPs had divorced or had 'poor' marriages, compared to 32 per cent among their peers. In Britain they are twice as likely to be alcoholics as other class one professionals, and have three times the rate of cirrhosis. (Thus, hostility to patients, and other sorts of personal and professional suicide, may be attempts to cope with stress short of real suicide.)

And many of these symptoms show before the strains accumulate. Students commit suicide, so do trainee GPs – or take to drink– as if aware early they are not temperamentally suited.

DR TRIMDON: 'It's funny – my trainee, who's an alcoholic. Now people smell our breath. I smoke; I never smell my wife's scent, you know. My sense of smell is poor. But everybody says she comes in steaming in the morning and I'm pretty sure she's an alcoholic. She's denying it. But she was absent from her place of duty yesterday afternoon, and again today, this'll be the last time. I'm going to talk tonight or early next week with the regional adviser. What I'm proposing to do with this woman, who's been difficult since she came, is not to sign her certificate of competence. I'm not going to damn her. I will advise that she be given further training experience. She's no confidence; she generates anxiety and no confidence. One of my partners won't even let her take his surgery. She can't cope with the stress, and she shouldn't be in general practice if she can't cope with stress.'

Solutions

DR TELSCOMBE: 'I play squash. Sometimes I play after a late afternoon surgery and it really is marvellous because all the sort of facts are going round in one's head; one gets on that squash court, and one comes off having forgotten everything about one's work, just being absolutely exhausted. It's a marvellous chance to take it all off.'

DR KINSHAM: 'Well, there's life at home, the kids. It's always a great pleasure to go back, particularly when they were younger. Delightful nine-year-old. Wife and friends who are not in medicine, having good holidays away – six weeks a year, go abroad. I think the average GP takes six weeks. Even single ones, I think so, yes. I suppose I try and shut off in the evenings, but not effectively.'

DR JANE EDSTONE: 'I think generally we should talk about more things. You see, doctors are ashamed of talking. One of the GPs came round to see me and he was talking an awful lot about himself and then rang up to apologize about it! I find that. There was a nice GP when I was in the west. He had an affair with a house surgeon, he was very important in the town, a pillar, so the house surgeon was shipped away and he had to keep up the façade of being an upright and virtuous man, and I used to go and see him. He always used to have a tumbler full of gin in his hand and when you went in he'd say, "Have a drink", and you'd have to drink it. In my last practice a lot of Catholic priests were patients of mine, and nuns. They were people I felt I could talk to a bit.'

DR DOLWAR: 'One of my partners, my new young partner; my work has been transformed again over the past two or three years by finding a partner with whom I can talk about my own emotional problems. I went for years thinking there was something wrong with me, about why we never seemed to be able to get down to things. And it wasn't until this new partner came, and I am now able to say, "I felt angry when you asked me to do that," or something like that. And when she comes in and says, "I'm really worried, or bothered about a patient," we can sit down and talk about it, that problem, until it's actually got worked out. Being able to do that with one of my partners has made a huge difference, really. Huge. And I think to work in a partnership where you can't do that kind of thing must be very, very, very difficult.'

DR KERRIS: 'It's really weird, because I've just been on holiday and got a terrible cold, but I think it's saying something, isn't it? The stresses are enormous, and anyone who denies it, I don't know what job they're doing but it's not the same as mine. I think it probably is possible to build into your job defences so you don't have to confront that stress too much – but it's just fantastic what people come and ask you, ask of you, it's ridiculous really. And people dying, and things like that.

'I've got a friend, his theory is that doctors have given up the bits that recharge their batteries, and one of the things was home deliveries. You can take a lot of the stress as long as you get the boosts, like home deliveries, or doing things yourself, even to stitching or small ops, things that give you a buzz.

'I mean, there are things like counselling I had to fight for. We *have* a practice counsellor – but I keep some patients that I can set aside an hour or so a week for. I want to do that, so I do it.

'And home deliveries – *really* nice. We've only just got ourselves teed up to do them. We had one last week – gorgeous. It also coincides with my political belief that women have the right to home deliveries, if they *want* to. And there are things like good deaths, too. It doesn't have to be a terrible scramble and failure and disaster. I can think of a couple of deaths, again, where there was a professional pride it was done as well as it could possibly be, although it was sad to lose those people. These things do recharge my batteries. You've got to get recharged like that.

'Another thing – we try to say nice things to each other. Doctors are terribly isolated if things go well – who praises them? Patients, but that emphasizes the status of them. "Oh, *thank* you doctor." And it's often the wrong people who thank you, actually. But when people who know, who you're working with, acknowledge it – that's recharging too.

'The other thing we have here is a doctors' group. Six or seven of us meet every fortnight. It's like a counselling group and just like we acknowledge the need for young mums to talk at depth about what's going on, we do the same. That's a good place to get out the stresses and strains. For instance, a young girl in the practice here died and that was just terribly traumatic really. And we went through the clinical side in detail, but also the sort of feelings it engendered.'

And it is on those lines, surely, that something should be done. Squash and the like are barely relevant.

The fact is the medical profession both acknowledges there is a problem, that it is serious, and behaves as though it almost weren't there. If this sort of thing was happening to Members of Parliament, say, if our safety, the running of the country, were at stake, there would be an outcry. Doctors have a suicide rate ten times that of MPs – and doctors are responsible for our lives and health.

Yet the BMA does almost nothing. The Royal College is meant to be encouraging groups along the lines described by Dr Kerris and by Dr Yetts (see 'Keeping up to Date') – but it is very muted. The Royal College of Psychiatrists has a service which, in complete confidence, allows doctors to say if they are worried about a colleague and they will then investigate and help. It is used 'a moderate amount'. I didn't find a single GP who had heard of it.

One trouble is that in one respect it is almost in the patients' interest for nothing to be done. The GPs under most strain can be the most conscientious. John Heron of the British Postgraduate Medical Federation, noted that the exercise of will and intellect 'Can lead to perfectly healthy control, but also to repression and denial of grief, fear and anger. And denied distress significantly distorts behaviour.'* One way is to dump it on patients, displacing it. Coping with and curing patients fools the doctor into thinking he is caring for and coping with his own distress.

A lot of GPs talk of sharing stress with partners and wives. In fact, the vast majority either don't talk about such things to their partners, or else do so in such a superficial way it is the same as not talking.

What is required is something radical and fundamental. I said earlier that in the TV film about stress, one GP chose a consultant as his example. But he didn't just say, as a GP might to his wife, how irritating the man had been. He *acted out* the rage he felt about him (and also no doubt about other facets of his

*Report in the *Guardian*, 22 June, 1983.

GP life); he yelled and screamed at the imaginary consultant, he thumped the table and hurled books; only then did he achieve catharsis. But there are all sorts of tried and successful methods of group or personal counselling that could be employed.

How much should they be institutionalized? A lot of the descriptions by GPs were superficial and were so because their stress was quite superficial, it was containable. After all, the vast majority cope. I don't see, to choose at random, Drs Warfield, Telscombe or Trimdon cracking up. On the other hand, Dr Thriplow didn't tell me about his stomach, his wife did. In fact, three years before he'd been seriously ill with an ulcer. He did nothing about it until he weighed eight and a half stone and was vomiting blood.

I think there should be some regular, organized system of confidential therapy or counselling which all GPs undergo every four months or so. Those that felt quite all right could do it fairly briskly. Those under considerable strain would find considerable relief. I am quite sure alcoholism, suicide, and the rest would drop dramatically.

I also think a lot of now scornful GPs would find the experience of value. I, in a small way, was the beneficiary of their habitual silence or superficiality on all these matters. I was often startled at the sudden sense I had of an outpouring, a release, the power of it. And frequently, it seemed to me, they were surprised to find they felt better, and often – though, bafflingly, there was nothing specific to thank me for, the reverse in fact – found themselves expressing gratitude for my visits.

Drs Michael and Lucy Veryan

DR MICHAEL VERYAN: 'We tried the very novel idea of de-stressing in the group; not everybody's cup of tea and mocked by an enormous number of the profession who found it really rather uncomfortable.

'Even with trainees, who have only been doing medicine three years, if you allow them to let their hair down and talk, you'll realize that the amount of distress they pick up from their patients, however they harden themselves to it, is *extraordinary*.

'For example, one trainee described the most distressing thing that happened to him was when – just two years qualified – he was in casualty looking after accidents that had come in. And a three-year-old was brought in who'd been run over and died in casualty, and he had to break it to the parents. You're never taught how to do this at all and yet it is always left to the most junior doctors to do.

'Well, the mother of the child just screamed and collapsed in a heap on the floor. The father was also obviously distressed, and he himself found this extremely distressing and he just couldn't cope with this woman. He just ran out. But, to compound things, another child was brought in ten minutes later, also having been knocked down, and who also died, and he had to do it a second time. You're not allowed to go weeping to colleagues about this sort of thing. So he just pushed it down, but when it came up and he was allowed to air it, and in a way re-live the distress, it was a sort of catharsis.

'You see, you can't do this. If you're very distressed and wanted to weep about somebody who had died, we've all been taught that big boys don't cry. You've just got to get on with it. John Heron at Surrey, who I've worked with, he is fascinated by doctors. He feels it is the most hierarchical, rigid, narrow, buttoned-up profession he has ever come across apart from the police, and he has been working with us for ten years. He has described a series of techniques which people used to avoid talking about things which hurt. He calls it "The League of Gentlemen". So what happens is that some doctors get together in the bar or something, to unwind after the day, and instead of getting down to the realities, the nitty-gritty, they all make jokes like, "I've had a terrible day, a real basin full, the bloody British public!" They talk in this superficial way about their problems without actually getting down to saying what really distresses them about what they have to cope with, and it's a sort of blinker effect.

'And it's quite odd. Psychotherapists, marriage guidance therapists, psychosexual therapists, all have a tightly-knit way of coping with this sort of thing. They go and share the load with a supervisor, who then has somebody else to share it with and so it's all dissipated in this way. Marriage guidance counsellors have been aware of this since they first started in 1937. Everybody who is counselling must have a superior, otherwise they'd just get broken in the end because they take on board so much family distress they could never manage it.'

J.G.H.: 'Why can't you evolve a method?'

DR MICHAEL VERYAN: 'We haven't and won't grasp the nettle. Because of this "League of Gentlemen". It's not admitted. Anybody who shows signs of cracking in front of his colleagues makes them feel very uncomfortable. "It's not done old boy." It's only when someone is really desperate, either attempting suicide as my predecessor did, or taking to the bottle – that, well in fact *that* is what happens. There's no one to go to. It's almost bred into you at medical school not to.'

DR LUCY VERYAN: 'I think an awful lot of the sharing of medical stress goes home to the wife. And the marriage break-up rate, again, is high among doctors.'

J.G.H.: 'But would you advocate some sort of institutionalized system whereby you could hold, say, monthly seminars, like your mid-course trainees?'

DR MICHAEL VERYAN: 'It would be very nice if we could do this, but it would take a revolution. The more diehard members of the profession would say, "This is absolute nonsense." '

J.G.H.: 'You don't do anything very organized in your own practice?'

DR MICHAEL VERYAN: 'No, I think there are two reasons for this, one is that we have a very sympathetic new young partner who's very much into this sort of thing anyway, and we can actually talk about our problems without this awful feeling we are letting ourselves down.

'The second thing is I've been toying with the idea of doing something for the whole practice. It's distressing for *everyone* involved – nurses, health visitors, staff. For example, a young man of twenty-eight who's got multiple sclerosis, and who's virtually paralysed, we have to co-ordinate, but it's very distressing for the staff to cope with this. I've been planning to get someone in to do something at greater depths like marriage guidance people with their supervisors. We've got a practice counsellor. We've done it for ten years for patients, but we don't do it for ourselves enough.'

DR LUCY VERYAN:'A potentially dangerous area, I think. It's easy to go too far. That would make me feel pretty threatened.'

J.G.H.. 'Threatened in what way?'

DR LUCY VERYAN: 'You'd get too deeply involved. The words and thoughts. You'd be bound to get personally involved with everyone's hopes and plans rather than concentrate on the problems in the practice.'

J.G.H.: 'Isn't it fears and feelings you *are* dealing with?'

DR LUCY VERYAN: 'Yes, but I have the feeling it would go too far, and if you go too far you make yourself vulnerable. Do you see what I'm getting at?'

J.G.H.: 'I do see, but earlier on we were talking rather about the reverse of that. The need was to be more open.'

DR MICHAEL VERYAN: 'But this is the problem with the profession as a whole. A lot of GPs feel there should be some method of de-stressing. But – and Lucy is far further along the tracks than most – but she is saying what the great majority fear or feel.'

DR LUCY VERYAN: 'I feel I've seen people being damaged by counselling, though I can't give an example.'

J.G.H.: 'If the problem is taking on other people's fears and feelings, and also raising these feelings within you; then if you say, "If we can talk about it we can let some of this out," isn't it a bit illogical to say, "We mustn't let too much out"? If you're trying to get rid of it, surely better to get rid of it all, face it all? Do you think you're really responding to the fear of what is inside you?'

DR LUCY VERYAN: 'Yes, I would 100 per cent accept that. It is fear of the unknown; fear of what you'd uncover. Especially in a group. We'd be overwhelmed.'

J.G.H.: 'How does it work with marriage guidance?'

DR LUCY VERYAN: 'More one to one with their supervisor. *That* wouldn't worry me in the slightest. That would be great. But that's not allowed.'

DR MICHAEL VERYAN: 'Oh no. The "League of Gentlemen" would be down like sixty tons of bricks.'

Dr Yetts

We have already met Dr Yetts on a number of occasions. You may remember his group of college GPs –'you bring a death'. More recently he came down strongly against any form of euthanasia. He made many comments typical of a good, conscientious, experienced, active, youngish College GP.

Yet Dr Yetts was not in the least ordinary. At the age of forty-four having built up the health centre practice almost from scratch, within two years of becoming the senior partner, he'd 'suddenly' resigned and taken a desk job in the Civil Service. The letter asking if I'd like to discuss this was couched in terms not unlike a master criminal at last ready in confidence to describe his crime.

They lived in a neat, moderate-sized house. Mrs Yetts was small, piping, busy in a perfect kitchen, all working surfaces and machinery, a good deal of it whirring. There were bright overhead lights, a burglar alarm, everything squared-up and precise – small prints in twos square on the walls, balancing two more, the electric fire with coal-effect base clean in the middle.

Dr Yetts was spry, tense and quick, with a face like a smaller, younger Roy Jenkins; he was balding with alert eyes, clever – not devious quite, but canny, sharp. He was entirely dominated by his three-month-old defection. Dominated by the excitement of this – there was the feeling of a balloon just released; also by the guilt – he really did see it as a defection.

DR YETTS: 'I suppose the main reason was the work stress. The thing that got me down in general practice was the unpredictability of life. You never knew what was going to happen in the next five minutes. And my personality couldn't cope with that – I'm a bit of a planner. I like to be able to see how the next few hours are going to be, next few days, months, years, and so into the future. And general practice just wasn't of that nature.

'When you're on call, I got extremely tense, not because I couldn't cope with the work, but because I was worried I might not be able to. You see the difference? In surgery, I liked to see a consultation through. I couldn't stand the telephone ringing, a major problem, a trivial one, stopping your train of thought and time with the patient. It was this sort of personality defect within myself that was the main thing. I've stood it for eighteen years and my thoughts were, "I'm over the top now, sixteen years to go." You know. Then – "crumbs, I've got to stick with this level of tension for the next sixteen years".

'We keep on devising ways to reduce stress, don't we? A one-in-six rota for night duty, then, as I said, some deputizing help for nights. But you never get away from the stress of when you're on duty and what might happen. Now the others cope fine with it. My senior partner laps it up. He creates his own stress. He loves having more than he can cope with, that's what turns him on. I'm just the opposite.

'And I wasn't very keen on the practical things – minor casualty, injections, things like this, even examinations I suppose. I'm quite happy talking to people, at a fairly superficial level – but you can do that as an ordinary citizen.

'And there's always the fear in general practice that you're going to make the most ghastly mistake and somebody's going to die or be permanently harmed because you've done something wrong. It happens to every doctor. But you feel guilty because you missed a strangulated hernia or whatever. I lost a child with diabetes. These are the things you are never quite happy about. My partners say I'm obsessional, but I'm not all that obsessional.

'Nevertheless, I couldn't cope. Everybody was amazed when I made the decision – including myself. A bolt from the blue. It was quite assumed – my senior partner retires in two years – that I was going to take over and carry on from there.

'I have mixed feelings – "Have I done the right thing?" I'm a civil servant now. Working with files about patients and not patients in the flesh. Quite a drop in salary. In '81, we were bringing home, after expenses, something like £26,000. Now, £19,750 – which is still quite a lot of money.

'But I feel completely different. When we were doing night work I used to feel tired all the time, as the patients say. But even when we stopped that, I still had a tension tiredness – I don't know if you understand what I mean by that – you're always a little bit edgy, which produces tiredness. Now I'm zooming about being energetic and things like that. The high point of the euphoria has gone. Will I still feel my life is as worthwhile as it was? But I've given twenty years of my life. Now I'm much more relaxed.

'I don't miss the patients. In fact, one of my new colleagues, an ex-GP, has a nice way with that. Every time he feels fed up he rings up his old practice and his old receptionist has got a list of names, and she just reads these out and he feels fine again.

'The main people who criticize me have been female and virtually all the males I've spoken to, apart from the senior partner who's twenty years older than me, especially contemporaries, have had a lot of sort of sympathy and, well, you know. "They'd thought of that sort of thing themselves, but . . ."'

Dr Yetts interspersed his account with observations about the speed with which it had happened, how this speed had amazed his colleagues, how it had amazed *him* – it was as though he had suddenly been attacked by some force and impelled into his extraordinary decision. Yet it became quite clear, when he later on went into the genesis of what had happened, that it hadn't been a sudden decision at all.

A few months before taking it he had come back from a holiday and felt more ghastly than usual about taking up the reins. He'd seen an ad for a Civil Service job, cut it out and put it in a drawer. A few weeks later he was working with a friend on a joint book, when he became aware of how relaxed he felt. He thought, 'If doing something away from the practice makes me feel like this, I must look into it. Perhaps I *don't* have to be a GP. Some time in the next five years I'll look into it.'

However, he in fact looked into it much sooner. He'd 'written around', and also replied to the Civil Service ad. Almost at once he was caught. Where, in his innocence, he'd seen hard-faced bureaucrats, he was met by wily tempters – 'Do you like milk and sugar?' 'They showed me where to park. All those years I thought that compared to marvellous general practice, the outside world would be drear and terrible – but no! It was *all right!*'

He got the job, resigned his practice. Then he made an odd discovery. 'Do you know, I found I'd sent off for the details of this job a couple of years ago. I'd forgotten about it. It was in the drawer, lost in the drawer. Exactly this stuff that came through when I wrote off, I'd already got, I'd suppressed it. Isn't it funny?'

So far from sudden, he'd taken active steps two years before, and it was likely, therefore, it had been in his mind several years before that, perhaps even from the time he began to appreciate what general practice was really like.

I think Dr Yetts had taken a courageous decision and the right decision – 'I've had conscious nightmares driving along the motorway and sort of thinking I was back' – but it was clear his wife minded and to a certain extent disapproved.

So did his eldest daughter. She was becoming a nurse on the strength of his vocation – 'always thought of me as a white knight' – and now he'd let her down. Whenever the subject came up, she went quiet.

By chance, one of the GPs I later spoke to, Dr Simon Kibane, had seen a report of Yetts's action in the medical press and, though for quite different reasons not at all content with being a GP, had expressed fairly pungent scorn.

It was very like someone who had left the front line with shell shock. People would allow it, but he secretly felt that they thought less of him, as he did of himself. And such are the stresses of general practice that doctors are not unlike front-line troops – this is one of the factors that leads them to protect each other, that binds them together.

But the stresses also operate on their wives and families, and here, though often cohesive, these forces can almost as often distress and strain and, sometimes, blow apart.

WIVES AND FAMILIES

DR JANE EDSTONE: 'He was teaching to start with, but he wanted a large family. I said I was quite prepared as long as he took an equal share in looking after them. But after Jenny, the fourth, he went into politics and said, "Ho, ho, you give up your job now and support me." But by that time I'd built up quite a nice little practice and there wasn't an awful lot of good marriage left, so things went from bad to worse. It was only the children that kept me going after that.

'And the practice kept me going. Because if you went and sat behind the desk there were people with worse problems than you had, so it evened out. From a general point of view, it's practice/children, children/practice, because they are the most dependent and your husband comes a sort of third.

'Also, I tend to become far too involved, but I don't think you can help people unless you're prepared to be involved. Some things do distress me, and probably that's reacted on my marriages because if I have someone who's having a tough time or who is desperately ill, I can't go to bed quite happily and forget about it. I tend to lie awake wondering if there's any more I can do and possibly that hasn't been the right attitude for the matrimonial bed. I mean, if I go to bed depressed about everything, I am not going to have a successful love life. If I'm all right, that's fine. But if I'm miserable, I'm miserable. So I missed out on husbands and they missed out on some things, because somewhere along the line the marriages cracked up.'

DR WARFIELD: 'I think women marry doctors because they think it's going to be a glamorous life, and they find it's a bit humdrum and the telephone's always ringing and they find it's very irksome. And when the kids need you for their homework and you're still doing your surgery at 6.30 at night. You can't commute the kids into school because you've got to start surgery at half 8. But I think it depends how philosophical they are about the whole business. If they accept the fact that your practice commitments come first. In other words, families have to come second, unfortunately. And providing your spouse accepts this then there's no great problem. But many women won't accept this and don't realize just what they're up against when they marry somebody who's a GP, or even worse are some of the more busy consultants who literally work their balls off.'

GP'S DAUGHTER (In Northern Ireland): 'School-goers would often bring him into the conversation and if I were to mention anything that I had done or was thinking of doing that was outside the normal conventions, they would say something like, "What would your daddy think of that?" Apart from the fact that my grandfather had been a big deal as a doctor, being a surgeon as well and one of the few doctors in the area for the first part of his life, so that my father had inherited a position of respect, he also had it automatically because he was a doctor, I think. Now that I consider it, it may have been due to personal merit.

'I know that during the Troubles in Northern Ireland he was always able to drive about and the hooded men would lift the barriers and give him safe passage although resentfully if it was a day of action or something. I remember one phone call in the middle of the night to our house where the woman said, "Doctor, my son's been kicked in the head and I think he needs stitching up." The call came from a block of flats nearby so my father asked the woman to bring her son to the surgery so he could insert the stitches there under hygienic conditions. My father said this and the woman said, "No doctor, I canne do that for the fellas that done him in are waiting outside the door." My father simply got dressed and went to the flats himself, casting a look of contempt at the young men waiting outside this flat door to do further injuries to the man inside. They didn't attack my father and I'm not sure whether he thought they might or not, anyway he said to my mother, "It's my job," and off he went.

'No wonder doctors drink when you think that at one stage he was on call literally all the time. I remember he sometimes got complaints that Dr O'Connell had been rude to his patients on the nights that he had been on duty for my father, and occasionally a patient would prefer Dr O'Connell and try and arrange to always get ill when my father was off duty so that they could see Dr O'Connell and vice versa.

'Sometimes I would meet a new person at school or talk to a person I hadn't spoken to before and they would look at me with a deep affection and say, "Your daddy delivered me."

'My sister was a pillar of respectability and has still never even held a cigarette in her hand or been drunk, or even had more than a total of two alcoholic drinks in her life. I was considered to be absolutely wildly out of control, doing things like hitch-hiking to Belfast, in a mini-skirt with dyed hair, thick make-up and a bottle of wine costing 7s 6d in my hand.

'The unfortunate thing about being a doctor's daughter in a small town was that everyone knew you even if you didn't know them, so sometimes, having lied to my parents that I was getting a lift with someone to Belfast, I would in fact hitch-hike and get a lift with someone I'd never seen before, who wouldn't mention the fact that he knew quite well who I was, then that person would come into the surgery and say to my father that he had given me a lift and my father would be angry with me. At one stage when I was about sixteen my mother told me that Dr O'Connell might have to leave the practice if I didn't stop behaving so badly because when they had made the contract to be partners there was a clause with something about how one party could withdraw without compensation if the other one brought disrespect upon themselves.

'After he had the stroke he became more sentimental and used to ask me to read out the death columns in the *Belfast Newsletter*. "Anyone from Kilkerry?" he'd ask in a doleful tone and he usually knew the person, even though the town had 20,000 people – I suppose that it has expanded and when he started there were only about 5,000 and he knew them all from doing duty for other doctors too.

'So when I read out the name of someone who was dead he would often say, "He owed my £100 – I'll never see it now", or some other figure. Although he was very restrictive about paying out money, seeing almost everything other than coal and food as an extravagance, he seems to have been always lending patients money and apparently it is a custom for patients in places like that to ask the doctor to lend them money – I suppose the doctor is the only person in the town like that with enough money to lend.

'He told me about one man who borrowed £50 (about ten years ago) and had never given it back except once my father had seen him in Main Street and the man had come across and given him a fiver, saying, "There you are doctor, I wouldn't want you to think I had forgotten about you."'

GP'S SON: 'Dad had a heart attack, then another, and was advised to take it easy – but he still runs the practice more or less from the shopping centre. As he's walking along ex-patients will come up and say, "Look, I've tried to get the doctor for my repeat prescriptions, do you mind?" He always walks round with a prescription pad in his pocket and he'll walk back to the surgery and tell them what he's done.'

POLLY LOCKING: 'You see, it's all right for the men. The women are worse for being on call because the men do their own thing but the women are always on *call* do you see? You're dying to go to the loo, as soon as you go to the loo the front door goes and you're sitting there, diving out of the loo and going to the front door, or you just get to the end of the corridor and the front door goes and it takes ages to get down. And people just disappear. Because it's a long way to come. I'm always burning things, you know. You get something on and people *always* ring when you've just got your pan on the stove or your hands in the flour, or you're tied up with the phone and you come back and the kids have tipped everything out of the cupboard or something. You know. It's very frustrating, but you get *used* to it.

'I remember last week Dolly Smeeton was ringing up on behalf of her sister Rachel. So I get a relayed message, a three-way conversation. Rachel had passed some blood, you see. This was the tale. "Could doctor come?" Now, it's about fifteen or sixteen miles and he'd had a busy day, and it was a nasty night, you know, and this old lady is known, well she frightens easily, so I said, "From where has she passed the blood?" You know, because there are various outlets where you could pass the blood. And she said, "Rachel, where have you . . . ?" "Is that the doctor who's speaking?" "No, it's a woman." I feel very indignant at being called "A woman", so in the end I said, "Look Dolly," I said, "will you please ask Rachel to come to the phone. I cannot carry on a conversation like this. From one to another." So anyway, Rachel comes to the phone and I said, "Now Rachel, from where did you pass the blood?" "From Fleetham," she says. That's where she lives, see. I said, "Rachel, have you been sick and passed the blood?" "No, not been sick." I said, "Well, did you go to the *toilet* and pass the blood?" "Well, yes I did. I went to the toilet and passed the blood." I said, "*Right* now," I said, "was it the right colour, Rachel?" "Eee, well, I don't know. I passed a lot of water as well. I don't really know." So I thought, Oh God, this is terrible. "Have you got any tummy ache?" "Nay, no, I haven't got any tummy ache. I wanted to *stir me bowels*," she said, "and I went to the lavatory to *stir* me bowels." You can imagine someone stirring the bowels. I said, "I'll tell you what – you stay with your sister and when doctor comes in I'll ask him to give you a ring so he can talk to you."

'So anyway, when Sam came in I said, "I'm not very sure about this, Sam. I don't know whether it's a call or not." I said, "It *could* be or it *may* not be." Usually I can tell but I wasn't very sure about this. So he rang up and he was chuckling when he came through. I said, "What's the verdict?" "Oh," he said, "I'm not going. Geoff'll be going next time on Friday." He said, "I've asked her to wee in her jerry next time she wants to wee" and she said "Eee, but I'll not be wanting to wee till about 10 o'clock", so Sam had said, "Well, drink plenty of water, Rachel." And we'd just sat down to a meal and the phone went and I said, "She's weed!" So anyway he went, and she had, and it was all clear. You know, but it is funny. It's funny in many ways.'

DR THRIPLOW: 'Many of the wives are working and the GPS seem to want a 9 to 5 job. But general practice *can't* be run as a 9 to 5 job. There has to be somebody at the end of the telephone, and all our children were trained from the age of five onwards to take intelligible and intelligent messages.'

ALICE THRIPLOW: 'Being at the beck and call of the telephone was difficult with the children. Trying to bath them at night and rushing to the telephone. There were, are, times when I feel like pulling the connection out of the wall. But I can't say it really bothered me on the whole.

'I quite enjoyed it in a way. It carries on from having been a nurse. One of the partner's wives wasn't and she finds it quite difficult when an emergency crops up. At least I can give advice. It's nice to feel you have some part. It's not just your husband that's part of village life, though it's a bit difficult when they expect your children to be better-behaved.

'What I've got used to now which I didn't like at first, I was never Mrs Thriplow. I was always Mrs Dr Thriplow. Why can't I be Mrs Thriplow? and not this Mrs Dr? But there again – you get used to it. The new partner's wife, she noticed it. "This Mrs Dr Hughes – do they do it to you?" "Yes," I said, "everybody." I think it's something particularly Welsh.'

Many of the GPs' wives described the same sort of lives – partly enjoyed, partly endured, partly resented. Mary Chathill was exceptional, in that her husband took great care of her when she was ill. When she had her children, he abandoned the practice to be with her.

Aside from that, she shared the telephone calls, in early days to the degree that the days and nights were a blur of tiredness. On two occasions they had to drive into a field to talk over some lengthy family matters. Like other wives, people tried to get at her husband through her – "background details, like the mother-in-law was wandering the house at night".

MARY CHATHILL: 'I'd just as soon have not done it all. I didn't realize, it sounds stupid for a GP's daughter to say, I didn't realize what it was like. I think there's a thing that a lot of women resent, clergymen's wives and people like that must resent it, is that you're not an entity in yourself – you're simply their wife. I've spent my entire life being Dr Woolaston's daughter and Dr Chathill's wife. Which doesn't matter of course. But – well they can waste my time as long as they don't waste his. I'm pleased they're not wasting his, but I don't see why they should take mine so much for granted.

'I think we are still expected to behave slightly differently from everybody else. One of the partners has had a lot of marital problems. In fact his second marriage has just broken down recently I believe, and somebody certainly said to me they thought it was disgusting and we should do something about it. And I said "Why should he be any different from anybody else round here? There are a lot of people with married problems round here."

'My mother was not a nurse and anything medical revolts her. She hated shop talk and had no knowledge and took a pride in not having any. She didn't like being a GP's wife at all. She hated it. She couldn't bear him being so important when she wasn't. I think that's why she went into the WI in a very big way. On one occasion, when she was being something or other, she was on the platform and the chairman introduced her and said, "We have Mrs Woolaston's husband in the audience," and that was the first time he had ever been "Mrs Woolaston's husband", and I think she practically had it emblazoned on her.

'I shall be most interested in knowing what the younger GPs' wives have to say. I'm quite certain that they don't expect to behave in the way we did.'

JANET BILSBY: 'I think there is a gulf between the older ones who gave up their jobs on marriage and who haven't worked since, and those of us like me and many of the younger ones I know who are professionally qualified in our own right in various things, and who work. After all, now that medical school intake is virtually 50/50 many doctors marry other doctors, who themselves wish to keep up a career. I think there is a big gulf between the different generations.'

JGH: 'What about your position in the community? WI, fêtes, clubs, when people come up to you and ask your advice or ask you to ask David something. Do you not feel you are some sort of figure in the community?'

JANET BILSBY: 'No.'

There are also stereotypes which could be abundantly but tediously demonstrated. GPs tend to prefer their families not to become ill and ignore them if they do – especially do they ignore wives. They like them to see another GP.

Many GPs marry nurses. It was quite surprising to see a cliché so strikingly borne out.

The children of doctors become doctors or nurses. This was so with nineteen of the GPs I spoke to; but then in a further thirteen their families were too young for any choice to be possible

And with this, one of the clear if reluctantly admitted reasons why GPs choose their profession, we move towards increasingly personal areas: their stands on moral issues, their attitudes to their own illness, to class, their cohesiveness as a group, until we reach the most personal of all, of which these are all manifestations, a loosely focused but vital centre of our subject – the characters of the GPs themselves.

32
WHY THEY BECAME GPs

DR CLARA ELLON: 'I knew what I wanted. Toddler stage onwards. My grandfather died when I was seven and a half and I always said I wanted to be a doctor like him.'

DR JOHN MARTHAN: 'I have always wanted to be a doctor. Even when I was a boy. But we are a medical family. My mother was a doctor, and three of her brothers, and one of my father's brothers, he was also in the partnership. And I have four cousins who were doctors.'

DR KERRIS: 'I don't really know. Well, it's not all that difficult, my father was a doctor, and my brother's a doctor and the whole family have just always been doctors as far as I know. There was a terrible rebellion – for a couple of years I wanted to be an architect, but I soon saw the light again, came back to the fold. No pressure, but it was just obviously around and I just became a doctor like everybody else.'

There is no need to belabour this aspect. There is a general tendency to emulate parents, and I explained earlier why I thought this was peculiarly strong among doctors.

This was borne out by a psychiatrist I spoke to on the subject. 'It's never questioned, never questioned. They don't have to say they're going to be doctors or "What are you going to be?" They are doctors. There is also the type of child who is told by the mother she wants a doctor in the family. "You will be a doctor and your brother a dentist." I had a case like that.'

This force means that doctors have carried into our advanced and complicated age inheritance patterns of an earlier period, when sons *automatically* became blacksmiths, wheelwrights, jewellers, or took over the farm or family business.

Self-respect, a desire to remain independent, often led to the roots being hidden or unacknowledged or fought, for a while.

DR TELSCOMBE: 'I don't know. I don't think there was any influence. It was just something I wanted to do; it seemed interesting. I mean, at the age of eight or nine one doesn't think about prestige or power or money.'

J.G.H.: 'What did your mother do?'

DR TELSCOMBE: 'She was a physiotherapist, except for that there was no sign of any medicine *at all*, and I don't recognize any influence from her.' (Further questions discovered a grandfather (maternal) and an uncle – both doctors.)

JILL, A STUDENT: 'My parents are, but that definitely put me off. I got so fed up with people assuming somehow that I would always end up doing that, so I thought I'd do the opposite. And when it came time to go to university, I thought, och weel – I knew sort of underneath that I did want to do it, so I thought I wouldn't let everybody else wanting me to do it put me off doing it. It was funny the way it worked out.'

A trainee GP, Dr Bonby, explained how it was quite prolonged hospital work that made him want to enter general practice. He couldn't stand the superficial, barely human relationship with patients, the hierarchical structure which required years of struggle, the need, often, to do things he thought medically wrong to further his career. It wasn't until the very end of the interview, as I was going, he revealed that his father, grandfather and great-grandfather had all been GPs. 'I suspect that's why I spent so long before I felt I'd like to be a GP. I didn't really want to be, you know, another off the production line.'

The familial links and pressures could be more diffuse. It was clear Dr Axmouth's ambitious school-mistress mother pushed him, but his father, who had died when he was eleven, had been a hospital administrator (a clerk) so it was in this direction he could be pushed.

Dr Locking said jokingly he wanted to be a bishop. Yet he was only half-joking. He had very seriously tried to become a parson. He had sufficient what would today be 'A' levels. He was baulked by the equivalent of Latin 'O' level, then essential. He took it three times, the third time gaining 0 per cent in one paper and 5 per cent in the other.

Dr Locking now recounted a horrific tale of *a whole year* devoted entirely to Latin. By these Herculean labours – 'And I really worked, I learned an entire crib book of Horace odes – *Ars Poetica* – off by heart' – he raised his marks to 31 per cent and 33 per cent. The door to a bishopric slammed shut. In a state that must have been one almost of shock, Dr Locking went to Ireland and, you will recall, took up a life of what, from rather shifty mumblings, I took to be smuggling. Then 'I drifted into medicine.'

Yet – drifted? It was quite clear that the side of him that had wanted to be a parson was the reason he enjoyed being a GP and was a good one. He was interested in, liked, even loved, his patients, 'and I think they like me'. His bluff and witty manner only partially concealed great conscientiousness.

And so, as one leaves obvious parental influence, motives become as superficial or chancy, complex or profound, as difficult to disentangle as they are for most human endeavour.

MARIUS, A STUDENT: 'Lots of people do medicine because they get very good 'O' levels and very good 'A' levels. Teacher says, "Oh, you're quite good. Medicine's difficult to get into; try for medicine."'

DR ABNEY: 'We had two GPs. One was splendid. David Bath, a *marvellous* doctor. We had great rapport. Very dapper little man. Thick set, but little, and I can always remember him. He was always interested in *me*, you know. I think he was a major influence.'

DR KINSHAM: 'I think I felt there wasn't sufficient challenge in geophysics. I always seemed to have done very well in exams and things. All too easy. So I went into medicine, got a job in a medical unit doing physics and medicine, with a promise of a consultant level job in three years.

'I had to go and get a reference from my old professor and I met a girl I knew in my year and she said, "Oh, come and have a coffee. I'm doing a trainee job around the corner," and I went, and I immediately realized that was what I wanted – a combination of humanity, dealing with individuals, psychiatry and the physical aspect.

'I was analysed. I find it very difficult to say what I learnt. I'll ask my analyst, "Why did I become a doctor?" There is a sort of feeling of guilt, I suppose, in why people become doctors. There's also a feeling of power. There's a sort of do-gooding element. I have a younger brother.

'Perhaps the reason I stay in the inner cities is because I feel I wouldn't be challenged in the country. I suppose there's a sort of guilt complex, to use these abilities, to do things for people.'

JIM, A STUDENT: 'I knew you were going to ask that. That is a really difficult question, because I've always wanted to be one, ever since I was really young. My father's a bricklayer of sorts. I'm not from a medical background at all. I don't know. My mother died early. I was about eight and she died of cancer and I don't know if that had any impact. I never had any second thoughts about it when I was doing my 'O' levels. Everyone said, "Don't be daft, you're being too ambitious. You're going to be let down," but I wasn't. I just knew it was for me.'

DR JANE EDSTONE: 'I was always interested in knowing how people worked. I was also extremely frightened of illness and my family would never admit to being ill, ever. I went around with a grumbling appendix for five or six years because it wasn't the done thing to be ill. I was terrified of doctors and I was very frightened of ill or deformed people. There was a blind woman and a hydrocephalic boy in the village and I would literally walk about three quarters of a mile round so that I didn't have to pass. I think I was so frightened that I was determined to build my knowledge of how people worked so that the two combined. I know when I had my children, I thought, this is ridiculous, so I deliberately took them into hospitals and nursing homes to see ill people. But the fact that I spent all my childhood being afraid of being ill or seeing ill people, a little of that, and the other was curiosity in finding out how people worked.'

According to *The Future General Practitioner*, one third of doctors questioned in a study said they 'just drifted into medicine'. People don't 'drift'. They meant they hadn't or couldn't or didn't wish to analyse what they'd done.

It's much harder for us. The deeper springs of human behaviour are not easily accessible after a few hours', even a few days' conversation. All we can do is speculate.

For instance, without exception the men and women I met were kind people. They responded instinctively and sympathetically to suffering. I always became conscious of this at some point and it was very warming.

Yet even kindness, without being devalued, has springs. A boy identifies with his mother. That part of him which is her, which is 'feminine', can still find it hard to express itself today; he enters one of the 'caring' professions – priest, social worker, doctor.

It struck me that Dr Cerney's childhood suffering (you will remember he was sent away from his parents, aged two) and its subsequent denial, had made him passionate to deny it in no one else – particularly among the underprivileged, who are symbolic children. Dr Jane Edstone also told me, 'I was so neglected myself as a child, I just used to be dumped here, there and everywhere.'

There was an element in quite a number of GPs, that is to say, one touched on in the chapter on stress, of having been wounded, damaged, and of wanting to cure the wounds of others – and by doing so, cure themselves.

At the same time, GPs are independent, they control themselves and their lives. A damaged childhood impels the need to make sure it isn't done to you again – that in future you will be in control. The student Jim probably also exemplifies these impulses.

And there is guilt. Dr Kinsham said he was guilty about his abilities. I don't think people feel *real* guilt about such things. There may be some bashful public-school modesty. But he mentioned, no more, a younger brother. Elder brothers bully younger brothers, and if unchecked this can produce proper guilt – for years older brothers try and make up for the damage they did when small.

I want, finally, to touch on two other motives I was aware of and which we'll explore further when we come to the characters of GPs. The first can involve guilt, though it didn't seem to, at least not obviously, with Sally

Finstock.

SALLY FINSTOCK: 'My mother is a doctor and it was assumed throughout my childhood that I would be a doctor. I really can't talk about parental pressure because it was both much less heavy than that and also much stronger than that. It was just a total assumption that that was what I was going to do. I think my mother feels that medicine is the only worthwhile thing to do in the world; it's the only thing that can give you a combination of human fulfilment in terms of the relationships you make with people, intellectual satisfaction and a reliable steady income in any country of the world in any economic situation.

'The feeling that I'm doing something that everybody's going to recognize as useful is quite nice. That's not, however, why I did it, at all. I've always been interested in sort of everyday sociology if you like. Given that I'm already a doctor, general practice is where I can really get into my interest in how people live their lives. I mean, for example, I'm fascinated by the way they speak. Every day I come home from work and talk about some other funny northern word that people have used about their symptoms. So that's one thing. Another thing is that I like to get close to people. I actually enjoy communicating and feeling warm with a lot of people, so general practice gives you good scope for that. It's a feeling of being down to earth, close to what is straightforward and ordinary.'

The final motive is one that leads straight into the next section, where it is surprisingly absent.

DR BRANE: 'Oh always, from the age of sixteen, I think via hypnosis, because I'd read a book, Bramwell's book on hypnosis, when I was sixteen. I was hypnotizing my girlfriends at sixteen and they were going out like flies, and I cured a boil on sombody's nose, Joycie, my current girlfriend. Joycie had a wart on her nose – no, a boil, a huge boil, and she wouldn't go to the dance. I said, "Come on Joycie, I'll send you to the dance", and I hypnotized her and there she was, dancing away with this huge boil, being the belle of the ball. It's a miracle, an absolute miracle. So I thought my purpose was to become a medical student; must be a medical student. But my motivation went deeper than that.

'The main thing was, I'd seen a dead child, a dead girl under a bridge in Westcliff-on-Sea and nobody could tell whether this girl was dead – I was seven, six or seven. And I knew the girl was dead because there were flies on her. Nobody else seemed to know. And then suddenly – it seemed like *hours* we were there – some stupid woman named Maude Sinclair had kept us watching this and looking at it, and it seemed hours that we were there. It must have been terrifying to see this child lying dead, without a coat or anything on, and then a car – a very large Daimler car, I remember it was a

Daimler – stopped, a man got out and he walked over, he looked very much like God and this is absolutely true. And he took his stethoscope out and put it on the child – he didn't need a stethoscope, it was obvious, at seven or six, I knew the child was dead. Now this is what he did, he put the stethoscope on to her, I thought it might be fantasy but I brought it up in analysis and there was no fantasy about it. He shook his head, got back slowly into his car and I remember thinking, my God, the *power*. I watched him, sort of absolutely staggered. He'd come out, said the child was dead, and then everybody disappeared. So we all went home!'

A Moral Stance: The Pill, Abortion

Dr Blairhall: 'I'm Church of Scotland. You know, I was brought up in the Calvinist tradition and the question of abortion . . . When I was a student and first practised, for a patient to *suggest* that an abortion might be done, other than for *strict* medical reasons, which would be me initiating them, was, you know, unthinkable. And then all of a sudden we get this, you know, the David Steele Act and the law of the country's changed. I just had to *accept* it. It's much more difficult to unlearn something you've been taught than it is to learn new facts. Very difficult.'

Dr Anne Uplees: 'I don't think it's right. But for years as a doctor I felt that I *must* listen sympathetically to people who feel they want one. Now I don't think I have to behave like that any more. And actually my partner's a Muslim and doesn't believe in them, so he often sends them to me. What I do is to tell them to go to the Pregnancy Advisory Service, so in a way they're no worse off.'

Dr Axmouth: 'Abortions, if they want them, I will not stand in their way usually. Occasionally I have said to a young married woman – now looking back I feel a bit ashamed, should I or shouldn't I? – I've said, if it was her first pregnancy and just arrived at a socially inconvenient time, I've said no, I don't feel I can refer you. This I leave to the Pregnancy Advisory Service who can refer, getting myself off the moral hook.

'The pill I just put them on if they want to. If they're under sixteen I want a responsible adult, not necessarily a parent. It only happened once and the sister-in-law came along, I knew the family situation and knew this was far the less of two evils.' (This was a case of incest.)

Dr Trimdon: 'I took a moral stand once, but I would rather have a termination than an unwanted pregnancy and I'll even give the pill to an under-sixteen-year-old, with or without her mother's consent. So although one's moral views haven't basically changed, you cannot fight against the permissive time – there's just no way.

'This morning, for instance, the young trainee had put down, "Wishes the pill; sixteen in three weeks; to use other contraception." Why split hairs about three weeks? But a young doctor would know that there have been things written about under-sixteen-year-olds and she'll play safe. So I suppose she was really doing the proper thing.'

DR THRIPLOW: 'Morality isn't our role. Advice is. I don't think abortion is good in principle. But you know them and sometimes you can say, "This is right for this family." I had one the other day. A woman had an extra-marital affair and is pregnant. If she had the baby it would certainly ruin her marriage. She wanted one desperately and I think I was right to endorse it. Again, there are girls whose hearts it would break, though it might be easier socially. It's usually the mother comes demanding an abortion, and the girl says, "No, I'd rather keep the baby." You have to try and decide who's going to be better off whatever you do.'

DR CHATHILL: 'It's their body, their decision, they're the ones who have to go through with it. One can advise, no, not advise. The art of counselling, a word I hate, is to get them to see what they *really* want. If someone is certain in their own mind of exactly what they want, then one has no right to take a moral tone. I think that would be totally wrong.'

DR BILSBY: 'I honestly don't know. I mean if marijuana was legalized I don't think it would do any more harm than tobacco for instance.
    'I certainly don't take a moral stance on terminations – I think it's the patient's right to decide that on the whole.'

There are more than 20,000 GPs and few generalizations hold good for all, or even for large numbers at a time. Nevertheless, certain characteristics are shared quite widely and numbers of these have already been demonstrated, often with some robustness, by the doctors we have met.

Like all jobs where the participant is the centre of attention – judges, teachers, MPs, policemen – there is an element of the actor in many doctors. I think of Dr Eastcourt striding into the panic-stricken house of the heart attack in the middle of the night, or Dr Locking with his bus audience of old ladies.

DR BLAIRHALL: 'And you see, going to a day-school in Edinburgh like Watsons, it had a tradition of producing doctors. I was keenly interested in amateur dramatics – rather a show-off. I was showing-off by writing to you! And out of that dramatic club one in three are now doctors. I've always felt that GPs in particular, they role-play. You know, we're acting in front of patients.'

Dr Blairhall's careful emphasis and dramatic timing were very evident on the tape.

A stereotype of the doctor – one much favoured by Glin Bennet – is of an authoritarian personality: identifying with the existing social order, right-wing or at least conservative, bad at emotions, taking moral stands. He said this was common among the students of the mid-sixties – but has 'all changed now'. However, many of the GPs now *are* these students.

I think Bennet goes over the top in this, as in some other respects. Nevertheless, if I found few examples (I can think of one) of the full-blooded stereotype, elements were there. For the mass of people, the GP is the most evident figure of the State's authority and also the source of its beneficence. Medicine by its nature is a profession of received knowledge, and operates by the application of rules and procedures. In social status the GP sees himself, and is usually seen, as above the parson and a little below the squire (if there are still squires).

Six of the GPs I spoke to were left-wing; the rest Conservative and SDP. I suspect this was atypical; but the large majority of GPs are certainly to the right (before the last election 75 per cent said they would vote Tory).

John Berger makes an original comment about this. So much of a GP's psycho-social load is due to social circumstance – lack of educational opportunity when young, poverty, unemployment, poor housing, 'the circle of deprivation' etc. – that it could occur to him that the most effective way of lightening his load would be to change society. For their job to become this as well as doctoring would be to put too great a strain on them, be too enraging. Only a Conservative can accept the status quo.

This aspect can burden GPS, make them callous and cynical. They become uncertain of the worth of the lives they treat – the drabness, the petty materialism, the small horizons, the paltry education, where telly substitutes for thought, endurance for experience, relief for improvement. This is what disillusions them.

Berger makes another original observation. The 'unconventional' GP is also traditional – Dr Nyewood's shambling tweeded figure longing for a glass of gin, though this has additional roots. Partly this is an indulgence licensed by the importance of his task. Partly an expression that this task puts him slightly outside the community. But it also shows that his importance derives *solely* from the task. It is *not* an authority backed by the establishment, not *society* being authoritarian. I would say that this attitude – whether or not accompanied by tweeded shambling – was much more common than Bennet's stereotype.

Minor mannerisms are common. A lot of GPS, after years of impressing indelibly on patients what they require to be done, had developed rather measured, even orotund deliveries, involving subtle variations and repetitions, and at the end of each passage there would a short statement, the message neatly summed-up. Hesse Sachs talked of 'the look'. They all had 'the look', even students. I wasn't quite sure what she meant. I never noticed a 'look' – but perhaps they looked at Hesse Sachs and me in a different way.

GPS usually have an exclusively scientific background. From the age of sixteen or earlier they have worked ferociously hard to pass difficult exams. Their medical training alone takes eight or nine years.

Mr Eston was a surgeon on the selection board of one of the large London teaching hospitals. Other aspects of his work took him to GPS far and wide.

MR ESTON: 'They tend to be, GPS, rather illiterate. It's so hard to generalize – there's so many of them – relatively illiterate. They're all educated and balanced in perspective, they know quite a lot of what's going on around superficially from politics to farming to the other things, but it's pretty heavy work and when they've got kids, as they usually have, and all that, there isn't much time. They never go to theatres and things like that, life's too full. Quite often they do have a mild interest in classical music and even occasionally play in trios, but very rarely. Much less often do they know anything about architecture or painting. They conform as to standard pictures on their walls, very few books – *The Third Reich* normally – as for poetry, not at all. They're pretty Philistine, yes.'

But there is a slightly more superficial but more subtle aspect to the difficulty or otherwise GPs have expressing emotions towards their patients and becoming involved emotionally with them. There are people, GPs included, who are shy and frightened at expressing feeling, yet who feel strongly and would like to express themselves, 'to connect' in Forster's phrase. The GP life can be, paradoxically, ideal for such people, because a certain distance is *expected*, the relationship is formal, almost stylized, yet at the same time the need and the response to it are genuine, warm, living, sometimes profound. I noticed that many GPs who were clearly bad at, and stilted when revealing emotion could express themselves through the medium of their job.

DR WYRE: 'It was a very enjoyable life. Because one had a sort of cross section of people to know, and there was always that excuse to know moderately intimately from the miners upwards, and equally one had an excuse to have a personal or emotional contact which one wouldn't conceivably in one's moderately shy way ever have achieved, if one hadn't got a professional justification for asking awkward questions.'

In this account, Dr Wyre touches on and moves us into a further dimension of our exploration – class.

Class plays a role in medicine, as in most departments of British life. We saw it briefly in GPs relationships with their patients. Class guilt certainly played a part, and not a dishonourable one, in the dedicated lives of certain inner-city GPs (that was probably one of the things Dr Kinsham meant by his 'abilities').

But there is a third aspect. Richard Hoggart in his *The Uses of Literacy* describes how in his northern working-class background the doctor was virtually the only representative of the middle classes who was able to, and who did penetrate and become accepted. (And accepted, incidentally, in a precise reverse of what Berger noted the GP himself feeling – as someone who was *not* a representative of society, of 'them'.)

But, equally, medicine is the road by which intensely curious, fascinated middle-class people can enter that strange, frightening, forbidden, unknown country – and find it, to their amazement, as real and human as their own, or even more so. Time and again I noticed this, quite unacknowledged, element. Dr Sally Finstock had something of it. Here is another.

DR WHEATACRE: 'The Hodsons were a particular family – absolute rogues – and my father conceived a theory that in fact they had gypsy blood in them. Small Chippings was the next village here. It was a great place in the last century and the gypsies came, and one of the Hodson's – several of the

Hodson family looked like gypsies – and they were extraordinary. They weren't very bright; they weren't very honest. They were capable of petty theft, but they had an enormous charm.

'Then the Maddoxes. The Maddoxes, one of whom became a jockey and was quite well known in his day; they were a shifty lot and several of them had been to prison. My father, who remained a great hand-washer because of the Lister influence of *his* father, always would wash his hands before even examining a patient – even in a slum – and they would have a basin of hot water for him. And he got home one evening and found that his ring had disappeared and he realized that it had probably come off somewhere and he thought he'd lost it. And that night, down came one of the Maddoxes who'd done time in prison for theft – for petty theft – and handed him his ring. Because they liked him and, you know, this is the kind of thing you'd find.

'And we'd go round and I'd think, this is rather an attractive girl; and he would tell me that indeed she was superficially, but that really her morals were disgraceful, but she was charming, yes. And I sort of learnt that people can be not just like the people at school who were fairly fixed, middle class people. A lot of intelligence. "There's *intelligence* in this family," my father would say, and I've seen it. The Hodsons have, indeed, produced not a university graduate, but somebody who's the equivalent of a sergeant-major in the RAF. My father saw this intelligence somewhere and this chap had a conventional secondary school education and then went into the RAF and rose through the ranks to be – is it a warrant officer, I think? Yes.

'And I could see this as a boy – I would go round on a Sunday. All the miners here – a lot of miners had pigeons; they would give us pigeons and the whole of our house – not the whole, but several bedrooms, my brother and sister, we'd have a box with pigeons in with a little spy hole and we could watch them through the window and the box would be tied on to the window sill. We knew all the local lads. It was *so* fascinating to see that there were people, real people, who behaved like characters in novels. There's many of my contemporaries of course had not lived in a pit village – they lived in the suburbs and they didn't have this experience of being, and mixing with miners. And also with somebody who knew them inside-out telling you all about them. So that I was, to some extent, hooked on people because of this.'

Dr Simon Kibane described how he found he missed his small son's crying at night when he went away. He *needed* his son's dependence. There is in fact a universal human need to be used, to have a function, for the sympathetic, loving, caring side of one's nature to be exercised and extended.

But this can get out of hand, and become an appetite; there is the, to a GP, fairly familiar figure of the patient-dependent doctor. I heard of several. 'They can't stop thinking about their patients.' There was one who went to the South of France and rang the practice every day to find out how Miss So-

and–so was, or Mr Blank. In another practice, the new partner, a girl, was refusing to take the other half of her holiday, badly needed, because of the way the patients had piled up, had suffered – 'They missed me.' The practice, the patients, become the only reality, source of love, life, feeling.

This can happen when a GP has unresolved childhood or emotional difficulties. He will project on to patients' fixations needs deriving from those felt for, or in relation to, parents, siblings, authority or guilt figures. This is very common; psychiatrists call it introjection. Doctors put themselves within their patients, projecting their problems on to their patients. (The psychiatrist I discussed this with said he'd wondered whether this wasn't more common than usually realized, and that the GP who refused to talk to or become involved with his patients might have, at some level, recognized the potential danger within himself.)

Yet another not uncommon figure, and not only in medicine, is someone whose distress is internal and deep but cannot be projected. These are the workaholics whose needs are only assuaged by the flood of work they take on, when its amount, their involvement, exhaustion and strain blot everything out.

In myth, and in different cultures, the physician is often the one who is ill. The Indonesian or Eskimo shaman is frequently epileptic or afflicted in some other way; so are medicine men in Africa. Asclepius was taught his healing arts, in Greek legend, by the centaur Chiron; but Chiron had a wound which never healed. 'Only the wounded physician heals.'

Glin Bennet argues that in some sense the wound must continue – or at least the awareness of it must continue. Just as the alcoholic talks more easily to the ex-alcoholic or the divorced to the person who is divorced, so the patient can speak to the doctor when he can see he is weak and human like himself (here is the more profound root of Dr Nyewood's shambling figure).

This does not mean the doctor must continue to *be* alcoholic or neurotic or whatever it is. The shaman often takes up his profession to cure himself. He owes his power and his prestige to the fact that he has done this. But his disease, his surmounting it, have given him his insight.

We have now, perhaps, sufficiently seen why and how the GP's situation – of which the wounded physician is a part – sets him aside. But this gives the profession, as it does to others similarly placed (the police for instance), tremendous cohesion.

This is reinforced at many points. Doctors don't just inhabit a different world, they speak a different language. It has been estimated that at medical school the student has to learn the equivalent of two foreign languages. And here, too, as Ferris says in *The Doctors*, they soak up 'their inheritance of tradition, ethics and common sense, which helps set them apart from everyone else. There are endless lessons. Doctors must not argue in front of patients. Beware of women who enjoy gynaecological examinations. "Arthritis" alarms patients but "rheumatism" doesn't. Do not, if possible, let a patient die on the operating table – move him out quickly if all seems lost.'

For this reason, doctors protect each other and are notorious for so doing. The most heinous mistakes are covered up, not just because there but for the grace of God might they themselves go – but because they are there already. In the end, *all* GPs have done something that has led to someone's death.

DR BRANE: 'If I go against another doctor, I've noticed there is immediately sympathy for him. If I am outspoken about some doctor whose attitude to medicine is extremely unprincipled, there will immediately be doctors who turn on me. It is almost as if they fear someone will turn on them. In other words, it is guilt that some of these doctors suffer, because they have all been in guilty situations.'

DR WHEATACRE: 'There is an organization, you see, for sick doctors, which means often "drunk doctors" or senile doctors. There are GP assessors in each region. I'm the one for this region. Well, I won't assess people here but anybody who's certified or thought to be sick, I will go down to wherever the region is and I'll have an interview with this chap and be expected to come out saying that this chap is not fit to practise. But it's noticeable that I've been one for years and I've never had more than my letter of appointment. Nobody is putting it to effect, you see. And doctors stick together, as patients often say, and I said to a student, "You know, you're in this profession, you're safe for life." Well, if you go mad, perhaps. But you can take to the bottle, you can take to drugs. The chances are that you'll never be found out. Your colleagues will do nothing about it. You're in a *marvellous* situation. Even the most frightful old drunks, their partners will say, "He's no bloody good, but what can we do about it? We can't shop him. He's got a nice wife and he's got children . . ." and so it goes on, you see.'

This also means that on the whole doctors are kind to one another, a kindness from which, due entirely to this cohesion, I benefited too. Dr Blairhall gave me an example of this and, incidentally, explained my position. He described how some years before, the then President of the Royal College – who only knew he was a fellow doctor – had gone to great lengths to get Dr Blairhall's son cured of depression. 'I'm grateful to that man,' he said. 'But then our Hippocratic oath says you should treat your colleagues as your brother.' It was at this moment that I said I'd been struck by how kind doctors had been to me. At which Dr Blairhall gave me what I can only describe as a very sweet smile and said, 'Yes, and the oath goes on, "your colleagues as your brother and his children as your children."'

When they learnt I was writing about GPs, people invariably said, you *must* meet this GP or my GP. They would often then add, after a glowing description, 'and he's very keen on music', or he 'has this valuable collection of old trains', as though to say, 'you see, this god is *human* too.' And I would then meet this perfectly amiable (or not so amiable) but quite unexceptional GP who had some Hornby trains in his garage or a few Haydn and Beethoven records.

The desire to deify GPs is very strong and adds to the considerable power, the *sense* of power, which GPs have already. This is another reason for their cohesion. The powerful, like the rich, tend to stick together.

GPs are aware of their power; and this puts a charge behind the role of actor since they are not in the strict sense, acting a role at all. It is for real, and the reality is often that of life and death – from whence derives the power.

Dr Warfield frankly admits what is quite clear the instant you meet this kind, frank, amusing man.

DR WARFIELD: 'Of course, a lot of GPs are ego. I think you've got to have a fairly high ego if you're going to be a reasonably successful GP. And this does give rise to a certain amount of – what shall I say? – dogmatic thinking. You can't say, "Well it might be this, it might be that, Mrs Smith, but I really don't know." You've got to say, "It is tonsillitis. It will get better. I will give you some tablets. That will do it." All straightforward stuff. You mustn't be airy-fairy. So I suppose GPs do tend to have fairly inflated ideas of their own importance, I'm afraid, inevitably.'

I discussed this at some length with Dr Veryan, his daughter sitting in and listening beady-eyed.

JGH: 'But to what extent is it therapeutically valuable to have people believing in the doctor as a god? Is there not an element of faith healing?'

DR VERYAN: 'It depends what you want as a patient. If you go into transactional analysis of parent/adult/child relationship, a patient may come to you as an adult expecting to be treated as an adult. A patient may come to you as a child wanting big daddy to help, coming in distressed – "Please help me, doctor." It depends very much whether you keep yourself on these parallel lines so that you react as the nurturing, kindly parent coping with the child or whether you act on an adult/adult basis. When lines get crossed and the patient is trying to be on an adult basis and the doctor's trying to be parental, then you get some crossed lines and things go wrong.'

JGH: 'I think that's a way of looking at the problem which isn't quite the same. Two adults can talk. Nevertheless, if you come to me and say, "Look, I've written a short story" we can talk as adults but on the whole you'll say, "He's probably right."'

DR VERYAN: 'But that's talking on a totally adult basis.'

JGH: 'It is, but underneath how you respond to what I say is the acceptance of me being "righter" than you, and the same is true surely of doctor and patient.'

DR VERYAN: 'No. I think that's a misconception of the transactional analysis definition. You can go and ask somebody's advice and receive it on a purely adult plane. But you can go as a supplicant saying "Doctor, help me! What would you suggest I do?" and the doctor says, "Well you take the medicine, you go to bed, you stay there," and gives a whole lot of sort of parental advice. And using the word "parental" in this instance is not a – it doesn't necessarily mean bossy. It means just taking the role of the parent and looking after a child who needs help. But on the other hand you could have a doctor who is bossy and wagging the finger; a really parental attitude, "You do this, you do that", and "I won't have this and won't have that", and this sort of thing. And trying to treat everybody as children. Adults don't like being treated as childen and therefore the lines get crossed and they dislike it intensely.'

JGH: 'What I mean by "faith healing" is if you say, "You will get better" people do get better.'

DR VERYAN: 'Enormously. I mean, the drug "doctor" is one of the most powerful drugs we've got. And what the pink or white pill is, is of less significance than the power which the doctor uses.'

JGH: 'Once you admit that, from that does derive a certain amount of authority and probably does derive a certain hierarchical situation in the grouping around that health care, which is why you're meant to lead.'

DR VERYAN: 'But on the other hand it depends how the doctor utilizes this. It is a power that's invested in him. I mean, he can misuse it.'

JGH: 'And extend that power into spheres where it shouldn't properly be exercised?'

DR VERYAN: 'Yes. You can see when doctors get out of their field they can become totally authoritarian in their statements and know nothing about the subject, so it really gets rather aggravating.'

DAUGHTER: 'It seems to sort of ring a bell.'

Towards the end of *The Future General Practitioner* comes a clear statement of what one might call 'the GP as artist'. So different, say the (largely GP or ex-GP) authors, are the possible diagnoses, the possible treatments, the ways of expressing and administering them, so personal and therefore variable are the contacts, that the GP's *character* is the only clue. That is:

> the doctor's experience of life, his personal philosophy, his tastes, his strengths and weaknesses, his characteristics as a convergent or divergent thinker, and so on. It is a very difficult thing for us, trained as we are in the scientific method, to face what seems an irrational element in our rational decision-taking. And yet we have to face that the personality of the clinician enormously affects the style of his practice – the choices he makes, the pathways that he follows through hypotheses, validations and solutions. Every doctor expresses *himself* in his practice of clinical medicine.

This is perfectly true. And it is nowhere more true – or at least it is nowhere more obvious – than in egalitarian, feminist and dual-role practices.

35

EGALITARIAN PRACTICES

I know of four egalitarian practices: one in London, one in a large city in the south-west, two in the north. The London one, at Limes Grove in Lewisham, is an all-woman practice, run as a collective, open to alternative medicine (herbal remedies, a consultant acupuncturist). I didn't visit it, nor the south-west practice. But Dr Sally Finstock, who was in the process of opening her own egalitarian practice, had worked part time in the south-west. The other northern partnership was that of Mike Kerris, whom we've already met several times, and Dr Nick Trull.

Dr Mike Kerris

The surgery was in what the man in the Post Office described as 'a very run down bit of this city'. I drove under a railway bridge, past about fifteen pubs, and came to the large, craggy building. In the windows were large CND posters and banners supporting a Health Service strike, then in progress.

Inside it was like a big comfortable ramshackle house. The waiting room was large, full of old sofas and armchairs, patients milling about chatting, smoking, making themselves cups of tea. Their children ('kids') playing with the toys on the floor; the receptionists, nurses, etc., also milling about and drinking tea. I recognized some from the leaflet I'd been sent introducing them (by Christian names). I'd noticed 'Jill' as she seemed to do a lot. She looked pretty formidable – trousers, wedge heels, tough face with a jutting nose, powerful plait down her back.

Mike Kerris soon arrived and we went up to one of several rooms to talk; again, house-like with easy chairs, three-bar electric fire. He was, what? Thirty-five? Forty? Beard, thinning hair more or less bald on top, sympathetic. He had a CND badge in his lapel.

Then, and especially later at the small practice meeting, I had the feeling – it was something he said in fact, but you could feel it – of a strong character deliberately striving to keep directing, managerial energies in severe check lest they swamped the democratic process.

DR MIKE KERRIS: 'It's run almost as a reaction, as a criticism of the way we feel other places are. *Really* it's to do with hierarchies, sort of doctors at the top, right or wrong, giving decisions and getting all the tangible rewards. Just waltzes in at his convenience to do what he wants to do, takes all the loot, and gets the rest to work to make life easier, while they're left scouring around, much less money and always feeling sort of resentful that they aren't able to do things that they want, basically, because the doctor's told them to do something else.

'We don't consider the money that comes into this practice as ours, that's fundamental. It's earned by everybody here. We *need* receptionists, we *need* cleaners, we *need* all the counsellors, health and safety people. So all the money comes into a pool and it's controlled by the practice meeting.

'We all get the same hourly rate. It's very complicated because everyone's on a different PAYE scale. But it's worth it, because everyone knows the doctors get the same. In fact, we take home more money because we are on call and we work longer hours, but I take home just over £800 a month.

'Then the practice meeting decides what happens to the rest of the money, and every member of the staff has an equal say. And of course it's *not* equal, because some people are very used to making decisions and dealing with thousands and thousands of pounds and other people just aren't used to that, so it's a slow sort of process. We've been going for three years now and I think it's getting to work. Certainly people are making demands now who weren't.

'I'm sure it works better, happier. It's very ponderous sometimes to be democratic and it's bloody annoying sometimes if you've got a project that you *really* want to do and it might take months and months because someone's got an objection, so you have to go through that. When we changed this building it seemed to go on for ever. It could have been done by one guy with a pencil, but it would have been unhappy for everyone except that one person. Now, even if it wasn't *exactly* what you wanted, no one's going to be so averse to it.

'It gives the individuals in the team more scope to do what *they* feel is important. I mean in other general practices I've worked in, the receptionists, or cleaners or other staff often have fantastic ideas, and they're often picking up resentments from patients and know more about it than the people who are making the decisions, yet they're not allowed into the decision-making. Well, you know the particular systems you need in reception – making sure patients are screened and recalled at the right time, and the forms to be filled in. All that has been worked out by the receptionists themselves, and they have a meeting each week to work out what they want to do.

'I mean, I worked in a practice where the opening hours were such that the doors of the surgery closed at 10 and the bus from the next village arrived at 10 past 10, and he just would *not* have surgery moved to, say, 10.30, because it was always 10. He got more and more annoyed at having to make silly visits to the next village. Well efficiency isn't the total end result, but it would have been much better if he'd left it to receptionists.

'Then elderly people in the practice. We have a nurse particularly to look after elderly people only. And all the staff, the nurses, the health visitors, have their people – so there are always people we can ask for help, who'll know that patient better.

'There's one person I get on with very, very badly, for instance, who gets on very, very well with one other member of staff. She's very angry with me now at the way I looked after her mother. Her mother eventually died and I'm to blame. She was always trying to get rid of her mother and there was this tremendous tension in the home. But now the mother's become sanctified – quite common. But I was always on the old lady's side so I can't grieve with the daughter and I can't really accept the anger against me as being justified. But she's also being seen and counselled by one of the other workers in the practice, this other worker always reminds me that, "Hey, behind all this anger and things, there is a person and this is what she's feeling," and that helps *me* to understand the daughter and not sort of just act emotionally against her. Now, if I were working on my own, that daughter would get a terribly bad deal from me.

'And that's happening all the time with different members of staff advocating for different patients and saying if someone's a burden to some one person then we'll discuss that. It wouldn't come to the big group, but we would seek out other members of the team who might be helpful and just go through it. We talk all the time – you know, lots and lots of times about people who are upsetting us, or something like that. And so, at that sort of level, you don't just have to talk to *doctors* – I think that's the sort of theme of this place. How come doctors have got all these insights into patients? It just isn't true. In fact, they've probably got less training in that sort of area than probably any other member of staff, I should think.

'It also makes it more fun: although it's tense, you get away from the boredom. You can't be bored, because if you are bored it comes out and someone will pick it up, and it'll come back to you like a shot.

'Just recently we got a report on a guy we sent for chest X-ray and it came back with a mass on his chest. Normal reports, everyone reads them then they're filed away. But with this guy we say, "Well, who will be the worker with this person?" both to tell him and follow it through. It's got to be one person. It isn't necessarily the doctor – there's a lady who's dying and one of the nurses will be the primary person for her. But *one* person is responsible.

'I knew him very well and really liked him, so it was my job to talk to him. So I just cleared one afternoon and by the time you've done that and invited yourself to see him they know really. And so he was asking questions, and that's all right. I mean, it's not all *right*, but I don't see how it can be better than that. He's about fifty-nine to sixty. Lung cancer age. But we stand a better chance of a good relationship now. And he's set himself certain tasks before he dies – to set his wife up in a bungalow and die is his sort of aim. And we'll help him in these things, but also pain relief and talking about the fears he must have.

'Reflect on my own death? It makes me reflect on my own *character* quite a bit. He isn't panicking and I'm finding this quite instructive. He's obviously very upset, but on the other hand, he's not managerial class, he's a steelworker. But he's a sort of manager, he's manager of the household for instance. I am a sort of manager. So I can take him as a model. I think if I was given the chance to die with dignity I think he would be one of the models. And so many other people I've seen die with honesty and openness.

'But they have a lousy consciousness of health round here. It's a class thing. A lot of people lead devastatingly unhealthy lives. Terrible, terrible, terrible lives, which they expect the Health Service to patch up really. To do with smoking and obesity and general levels of fitness. I mean, the diet is just so terrible. On our holiday we stopped off at a transport café on the way there. I'm just not exposed to it because of the milieu in which I live, and our family eating habits and things. But it was *terrible*. The people from their big Scania trucks or whatever, they stop and have white bread, dripping, bacon, white bread – you know, really, a three-tier sandwich – dripping with dripping and white bread and that was all. Nothing else. And then they get back in their trucks and that's it, a cigarette stubbed out in the corner of the congealed fat. Yorkie man, you know. But it's *terrible*.

'I suppose it began when I was a student in the late sixties. Also my father was not all that different from me, although I thought he was. His attitude to his team was more that of friendship than hierarchical. And because of the sixties politics, a lot of my friends are to do with egalitarian politics – and that includes the few doctors I mix with. I realize when I do meet other doctors how upset they are by egalitarian notions. Quite a lot of aggression. We hear sorts of stories about what people are saying about this practice. But that's it. It's too bad really.

'You see for me it's a paradigm if you like of what I feel about what's going on in the rest of industry. I mean, in a steelworks we get people coming to us under all sorts of tension. It's not just that they might get steel splashed down their boots or something, it's also this tremendous tension on the shop floor because they feel they aren't part of the machinery. They never have access to the people telling them what to do. If we're going to move into the community and be fiercely critical of the way the steelworks is run – because all this tremendous resentment *causes* ill health – and we say, "Your workers haven't got a say in what goes on," then we've got to be doing the same in our practice. So it isn't just a sort of empty theory, not just differences for differences' sake. It's a way of thinking about working people's lives.'

Industrial democracy isn't easy, whether in a steelworks or a GP practice. I sat in on one of their meetings later, and got an inkling of the enormous amount of discussion that had to go on.

HEALTH VISITOR: 'I mean, I've been at a meeting till 11.15 this morning with a group of social workers, trying to share with them the work that gypsy health involves me in. And I come back, to do two quick visits and start another meeting – this meeting – go off and do my work, and then go to another meeting after half past 4, until well after work should have finished, with another set of professionals about care and duties. Thursday's getting as daft as Tuesdays.'

There were other difficulties. The Limes Grove practice came up and the health visitor (the same one) said the only comment she'd heard was that their democracy worked better because they were all from the same social strata. She said that in this practice democracy *could* not and *never would* work. The staff were multi-layered class-wise; some middle class, well educated, articulate, with a 'good esteem' of themselves; others working class with very little self-esteem. It simply wasn't possible for them to play a dominant role. They just didn't feel on the same level. They just pretended they did.

It wasn't clear where she placed herself. She said she couldn't possibly ask for money, for instance, for them to afford another health visitor which was clearly needed; and did, it seemed to me, by the very act of *not* asking, ask. Dark hair like a wimple, a pleasant face with lines of bitterness, she was extremely articulate and, I thought, *well* able to get her way.

But there undoubtedly was a different atmosphere from all the other practices I saw, no matter how friendly – a lack of deference, a feeling of ease, familiarity, of community, a feeling of freedom.

Dr Sally Finstock

Dr Finstock was small, fuzzy-haired, in trousers, looking much younger than thirty-five. A bit defensive at first, giving forth fairly strong anti-charm signals. She was in a hurry – a depressive she had to see at 2 o'clock. But she warmed, and was intelligent, assured, merry, honest. Her middle-class accent had been slightly flattened – words like 'bloke' incorporated – but far less than is often the case. Very articulate, from which she got pleasure. 'Where was I? I've lost the thread. I was about to reach my *peroration*.'

We spoke first of all about the egalitarian city practice in the south-west.

DR SALLY FINSTOCK: 'It was very exciting working in a collective and so forth, but the practice population was a bit skewed. Partly because some of the patients sought out that practice and particularly those who had been there from the beginning, it was mostly younger people who came to register and a predominance of women.

'But the atmosphere there was completely different. Everybody who works there is known by their first names, which, well it's rather like a hairdresser's really, just to know people by their first names. It's all interesting. It makes people think, I'm sure. The waiting room is scruffy and informal and people can make themselves cups of coffee and are kept waiting for hours.

'There were four theoretical rungs. One of them was feminism. The second was a social strand, an awareness that working–class people get a raw deal out of the Health Service and to improve that. And also to treat patients as equals. One of the things we did was making it possible for patients to read their own notes if they wanted. In principle me and Paul do that here, though fewer people are likely to ask up here. There's still a surprising amount of old-fashioned respect for doctors.

'The other thing about equality in a group is collective decision-making, and of course you have to be terribly careful about this because it's terribly easy to have a sort of collective in *name* but actually still have the doctors pulling all the strings.

'Well, I left because I wasn't happy in the actual city. Also, the practice was pretty chaotic – but it was more personal, really. I felt fragmented there. Also there was something a bit unreal about the practice, so consciously part of the radical alternative trendiness they had there. I wanted to test out the ideas, about feminism and socialism and equality, with a completely ordinary population.

'And then I saw this advertisement Paul had put in asking for a feminist doctor, so that was immediately appealing.'

JGH: 'When he said feminist, what did he mean?'

Dr Sally Finstock: 'He meant . . . well, he obviously implied that he wanted a woman but he meant a woman who was – I wonder what he did mean, we would have to ask him – but what he meant I think was a woman who was committed to the Women's Movement and would approach women's health in feminist terms. Now, trying to define that is something that I'm now so deeply into that it's hard to actually define it. I think to do with seeing women's health in terms of women's position in society, and being prepared to take the social position of women and the sort of role expectations that men have of women and all that stuff into account when dealing with both women and men patients. I think, meaning a political attitude.'

JGH: 'Meaning that you would try and change that?'

Dr Sally Finstock: 'Well, that's an interesting point. I think as a GP you don't change much – but you can try and help people to try and change things in their own lives and try to help people to be more aware of the things that make them ill. If a woman comes with depression because of her social situation, because she's being oppressed by her husband or is on her own in a high rise block with small children under five, or whatever it is, we don't label it depression and assume it's her individual fault, but you help her to see the factors behind that and possibly help her to find ways of changing her situation, or living in her situation with a different awareness of it, even. It's the antithesis of just giving them tranquillizers all the time.

'I don't know what it was that Paul had in mind, but I can tell you what it is that I'm doing. I suppose I'd want to see myself as sitting there with the person and trying to put our heads together about how their social situation affects the way they're feeling, so there's no point in me, with my middle-class, southern ideas about what *I* would want in a relationship with a man assuming that because someone, a bloke, doesn't talk about his feelings, goes to the pub every night and expects his wife to do all the housework, that she's actually oppressed. She may very well not be, but she might be. But, I want to hear what she's got to say about it and understand her point of view rather than imposing mine on her. The more experienced I get, the more I recognize how important it is to listen and tune in to where the person themself is, and make it possible to express those things.'

JGH: 'Even if they turn out to be, well, on either side, a rabid chauvinist?'

DR SALLY FINSTOCK: 'Yes, I think you've got to hear what people have got to say. That's interesting actually, because I mean mostly I find that talking to women we get to understand each other quite easily, and if I'm open to what they've got to say – women of all ages really – we find we've got quite a lot of understanding. What I find difficult is dealing with youngish men. If they do talk about their feelings – which they *do* sometimes, because I think I'm quite good at getting people to talk about their feelings – then they'll say things like, "I don't know what else she wants of me", "I have always brought in a steady wage", "The children are always well fed", or whatever it is. I mean, it's such a mind-boggling thought, because I've got a very good idea of what else she might be wanting of him. I mean, one immediate reaction is, "Why don't you ask her?" But I haven't yet found a way to kind of explain it. I mean, it's difficult enough with the men in your own life, let alone those that walk into the surgery.

'But, what else might I say about being a feminist doctor? What I've just said kind of moves into that, but I don't only want to treat women. The thing that I love about general practice is how you have to see everybody in all sorts of situations, all ages, all kinds of illness from the trivial to the very serious, from the very physical to the very psychological to the very social. And I like the feeling of being accessible to everybody and seeing people in their context, and so forth, so from that point of view, seeing and treating men is quite important to me. Also, I've got quite a strong intellectual interest in medicine. I'm actually quite interested in the diseases and all that, so you've got to see everybody really.

'I actually think I might be bored in another branch of medicine. It's partly the variety. It's partly that you don't know what's going to walk through the door next. Very often something like, "Why did they come today?" is absolutely fascinating. I mean, somebody who has a pain, or a lump, or whatever it is, three or four weeks, what was it about Wednesday that made them walk in with it? You can keep your brain busy with that for some considerable length of time.'

Dr Finstock came north and joined Paul. Their surgery was two Portakabins – very small, cosy, like being in a boat. She said the smallness meant an intimacy between patients, receptionist and doctors. Showing me round, 'Our predecessor kept his whisky there', pointing under the table in the consulting room. It was fully equipped, with two basins, heating, lighting, facilities for treatment, a feeling of efficiency. They were planning a new surgery.

'I found that relationships between doctors and patients are much more sort of traditional and respectable up here. I mean, suggestions that people call me by my first name were really out. I did, when I first arrived, tell a few people they could call me Sally, and this unsettled them. And it was silly. This bloody trendy, southern middle-class idea. I should have kept my mouth shut and waited to find out what was really appropriate.

'Working with a collective of four people is delightful compared with working in a collective with fourteen people. It's *much* nicer working with fewer people. That thing of the doctor pulling the strings is helped with us by a rather curious circumstance, which is that one of the women who does reception is actually married to Paul, and the other one is her sister. There are disadvantages, but it does mean they are much more ready to challenge the doctors, seeing themselves on the same level. And of course, genuine equal pay, equal hourly pay, that stops a hierarchical practice. So I take home about £8,000 a year after tax.

'I like the people here. I enjoy the sense that they need so much that whatever I give them is welcomed. That's very personally gratifying. I'm not sure that it's very politically correct.'

JGH: 'I think one's allowed to be gratified in a socialist world.'

DR SALLY FINSTOCK: 'It isn't that. It's more the feeling of enjoying working with people who have very little in life, because you enjoy the illusion that you're giving them something. It seems a bit suspect.'

JGH: 'Why is it an illusion?'

DR SALLY FINSTOCK: 'I don't know if it's an illusion or not, that's the answer to that. I don't know how much difference I'm actually making to their lives. Possibly I am. I went to the dentist the other day, had a really horrible time and felt humiliated and distressed by his attitude to me and felt that it was actually a very salutary thing to happen to me because it made me realize how some people feel when they go to doctors – that sense of powerlessness and of being patronized. And in fact I was being slightly flirted with and it was most offensive. But quite intangible, so that one couldn't have made a formal complaint of any kind, but it was just really hurtful. And I think a lot of women particularly, but I think people in general, actually experience that with a doctor. Being a bit patronized, a bit glossed over, a bit not heard. It was interesting. All I was trying to say was, that perhaps being the sort of doctor, I hope, that does hear people and does respect them, I maybe did give people something.

'Incidentally, Paul and I both work about two-thirds time, and we're not going to work more even when we've room to work simultaneously. The hours that are expected of GPs at the moment give a sort of role model really of a male GP with a wife who is really pretty much a full-time support system for him. And I think that's wrong. And I think that if having more women in medicine means that men are actually able to do more part-time work, participate in the care of their children, if that's what they want, and it's what an increasing number of blokes my age want, and younger, particularly on the Left, I've lost my flow. That was going to be a good rhetorical sentence and it's fizzled. Yeah, I think blokes should be able to work part time. I think we should *all* be able to work part time and I think we should all be working towards a more harmonious balance between our working lives and our lives outside work and traditional general practice is a bloody awful model for it. It takes up far too much of people's time potential. So my answer to that is that everybody ought to be working part time and the blokes with young children ought to spend time looking after them.'

36

A Shared Practice:
Drs Simon and Janet Kibane

Janet Kibane, about thirty-two, buck teeth, full lips, a bit skinny, with a mop of frizzy hair, attractive, confident, relaxed, intelligent.

Simon Kibane, thirty-five, a beard, a strong, handsome face, a more difficult character. Had worked his way up through grammar school. Extremely clever, he had wanted to be a scientist, but partly absences – long, adventurous trips up Everest, across America – and possibly something prickly in his character – had made that impossible, and he'd taken to GP life. She gave the feeling she was with someone tempestuous, ready to follow him anywhere.

A pleasant, untidy house, a familiar mess of children's nappies, toys, the two toddlers running about.

DR SIMON KIBANE: 'Well, a normal doctor would be in every day doing two surgeries and visits and what have you. Well, we do the same but she does one surgery and I have the other. In between times, I do all the visits and whatever else there is to fiddle with, and I do the night calls.

'That is, I'm at home two mornings a week and one afternoon, Janet's at home one morning and three afternoons and all day Thursdays.'

DR JANET KIBANE: 'Because Thursday is our half day so that only Simon goes in on Thursday mornings, which is why I have all Thursday off. Really we do the childcare between us – Friday is the only day when we need someone else, when Simon's doing this hospital job.'

DR SIMON KIBANE: 'I do a clinical assistant's job in the local hospital.'

DR JANET KIBANE: 'He does lunch on Mondays. But one of the main reasons I do mostly mornings is because it's more convenient for picking up children in the evenings and doing the evening meal. Lunch is a scrap meal in our house anyway. I mostly do the evening meal. He'll do cleaning and bed-making. A bit.'

DR SIMON KIBANE: 'I don't do a lot.'

DR JANET KIBANE: 'Not a lot, but he will do things, especially if I've not had time for them.'

DR SIMON KIBANE: 'Especially if left a list.'

DR JANET KIBANE: 'I suppose I must do most of the house when it boils down to it. But then, he's doing other things in the house, like he's doing *most* of the financing, so I consider it fair.'

DR SIMON KIBANE: 'Each separate doctor has 2,000 patients, and we share 2,100 between us. It's quite rigid. If you are our patient you see one of us, or either of us. You don't see one of the partners. We are, essentially, one doctor.'

DR JANET KIBANE: 'We try to make it that anyone who wants it has access at least on the phone during the day. I'll take calls in the morning for anyone who wants a doctor and often you can reassure them. And Simon has this access at 4 o'clock every day when people are told to phone and speak to him.
    'When they first come we say, "We would *prefer* it that you choose one or other of us, especially if you have a chronic problem," and by and large they comply. There's a list of people sees me and a list sees Simon and of course, anybody with just a cold or sore throat, either of us can see.'

DR SIMON KIBANE: 'It's certainly an advantage to the practice, because we're both paid this magic thing called the basic practice allowance, which is £7,000 before you even start working. But we each get it, whereas if there was only one doctor then there'd only be one lump of £7,000. On top of that is £2,100 we both get, supplementary practice allowance. Then supplementary capitation fee for being on call – which we share.
    'As for talking out stress problems – and there certainly *is* a hell of a lot of stress – we've no room for talk, as they say, because we've got a split practice and we share it. At 12 o'clock she can bugger off and someone takes over, you know.'

DR JANET KIBANE: 'But it's one of the reasons why we're *doing* it I think. If we would admit it, that we are sharing the potential stress and making it easier for both of us. I mean, we don't have that *continual* strain of people coming with their problems. It's diluted.'

DR SIMON KIBANE: 'Well, of course, there's certainly less of it in the way.'

DR JANET KIBANE: 'And another reason was this friend of ours who's Simon's age. She lives in America but we see her regularly and her father is a family doctor in Connecticut, and she said they never saw their father, because he was working so hard. And a busy GP here could do that, he might hardly see the children if he left at 8 and didn't come back till 7, which is what our day is. For *her*, it was a very great emotional point in her life, and it was something we didn't want to do, to have happen to our children, which is one of the reasons I don't *ever* want to work full time. I'm very happy working part time, and I can't see myself necessarily – I might do *more* hours than I'm doing now – but never full-time work.'

37
WOMEN GPs

PROFESSOR CHARDSTOCK (dean of a medical school): 'I think medicine is going to be disadvantaged by women in medicine and that woman is going to be disadvantaged by taking up a medical career and I don't think there have been enough people who have said this loudly. Because medicine is a very demanding career. It's a demanding career first of all in the training thereof, no matter what branch you go into. And it's a demanding career once you've reached your career goal. And it's demanding in terms of time; it's demanding in terms of application; and it's also, as you said earlier on, it is in fact demanding in terms of stress and I think that many women aren't suited to that, for a number of reasons.

'First of all, if a woman wants to undertake a career and have a marriage, then there's conflict, and given our social structure, most men expect their wives to be wives and not professional partners as such. Most men would want to have a family, and I guess so would most women, and so it throws a considerable strain on a female which many females find a great deal of difficulty coping with. And so you find an intelligent woman who also wants to be a mother having difficulty in practising proper motherhood, short of using crêches or nannies, or grandmothers, and never seeing their children, and again, my belief is that that's bad for a whole generation of children growing up in intelligent, professional households who are not subject to the kind of mother care that I would think would be appropriate in the first ten years of life. So that's one thing.

'The second thing is that if you do try and act as a mother, then you can only do part-time work in the hospital or in general practice, and our structure of medical training is unable to cope with that.

'I have a third view – at least, I have a third point to make – and that is that I think women are temperamentally disadvantaged. I just haven't in my career – I've worked with a number of women – and I can see them having difficulties in making logical, cold, calculating decisions which is what a doctor makes. When they're faced with difficult situations – a sick child, a dying relative – a woman would often, because she's a woman, think in a slightly different way to a man, and would often become emotionally involved, which a man doesn't. Now people say, many people say I'm talking nonsense, but I have happened to work for three women at a consultant level, and all of them I thought were guilty of reacting in that sort of way.

'I can think of a woman having problems with a child. I worked for a woman who was a radiotherapist, and children who had leukaemia and that sort of thing. You could see her great difficulty in coping. Whereas I think men come to that decision much more easily.

'I have a lot of sympathy with women in medicine and I think a lot of them end up by not really achieving career goals which males would normally do, and they are subjected to a great deal more stress. And it's going to become worse. And the reason for this is that because there are a lot of women in medicine and because the women tend to marry doctors on the whole – I mean there's a high incidence – then, whose career comes first? And you know we are still in a society where the husband's career, on the whole, takes preference, precedence, and then the woman is dragged along and has to try and find a job, and can't. And I see this very often on selection committees. The first thing you do when you have a prospective candidate: "What's your wife do?" if she's in medicine, "What branch is she in?" and you say, "Well, I'm sorry, we won't be able to fit her in for a job," and they've got the difficult decision of bringing up their wife who can't find a job. And I think that there are all these subtle strains about it.'

(48 per cent of the medical students at the dean's university were girls.)

DR CERNEY; 'One of them [among the trainees to whom he lectures], who I know well, said last week she was expecting to complete training, follow her doctor husband around at work doing this or that – a part-time, temporary job, have children and then look for a definitive practice, perhaps when she was forty – and that's fifteen years' time. It seems a great waste and there was no sense in her conversation that I could get that *she* might in fact be the one who does the moving around while her husband goes for part-time jobs.'

DR JUNE CRESSING: 'It can break up relationships. I had one friendship break up because one friend couldn't divorce the fact I was a doctor and the fact I wanted to be a friend. We had this tremendous argument, about the handling of children which is what women always argue about. It was my attitude towards her son, which I had thought was a pure, simply "Hello Robert, how are you? Lovely to see you" attitude. It's too involved to talk about, but I think that being a doctor had something to do with our estrangement. And it made me think very *hard* and is one of the reasons why I now don't go to mother and toddler group because the incident started there, so I thought, well, if she's doing that, maybe other people are thinking that and analysing things too closely. I'm just a mother too.

'It's easier, I think, for the wife of a GP in the community than for a woman GP in a community, in fact. Like clothes. My dungarees and all that. I don't think it's easy at all. I have my female GP wardrobe which is very conventional – knitted suits, skirts. I do wear trousers to work but they're my brown velvet cord ones, or my black, fairly tailored ones. But usually very conventional clothes with high heels. You know, completely different from my image at home. But I'm obeying a convention, really. People might say that I shouldn't be; I should be myself, and I should be turning up in my dungarees. It's very difficult, because people of my mother-in-law's generation *expect* me to dress like that.'

JGH (talking to Dr Wheatacre): 'Do you think those qualities of mind – I mean, I take it that your argument is that general practice is about people and that you've got to be interested in people? Some people might think those are feminine characteristics *par excellence*, so it is interesting that something like 50 per cent of the students are now women. Do you think that's a direction general practice will go?'

DR WHEATACRE: 'I think it will, but of course the women who come into it are often the wrong sort of women. They are often scientific, *hard* women. There are not enough soft women. You know, they're determined women who've decided they're going to get their three 'As' and they've got 'em. Not all, but there are quite a few like that, who aren't going to be good GPs and who won't want to go into general practice. But, oh yes, quite a lot are good.'

A number of people said this to me. It was not substantiated by any of the women GPs I talked to – nine – nor by any of the quite numerous girl students. There is some statistical evidence in Cartwright. Patients of women GPs were more likely to say that their GP hurried them – 29 per cent as opposed to 13 per cent; and less likely to consult on personal problems – 15 per cent as opposed to 32 per cent. The report speculated that this might be because of the conditioning of medical schools, and that taking up a male profession in a male world led to the assumption of excessively 'male' characteristics.

DR ABNEY: 'We've got half a woman doctor. Great. I like them. She's great. Looking around, the only woman in the practices here who is full time, she's the girl along the road who does psychosexual what's its, and she's single, well ostensibly. But I don't think full time is possible for a married one, or the family would suffer.'

DR SUSAN GLYNDE: 'It was difficult when the children were very small and I think still now. My children are now twenty, nineteen and sixteen. One at home, two away. Still the differences between us and between men is that our priorities are different. I think men put the job first and come back to families tired and without much time for them; but I think all the time, if you're a woman doctor, to be honest, at the back of your mind is, I wonder how the children are getting on, and I wonder what we are going to have for supper.

'But I also think it helps a tremendous lot to be a wife and mother because it puts you straight away on the same wavelength as most of your patients, and they seem to have confidence in you and they find you easier to talk to, they think you have been through it. Someone with an unhappy marriage will come along and talk to you, not because they think you are unhappy, but because you know what it is like with a husband, what husbands can be like. And what wives can be like, I suppose, too.

'Men want to talk to you, but they don't know how to start. You really have to lead them on and then, once you open the floodgates, out it comes. They don't go and talk to people in pubs about how awful their marriages are, they bottle it up and it all comes flooding.

'I try to tell people to stand up for themselves because so many women just don't. They just let their husbands ride roughshod over them, and it doesn't occur to them to put their foot down and say "No." It works – sometimes.

'If a husband is interested it's easier; but if – well, I'm always there, I just manage to slip in and get the food ready. I don't think he would be too keen if the food wasn't ready for him and the house straight.

'I wanted to be a paediatrician very much, but I got married and that was the end of that. I do regret it, I suppose, but then I wouldn't *particularly* encourage a daughter to be a doctor, I don't think. In fact, neither of mine is going to be. Because, if I'm honest, I have to admit it's a man's life. You can be very happy being a woman doctor, but I don't think you can be totally dedicated, and it's jolly hard to get the better jobs.'

DR EASTCOURT: 'Of course it's worth it – for a group of three GPs like us to get another female doctor. We say we'll give her £10,000 a year. She gets the basic practice allowance – £7,000. So it's only costing you £1,000 a year out of your own pocket. Take off your tax – £500. So £10 a week and you've got an extra female hand. Take another man, and you've got to find another £10,000 or £12,000, you see.'

DR AXMOUTH: 'We're both very much in favour of our next partner being a woman. But you've got to watch the flexibility. In my training practice we had a fairly pleasant girl who did indeed take on a part-time commitment and then went off to have a baby and was then back in the surgery sneaking off to the doctors' common room to breast feed this infant within weeks. I think it worked but in a slightly unhealthy sense in that I thought she was rather the practice mascot. She would probably hate me if she heard me saying this aloud, but with all the GPs, some of them slightly fancied her and some of them rather fathered her, I'm not quite sure whether generally the patronizing air – to which she played up to some extent in order to survive – is what I would want. If they're coming in as partners, they jolly well ought to be equal partners. You ought not to be patronizing them or carrying them or fathering them or fancying them, or anything else. They ought just jolly well to be there as equals. For everybody's sake.'

Drs Henry and Mary Trimdon

DR HENRY TRIMDON: 'A single lady GP is no use. I had two lady partners who cracked up under the strain. You see, I could blow a fuse, where they were going home to empty houses and not organized. I mean, with thought, they could have had their mince in the deep freeze.'

DR MARY TRIMDON: 'They've still got to make it one day. It doesna' make itself every day.'

DR HENRY TRIMDON: 'Well, if they had a session like you and filled the freezer. As I've tried to tell them, in my funny little way, but they both cracked up; so in my view you've got to be married to be a lady GP.'

DR MARY TRIMDON: 'What about Lizzie King? Look at her. I mean she's managed fine all these years, she's single. She'd a housekeeper.'

DR HENRY TRIMDON: 'It takes someone pretty clever to run two shows. You know, she's going on her calls, she's bound to be wondering about the mince.'

DR MARY TRIMDON: '*Me?* Not at all. When I'm at my work I don't think about the house. That's why there's such a panic when I'm shopping at the weekends.'

DR HENRY TRIMDON: 'Well, OK, so the house is not run properly then.'

DR MARY TRIMDON: 'The *sack*! You'll have me out on my neck.'

DR HENRY TRIMDON: 'Well, there you are.'

DR MARY TRIMDON: 'Of course it's run properly. When did you ever go without a meal or a clean shirt?'

DR HENRY TRIMDON: 'That's why you get in a panic, worrying about the mince, because you canna take it all in your stride.'

DR MARY TRIMDON: 'I can fine take it in my stride. I'll take you in my stride!'

DR HENRY TRIMDON: 'Nooo. I mean she's very good, a good administrator, a clever woman. I mean they don't get the same chance if their attention is divided. I mean at lunchtime today I cased *Pulse* and the *General Practitioner*. Well, they're not worth reading, but at least I paid attention. You don't even do that. You haven't time.'

DR MARY TRIMDON: 'Of course I have time. I read the BMJ [British Medical Journal]. I read three articles today in the BMJ.'

DR HENRY TRIMDON: 'But you get the point I'm trying to make? They haven't the same time to devote to their work, so therefore they're bound to know less.'

DR MARY TRIMDON: 'I wouldn't say we know less. We may not know as much practical medicine as you do. But mind you, I see as many patients in the time I spend. I've as much patient/doctor contact, or as many, as you do in a week.'

DR HENRY TRIMDON: 'But it'll wear you out more than it'll wear me out.'

DR MARY TRIMDON: 'Because I have to work twice as hard, twice as fast.'

DR HENRY TRIMDON: 'So really there shouldn't be too many women doctors.'

DR MARY TRIMDON: 'A practice likes a woman doctor. A practice needs a woman doctor. The ladies in a practice like a woman doctor and some of the funny old men do too. I've a very large clientele of men. There should be as many women doctors as possible.'

DR JUNE EDSTONE: 'I've had five children and it was really never too difficult. We always had a big house. When we first started off I used to farm Daphne out on neighbours. But afterwards we had a big house and divided a flat off so we had other people living in. If I had to go out and couldn't take them with me, I could say, "Listen to them." But I liked to look after my children myself. I breast fed them, fed them at mealtimes. I like to be in control of my house and don't like too much interference. I couldn't cope with a nanny. And it was quite possible to run the practice and the family.

'I had to have somebody in the house if there was a real emergency, which doesn't happen very often. 99 per cent of the time it works out OK. When they were small they used to come round – do my rounds with me and play about in the car; go in and see old ladies and old gentlemen. I'd take them around nursing homes and I think they gained as much as anything else. They've all done very well.

'A lot of patients have said how nice it is to have someone who has had children and knows what a pest they can be. This is an area where, yes, a woman doctor scores. Men can very easily divorce themselves from the most problematical side of bringing up children – if they want to.

'I found when I was fed up with the children, the surgery would give me breathing space so I didn't kill them, and equally, one could relax with the children when you were fed up with patients. I think it really marries in quite well. The fly in the ointment is the husband. He doesn't play ball. Husbands don't like telephone sitting – nor does anyone.'

Dr Axmouth had a theory about women GPS. As regards the hospital side of the NHS, it was necessary to have an abundance of doctors struggling to be consultants so that you got, through competition, the very best consultants; and also so that there were always enough consultants to keep the hospitals going. This surplus should also eventually be capable of dispersion, to let in new blood and to get rid of the disillusioned. In the past, the dispersion had taken place into general practice or out to the colonies. Now, because general practice had become a specialty, it was increasingly a focus for the ambitious. The colonies had gone. The solution was lots of women doctors who really turned out to want children. They would thus be unable to become consultants – since these were not geared to dual-role figures – and would have to become GPS. But since they would all be part-time GPS, there would be plenty of room for them, and also for the male full-time GPS. If a great many women wanted real careers he foresaw a chaos of doctor over-production. The women would also have to do a lot of doctor dogsbody jobs.

I put this argument, which seems to me to have some force, to Dr Thurston Riard, who had been Professor of General Practice at a large teaching hospital.

DR RIARD: 'There is an element of truth in what he says, which is worrying, and that is general practice by and large has been quicker to adapt its practice and its teaching to the needs of women than the specialties, and there is some evidence now that women are going into general practice, not because that is their career at first choice, but because it's easier for them to do it than go into a hospital specialty and that will be, I think, bad for general practice and bad for the women involved. It's a kind of price that general practice is paying for having been a little more liberal in recognizing that women have different social obligations from men. My view is quite simple. I believe that any society, if it wants to give its women the kind of equality of opportunity it's always talking about, they've actually got to do it, and that means it's uncomfortable and difficult and sacrifices have to be made. But as long as it is women who have the babies, and who are going to bring them up in the first few years, we're going to have to reconstruct our professional pathways to take note of that. It seems absolutely nonsensical to talk about it, but to erect barriers.'

38

AN INDUCEMENT PRACTICE: DR JIMMY COLKIRK

Dr Colkirk's was the last practice in which I stayed a number of days. It came after the slum practice and could scarcely have provided a greater contrast.

I set off north after an early breakfast. It was snowing hard and lying on the hard ground. Gradually, as I drove, the scenery increased in beauty and grandeur until, after about 100 miles, I was driving through the Highlands – great mountains on either side, their tops covered in snow, flanks bare, bracken and heather, or else cut by drainage where the Forestry Commission was planting. There were quite a number of young woods, young *forests*. The Commission is transforming Scotland, for the better I think. They would improve it by releasing packs of wolves.

By 3.30 it was already beginning to grow dark. I drove through glen after glen, some wide, some narrow, burns belting down them, alongside long twisting lochs. The sun was sinking blazing ahead; it looked as though a huge ball of light was held, cupped, by the mountains in front of me, the light spilling over the rim.

I arrived in darkness. Elizabeth Colkirk, about thirty-four, was plump, dark, good-looking with full red lips, dark hair, red cheeks, all round and strongly coloured. Jimmy Colkirk was smallish with a tuft of grizzled beard on his chin. He looked like Lenin, but more boyish.

The tempo of his life and work was extraordinarily relaxed and slow – and continuous. Leisurely surgeries, Dr Colkirk gossiping away (gossip was the clue to his practice); leisurely mornings while we drove twenty, thirty or forty miles a see a distant patient. The mountains incessantly varied as weather flowed in from the west – now all clear and sparkling, a quarter of an hour later clouds had descended or it would be snowing soft snowflakes as big as sparrows. There were eagles, a buzzard on the telephone line. While running up behind the house I saw three grouse. The glen below his house was very wide, too wide to be a glen – in the middle a magic loch, with tiny islands.

The First Evening

Indeed, I began to get the flavour of the practice almost immediately. We were just sitting down to high tea, when the telephone rang. A mother about her little boy. 'Acute' pain in the legs. He could hear him crying in the background as she explained.

It was 6.30 when we set out and had already started freezing. It was about four miles. This was a shepherd, she his second wife. Well-covered girl, Jimmy said, mid thirties, shepherd perhaps fifty. As we came along the road above the loch a deer in the headlights. 'They come down to feed when it gets dark, once the snows start.'

Low, white house. Sheepdogs in the pen running swiftly up and back the wire.

In the little living room, a bright coal fire. Two toddlers, the boy five, girl about three; red dressing gown, green pyjamas. Running about and giggling. She said, (well spoken), 'Of course, it's better now.'

Doctor examines. It doesn't seem to hurt anywhere. Lots of giggling. 'Sometimes it hurts in the knees,' she says. The shepherd has a fine, narrow, sensitive face. Watches as the doctor massages in some cream. Little boy insists it *doesn't* sting. He coughs suddenly. A cough he certainly *does* have. 'Who's cough is that?' says the doctor. 'I think it's me aine cough,' says the little boy, seriously. The doctor examines.

Wife: 'He's had these leg pains since he first started walking – after exercise. Perhaps they're just growing pains.' Doctor: 'Intelligent woman – exactly.' Gives some medicine for the cough.

I note, as we leave, that the dogs don't bark. 'They never bark when the shepherd's home.' The moon is coming up in a clear sky as we get into the car.

Mrs Davis: After high tea and some telly, we have to walk across the way to see a neighbour. Jimmy explains she's a widow, seventy-four, very apprehensive and particularly upset by 1) snow, 2) frost, 3) wind. She can't drive now. Her neighbours drive her, borrowing her car, but since *they* drive, they decide where to go. That very afternoon they'd taken her all the way into the town when she was expecting just to go to the nearby village. This has so upset her, along with the snow and the frost, that she's appealed for a call. She's a terrible gossip.

Actually, not so much gossip as a talker, a conversationalist. Small, plump, twinkly, a woollen hat like a tea cosy on her head; small, untidy room with a coal fire, plants on the table. The numerous very loud clocks unsynchronized. (I suddenly wondered if old, lonely people sometimes had clocks for companions.) She explains at great length how the unexpected journey upset her, that her heart suddenly went bang! bang! bang! beating her chest. 'I couldna settle at all!' She can't take pills. He gives her a liquid sedative, which she slowly sips from a tablespoon, talking all the time.

The retired sheep farmer who lives nearby. He's ninety. She goes and feeds him and talks to him. 'I clean him up. He gets in such a *mess*.'

Mrs Davis, she's called. Bright as a button. He asks about the damp. She chatters away, one drooping eyelid, Fairisle jersey, sipping her sedative. Sudden loud bang as it strikes 10.

She tells of a boy she knows, from the town. He took all the exams and became a policeman in London. A raid on a Woolworths, and they caught the thieves red-handed; literally – he had one in his grip. He asked him his name. The thief gave one – something. 'I canny recall – Smith. "You're a lying rogue. Your name's John McCullen and you were in my form at school." Out of all the men in London,' she ended. 'It was they two met. It was a *singular* thing that.'

We left after twenty minutes, her much soothed. 'It's loneliness and old age,' said Jimmy. 'She absolutely refuses an old people's home.' Freezing hard as we walked back to the house.

First Morning

Marvellous day. Clear and cold, the tops of the mountains capped with snow, as they'd be now till spring. Broad flanks of their heather and bracken brown sides sweeping down to the loch. It was Wednesday. No surgery, just visits. We set off early after breakfast. As we drove, he pointed out houses, and told me about them.

'There's a lad in that cottage – his father works for the hydro-electric. It's this girl from Newcastle. He was going to marry her anyway, but she suddenly got pregnant, so they're hurrying it up. She came for her ante-natal. Let on she'd had one or two affairs in Newcastle. Then what did I find – a tattoo on her thigh.'

We'd been speaking of inbreeding in the Islands and Highlands. I said she'd bring in new genes. 'Aye, and perhaps syphilis too. There's sailors in Newcastle. You have to think of this – I wouldn't have known but for the tattoo.'

People waved as he passed. 'That's the man who upset Mrs Davis yesterday. He's had two heart attacks. He's on a knife edge. All he can do is drive two old women about now.'

He said the practice had 804 patients. 'You've got to be terribly careful about who's related to who.' About 8 per cent were English; 40 per cent natives of the area. The rest from other parts of Scotland. The workload? Well, perhaps *slightly* smaller than a big city practice (and he knew, he'd been in one seven years), but it was *constant*. A steady forty miles an hour. Where a city one was all short bursts. Here, a visit could mean an hour's drive.

WIDOW OF EIGHTY: In fact we've now been driving for twenty minutes, gone about ten miles. It is a completely empty glen, up which road and rail run side by side. The widow had half a bungalow, underneath the mountain whose sides are dark with Forestry Commission planting.

She obviously lives in the kitchen. A 'Royal', a Rayburn-type stove, chaotic and pretty filthy, piles of washing-up. An old range kettle. A fiercely growling dog put out when we came in.

Tough, spry, amused. Chat; then she explains about her 'turns' – panting, knocks her out, dizziness. He listens to the thin old chest. 'Sleeping well?' 'Very badly. After three – that's it. But I don't seem to need it. I feel fine – except for those turns.' Is she taking the pills? Yes. She asks if it's all right if she has some sips of brandy when these turns come on, as that seems to help. Doctor says yes, fine.

We have to force an exit. She longs to talk. She's going to America in December. 'I just live here to get away,' laughing.

'It's old age. Nothing I can do. She's one of the few who realizes that.'

We drive off up the glen. Hers is the only building in sight – her half-bungalow, which is really just a shed.

We have another twenty miles to go. Jimmy tells me how he is paid. He is paid a fixed sum of £15,620, something like 85 per cent of the average GP's salary. This is an 'inducement' to get GPs into sparsely populated territory. In addition, he gets two cars as practice expenses, since the isolation means he can't afford to have only one and that break down.

The system filled Jimmy with a sense of deep injustice. The salary was fixed at £15,620. It took much of the zest that, say, Sam Locking had felt, out of dispensing, because if he made enough money to raise his salary above the inducement level, the amount was cut to bring it back. All the dispensing did was to tie up about £4,000 of his salary in stock. He felt the real average of GPs was probably higher, but was pulled down by inner city GPs who earned £10,000 on the NHS and then £60,000 on private. (I doubt they are numerous enough to seriously affect the average.) He said when it came to donations to local funds, 'They're not going to be happy with 20p. It's fivers they're looking for from you. Pennies from other people.'

But he preferred living there? 'Certainly, but that's a bad argument, always advanced about remote areas. If roads are bad, communications bad, electricity costs twice as much, coal three times as much – you pay your taxes, you complain to central government who are meant to be levelling out things over the country, they say, "What the hell are you doing living there? Come to the centre of Glasgow, you'll find better facilities." The only thing fair in this country is the post.'

Nevertheless, I persisted, £15,620 wasn't bad (my humbler writer's position perhaps skewing my view here); and he *did* prefer it, the peace and so on, didn't he?

Well, he did. 'And you know all the people personally.' He waves out of the window. 'That's the road gang; they're all my patients. There's a certain friendly feeling you couldn't get in a city.'

GILLIE'S FAMILY; WIFE, NEW BABY: We crossed a bridge, and the road narrowed to a single track. Great mountains rising smooth to the right; in the distance, top in cloud, Mount Everest. Thirty-three miles from his surgery. The road ends and we bump along a track. It had been almost impassable, just boulders and rough fords over burns. 'Old Jamieson – sold a wee patch of land at the very end to the Forestry Commission. Cunning devil. They did up the road.'

A green hut by the track. 'They call that the larder. After shooting the deer they bring them down to butcher them.'

At the end, a long low whitewashed building, barns at the end. Two toddlers playing. Into the front room – cheerful, wood-lined, fire in grate. The gillie and another one in deerstalkers, boots, gaiters, sitting having coffee and cakes. We're given some by cheerful young wife.

All of them intelligent. Talk about the Gaelic for TB and for rheumatism. Delicious cakes. The second gillie has a drinker's face. The old father appears – he's a retired gillie, seventy-three. Indicates he wants the doctor to see his tooth, and goes out again. Chat about my book. They say the plaster on my chin is where the doctor struck me for asking an awkward question. The doctor goes and picks up the baby; three months, doing fine. Then slips out to see to the grandfather.

The two gillies go. The young wife tells me how useful the grandfather is – he tends the chickens; minds the children if she and her husband can get away. He doesn't mind doing it at all. Hates his retirement in some flat in town and is dreading going back. They get their supplies monthly for a deep freeze. In the place they were before, still further north, the old gillie used to hang the deer up in the wind. It would form a sort of crust and turn black, but if you cut through it, it was quite fresh.

Doctor returns, gives her penicillin for the old man's tooth, and we leave. Half an hour.

FRENCHWOMAN MARRIED TO A SHEPHERD: As we drove, I remarked that the marriages seemed fairly stable. He agreed. He could only think of one really unstable marriage; 'perhaps a few simmering under the surface'. He described them at some length, while we took a narrow road through a vast private estate. The mountainside beside the road was alive with deer. At one moment a group of six stags; at another, one old stag and seven hinds. 'The culling of the hinds will start soon.'

The visit is to a Frenchwoman, now thirty-eight, the daughter of a smart Parisian, who'd married a shepherd. She could get depressed and he called from time to time to check up. Another square house, Land Rover outside. He parked the car so it wouldn't be seen from a house half a mile away. A recent widow. If seen, we'd have to go in. Once in, have to stay.

The ex-Parisienne was cheerful and well. I noticed a string of garlic on the kitchen wall.

THE POSTMAN: Jimmy gave me the long history of the next call as we drove. Heart difficulty, only fifty-nine, but it definitely wasn't right. Bronchitis had revealed it. He was going to have to retire from the Post Office. But he'd break this gently, let it sink in.

House by the burn near the hotel. A gentle, sad man, in trousers and braces, his wife out. A quiet resigned meeting, the doctor gentle too. Listened to heart. Talk of pills; postman panting when he returns from getting the box in his room.

THE EMERGENCY: We leave in some hurry, because the postman has had two calls from the doctor's wife. This is an emergency, though a mild one. We start to drive fast, through a rapidly changing scene – clouds descending, the mountains darkening.

Jimmy explains. 'She has Hodgkins disease – had it for five years. It's been arrested, but she has only just recovered from the recent chemo-therapy. She's thirty-five and gets into a panic at the slightest symptom. It's a dilemma. There's an 80 per cent recovery rate from Hodgkins disease. She's being seen every six months. (It used to be every three.) To send her to hospital for tests costs the state a lot of money. These panics are for nothing – just fear.' He feels, as a representative of the state, he should say 'No'. And in a town he could. She'd probably refer herself. But he knows by the time we get there she'll have built up such a head of steam, she'll *insist* on going. You can't just say 'No' in a small community. 'I've got to look after her for years. It would be a terrible loss if I lost her confidence.'

He already knows it's a panic and already knows he will give way to it.

So it turns out. A pretty, but determined woman, a bit haggard – panic subsiding. In bed, sharp chin. She rushed through her symptoms – dizziness, terrible pains at the back of her head. She is twitching. Says, 'Could we have a scan done? To see what they come up with? If you *wouldn't* mind?' A lot of talk of Dr McW. 'He doesn't let you dangle about – he deals with you at once.' She ends, she doesn't think her husband can take any more.

He acquiesces.

In the car he says, 'She hadn't even taken the pain-killers. She'd made up her mind – even down to the name of the consultant. It's the transfer of support. When your life's threatened, your husband can't help you. So he gets sick of her moaning – says, "We've *got* to do something." Nor can your GP. Only your consultant, the man who saved you at the start, will do. Last time she went in, she only got to see the registrar. I've seen this coming for a week or more. Only seeing the consultant will calm her.'

We get back – to find her consultant has retired. No one contactable in the hospital.

The Afternoon

Into the local town to buy more drugs for the dispensary – £300 or so. We talk all the way about various things: his experiences on the Islands, a spell on the

Falkland Isles, his practice in Edinburgh. He has terrible battles with his nurse who seems more or less uncontrollable, a virtual 'Bolshie'. 'I think, I'll get nurse to do this, then I remember she's on one of her six days off as usual. So it'll be the relief nurse. And then I don't want the relief nurse involved because she's a fearful gossip. I end up doing most of the nursing myself.'

When we get back it is growing dark and raining heavily. The grand mountain vistas glint behind the cloud and the driving rain. This is his 'easy' day (no surgeries). We've driven 164 miles.

His wife has talked to the new consultant's secretary. The woman can go into hospital tomorrow to have her scan.

The Evening, the Night

Nothing. It is 'free' till 10 o'clock. (Dr C. fifteen miles away takes calls till then.) So we can drink whisky, which we do. He writes a long letter to the cancer consultant, which he shows me. Patient is neurotic but that only he, the consultant, can calm her; all a bit veiled in case she should open the letter, which she has to take with her tomorrow.

Telly announces approaching depression – mood-swings from the Atlantic – and during the night the running and drumming and splash of rain. Stopped towards dawn. When I get up, snow lightly everywhere. Large wisps of cloud, scarves of it, round the mountains below their snow-covered tops.

Morning, Second Day

This is an 'appointment' day, but there is no one till 11 o'clock.

We are called out at 8.45 to an old couple – aged seventy. Both refusing to *consider* old people's home. (It seems to me Dr Colkirk is rather keen on these.) She is becoming confused and he is often called out just *for* this. She has forgotten why. The old man has had two coronaries. He has to go to them because the old man tends to play things down. Then – it's a coronary.

Little old lady, little old man, in two-storey council house away in hydro-electric area about four miles down the road. She is in bed, white hair, round face, spectacles. 'It's a very sore knee.'

He feels, his face suddenly attentive. Something wrong. Swollen. He gives her pain-killers: 'I'm nae tay guid at swallowing.' Tells her to stay in bed, he will send someone to bandage it. She complains, but he insists.

Doctor to the husband, 'Get a box or something to put under the blankets.' Husband: 'I'll ask Donald.' Doctor: 'What am I saying! His son's the shopkeeper. Aye – get Donald to give you a good stout whisky box.'

We return to the surgery. This is attached to the house and reached through the rarely used dining room. A built-on neat, square, modern block, with rather too much plate glass for this latitude. Small receptionist's area, with telephone, and, like most of Scotland and virtually none of England, the new big clean record files. Waiting room, about 18 foot by 10 foot; more glass, an aquarium. Next door, his consulting room, with the dispensary and a little treatment area off it. All light and airy. He had a good deal of equipment, including the Japanese blood pressure machine. There was another Japanese instrument for ears with which we found I was, in one ear, to all intents and purposes stone deaf.

On Wednesday there was no surgery. On Monday and Friday there'd be no appointments and he'd see anyone. Tuesday and Thursday – appointments. On appointment days, three or four would make an appointment before, a few more would ring up on the morning, some would just turn up.

We saw four cases together, one he thought he ought to see alone. This was a 'social' case, a family matter. For years two brothers had run a farm together. The elder was very dominant. The younger one and his wife had become increasingly aware how well off the elder was: with two cars, a video machine, holidays abroad. Meanwhile, they slaved in poverty. Resentment had seethed for years. Finally, a year ago, the brothers had fallen out. Under the wife's impetus they'd got a lawyer. Each step of this dispute she liked to discuss with the doctor. He couldn't take sides, of course, but he listened, and sometimes said, 'Well, I'd wait a week or two . . .'

WOMAN AGED THIRTY-NINE: Long, fair hair. Yorkshire. She and her husband had just bought the hotel up the way. A terrible rash. 'Everwhere, my back, back of my legs. I hurt. I itch. I was just *alive* last night.'

They go behind the curtains for him to look. She'd got back from Spain last week, perhaps it was something there. (In fact she'd told him that when she came in, but he wasn't listening.) Could it have been the venison she had on Friday and again on Monday, for the first and then second time in her life?

He'd clearly decided food allergy when she came in. He explains that her body probably said, 'Here, this is nasty' on Friday. Built up an allergy which reacted when she had it on Monday. Goes out into dispensing room and gets her anti-histamine pills and cream. (Ten minutes.)

RETIRED WARRANT OFFICER, RAF: Before he comes in, the doctor explains he's English. 'The most irritating type of Englishman. You know them – often questions my decisions. Tells me about his life in the RAF. Complains. Married to a very submissive wife, a chronic bronchitic and bad rheumatism. Heavy smoker. He's come for her pills. But they're a self-sufficient old couple, over seventy. Won't *hear* of an old people's home,' he ended, somewhat wistfully.

The RAF man is small, brisk, from the Lake District. Complains about his wife. She wheezes and coughs when she wakes up. 'By the time she's up – she's absolutely jiggered.'

Doctor gets pills from the dispensary – distalgesic, Ativan. Then, for my sake, draws the littled lined man out about the RAF. He'd been in from 1929 to 1966 – thirty-seven years. 'I just about owned it when I'd finished. It was a good life.'

When he'd gone, Doctor said, slightly disappointed, 'He usually complains far more.' (Six minutes.)

Quite a long gap. It is all leisurely. The doctor fills in forms so that the builder can get paid for mending a door handle. 'I can't put up a coat hook without asking the Ministry of Health.' He shows me the agreement he signed. He gets his large, four-bedroomed, two reception-roomed, dining-roomed, centrally heated house for £88.50 a quarter, less £23 for the surgery. That is, £258 a year.

GIRL FROM HOTEL: Sharp, pert little piece from the hotel up the road. Dr Colkirk rather stimulated by her. ('She's social class four, I'm almost sure – but she's innocent in a way. Swears away – doesn't see anything wrong,' he'd muttered rapidly to me before she came in.)

Didn't seem particularly innocent to me. Just back from Tenerife – 'Sunbathing, disco, swimming.' A cough that wouldn't go. *She hadn't smoked for three days.* He gave her a mixture. Told her to finish the penicillin he'd given her before and of which she'd only taken one tablet. 'I don't have to pay for prescriptions. I'm unemployed the noo.' (Five minutes.)

THE ROADMAN: Curly, grey beard, strong face, fifty-five or sixty, in his orange roadman's uniform. 'He keeps the snow off our roads,' says Doctor Colkirk. Come to get diarrhoea pills for his daughter. Stands the whole time. Some talk of his wife and how she's taking the strain. Very nervous, it seems. Her favourite brother and mother died recently within a few days of each other. Some talk about whether she should go away. He leaves. 'Thanks very much, doctor.' He looks strained too. (Five minutes.)

'A very interesting man,' said Dr Colkirk. He'd built up a very big road haulage business. An executive. Then he'd taken to drink. His wife had left him. Business had started to collapse. Brother had taken over and insisted he get cured. He did. Came back, but brother difficult. So he'd suddenly said, 'Bugger you', and came here. Married again and had this daughter. Joined the road gang and became foreman. Frustrations of ex-executive fighting red tape. Now a chance the council would ask for private tenders – he'd jump in. A tough man.

That was all. He was ten minutes with the social case, and then we were all having coffee in the kitchen. It was 11.40.

While we drank, he told us the latest instalment of the two brothers saga. As he suspected, she'd brought him three letters: from the lawyer, from the dominant brother. The brother had given the accounts of the farm. He said he'd paid her £29 50p a week, and his brother £60 a week. 'She hadn't had a penny; and her husband never had that, nor anything like.' There was going to be a lot of back pay. Letters had gone out, demanding the new scale at once. And it meant that for years the elder brother had been defrauding with declarations of false income tax – and more. 'He'd say, "We'll send 100 sheep to the market," then take 150. The younger fellow couldn't tell out of 3,000 all over the place.' Elizabeth said it was foolish to leave all the running to the elder brother.

'But it started fifteen years ago – and the younger was alcoholic at that time.' Since ten years he hadn't touched a drop. The row was common knowledge up and down the glen. 'It's going to go on and on,' said Jimmy with some pleasure, looking forward to it.

It was 12 o'clock. There was nothing else to do. The doctor vanished. Before lunch there was one phone call, booking in for the afternoon surgery.

I wrote up my notes, among them this one: 'The interesting thing about the family row saga, which must have been extremely stressful for all those concerned, was the effect on the wife. For years she'd suffered from severe depressions. Since this started, they'd vanished. She'd never felt better in her life.'

The Afternoon

RAILWAY WORKER'S WIFE: We had time for a quick visit before afternoon surgery. Rain had washed the snow from the mountains. Puddles everywhere.

This was a railway worker and his wife. She is sixty-eight, had breast cancer and the breast off five months ago. All tests good and she seems to have recovered. A visit to reassure her and report latest tests. Problem is, she's going ga-ga. You don't notice, but he gets his meals at all hours. He doesn't complain, but it must be difficult.

We arrive. Very large fire, *logs* of coal. Doctor: 'Your tests were fine.' Her: 'I'm feeling grand.'

Lots of jokes and talk. She does seem quite all right and perfectly sharp. He has a sensitive face, kind, humorous. We stay fifteen minutes. (He *enjoys* talking to them all.) She says that at the hospital, 'They said "You've a very good doctor in Dr Colkirk. You've no need to come in here." Oh yes – they like you there.' He looks pleased. She goes on, 'That's a nice feather in your cap. I'll have to be plucking one out soon.'

As we leave into the pouring rain, she says to me, 'Very good to see you round again.'

We get back for the 2.30 surgery. Five people have now booked in.

FIFTY-YEAR-OLD HIGHLANDER: From the hydro-electric works. A piper. High blood pressure. Doctor takes his prescription money. He has only come to get his blood pressure pills. Doctor talks away in his garrulous way about piping, and the man – very big and proud of looking younger than fifty – has to actually stand up and walk out to get away. (Ten minutes.)

SCHOOL MISTRESS: Rheumatism, eyesight, sleeping pills. Again, doctor gossips. The point is, it is the gossip, the talk, that is often the important element in these consultations. He checks that the pills are working, how long they've been on, etc., but it is the *talk* that interests him. In fact, they are what make these meetings not just possible but enjoyable.

Also valuable. It is from them that he has got his huge background knowledge of the families and the various set-ups. That the blood pressure man, for example, *dotes* on his twelve-year-old son, and his concern with his own health is that he is nervous he may not remain alive long enough to see him started. At some point, this could be useful. (Fourteen minutes.)

ELDERLY LADY FROM THE ISLANDS: Gentle, in green wellingtons, she is given a new asthma inhaler.

In the middle a long telephone conversation. It sounds to me as though it is with the consultant about the woman with Hodgkins disease and that he is agreeing with Dr Colkirk's diagnosis. Thirteen minutes, seven of which are on the telephone. He chats to the old woman about the Isles, partly to make up for the interruption.

RECEPTIONIST'S MOTHER-IN-LAW: Comes for pills for herself, and for her husband – Dick. Plump, in scarf and nice red coat. Dressed up. Dr Colkirk gives Ativan for Dick – he takes half at night. Is he using his inhaler? 'Not much.'

He takes her blood pressure, using his fine new electronic Japanese machine. She bares her big, soft, white, pastry-making Scottish forearm. The machine makes computer-game noises. He does it again, adjusting the wide rubber band. 'A bit higher than usual – you're taking the water pills?' 'I'm feeling fine. Yes.' He gets pills from dispensary. (Ten minutes.)

BODY-BUILDER, SIXTY AND WIFE: He has time to tell me Mr Smart was deaf at sixteen. He took up body-building. Recently, had an orthopaedic operation on his back, and his muscles went. This made him rather resentful. His wife is thirty. Working class. Always talks.

They come in. I notice a curious smell of old biscuits in the air. She translates for the tall, still strong, deaf man – chesty cough, difficulty swallowing, sore throat. Sits with his large hands open, looking at his small, intense, round, white-faced wife. Gets his pills.

She then launches into various channels of conversation, her little head with its woollen cap bobbing with the intensity of her talk. First, possible rheumatism – he reassures her that nowadays you can keep it well under control. Then long, long saga of her brother, a jointly owned house, how he won't pay.

After fifteen minutes, Dr Colkirk brings it to an end. 'So sorry for taking up your time.'

But now (once again encouraged by him, he draws her on), she describes her work for one of the hotels – £30 a week, 100 hours. 'It's like bloomin' Victorian times.' Another ten minutes and they go.

SPOTTY BOY: He is in for pain-killers for a bad tooth. (That is, people come in and use Dr Colkirk as the chemist, which of course he is.)

'What are you doing at the minute, Jim?'

'I'm unemployed, actually.' He leaves.

Nothing is what it seems, even this. The parents are rich. They have two children of their own, but have adopted three more. The adopted ones always seem to be duds. This one they apprenticed to the local plumber. But are they *really* duds – or made so? For instance, the latest was a severely handicapped seven-year-old from a home, with very bad skin trouble. Do they *choose* duds to set off their own children? The father is a typical junior army officer. Thick.

'And they're *rich*', says Dr Colkirk. 'Fancy apprenticing him to the plumber.' (Six minutes.)

WOMAN, FORTY: This is a case he wants to see alone. She has attempted suicide three times. He is with her half an hour.

While this goes on I go for a run. Dusk is falling. Down in the wide valley mist wanders like smoke among the pines. I look across to the mountains. The rain has in fact only cleared the snow to half-way; above that there is still snow, indeed it probably fell as snow. Clouds cover their tops. They are manacing, remote – slabs of black rock out of the snow, very lofty and distant. I run up the wet, winding road which goes steeply through the new-planted wood. The mountainside is gushing water, loud, pouring down to the loch. Two grouse whirr away. Crows flap above me towards some birch.

I get back, have a bath and tea. While we have tea, Dr Colkirk talks about the suicide, a complicated and sad case. She had, which was rare, talked freely. He also says the telephone conversation *was* the consultant, and he completely agreed with Dr Colkirk. He was, however, going to do a series of scans and tests to make quite sure, and also to reassure the patient.

Dr Colkirk does paperwork till 5.30. Then he has finished. He says he feels quite tired. The talk with the suicide tired him. The only other time she'd talked like that, she'd taken an overdose that very *night*. Perhaps we'll at last be called out to a proper, after-11 emergency.

And so it went on. The next day, with the non-appointment surgeries, wasn't very crowded. We drove forty-five leisurely miles. He does about

23,000 a year.

It seemed peaceful and, compared to many practices, quite gentle. Yet it was, as he said, continuous and, no doubt, cumulatively trapping. The house was strewn with various radio sets and intercoms and bleepers, all tried and all to no avail, to let him get a few miles from the house and still be contactable. To fish or boat on the loch or even just go for a walk further than a mile. Each time, the mountains blocked off all sound.

He'd been born and lived on one of the Islands, spoke fluent Gaelic. You'd need that background and training to endure. I also thought that, though GPs impose the patterns of their character on their practices, the reverse was also true. Dr Colkirk had a leisurely, almost meandering style of talk, derived from long winter evenings, long drives to isolated crofts. I could see how the saga style developed.

As I drove away on my journey south, clouds were coming down and obscuring the peaks, making the glens little valleys. I felt I was not only returning over space but over time. Given obvious changes, there was not a great deal of difference, the feeling was the same, as the life Dr Stane had described in his practice in Fife over sixty years before.

39

THE TRAINING OF GPS

Anyone can call himself a doctor and practise without being qualified. National Insurance, in deference to an individual's right to be treated by whom and how he likes, will recognise certificates signed by herbalists or acupuncturists.

But a non-qualified doctor can't sign death certificates, can't prescribe drugs or operate within the NHS. He may be prosecuted for manslaughter if a patient dies.

To qualify, a GP now undergoes eight years' training. After five years registerable qualifications are awarded by a university medical school. There are two sets of initials: MB (Bachelor of Medicine) for the 'physician' part: chB, BS or BCh (Bachelor of Surgery), for the 'surgeon' part. Another route is to take the conjoint exams and become a Member of the Royal College of Surgeons and Licenciate of the Royal College of Physicians. The doctor can then write MRCS and LRCP after his name. These are no better than MB or BS. Some people take both sets of exams and could have huge imposing streams of letters after their names: MRCS, LRCP, MB, chB. To which a number, and they are growing, add MRCGP – a member of the Royal College of General Practitioners, achieved after yet another difficult exam.

General practice is now regarded as a specialty in its own right, and after these basic exams, the would-be GP still has three years training to go. Two are in hospitals, where he or she will choose (usually four) suitable courses. They might be obstetrics, geriatrics, paediatrics and psychiatry. There remains a final year where the young doctor becomes apprenticed for two periods of six months to two GP trainers.

We shall look, fairly briefly, at three aspects of this process. It is interesting to have a vague idea of student life, though elements are like all student life and need only be referred to, if that. (Janet Bilsby: 'The main tradition among students at the Royal Free that I could ever see was fornication.')

But other elements are unique. For many years it was the fact that consultant specialists did the teaching, and these had a very low opinion of GPs, which gave general practice its low status in the medical profession. Though this is waning, it is by no means dead – particularly in older medical schools. It has also been suggested that the abrupt confrontation when so young – at eighteen, nineteen, twenty – with sudden death and intense suffering, leads to that emotional withdrawal which can damage a GP's effectiveness with the patients. Also, that this toughening-up process is deliberate and encouraged.

We shall see if their selection and training as *doctors* is appropriate for people to become GPs. There is controversy here. It is the most important part of this section and is the reason I have put the section itself at the end rather the beginning of the book, which might have seemed more logical. It would have been impossible to judge if the selection and training were suitable for their life and work until we knew, as fully and deeply as possible and in all its aspects, what the life GPs were going to live was like.

Finally, we shall look at the trainers and trainees, something that has existed for some ten years, but which became mandatory in 1982 and, it is hoped, will transform the face of general practice.

Student Life

JACK, A STUDENT: 'It's difficult to come out with a typical sort of consultant, but they just tend to be so pompous and look down on you. You can always tell by the way they walk – the hands behind the back, the swaying.'

SUE, A STUDENT: 'The nurses are much more primed to cope with these things than we are. It's completely wrong. You go on to a ward for say the first time, and they'll ask you to take blood. And there are nurses there who have been there for thirty years and they're not allowed to take blood and you go along and say, "I'd like to take some blood please." You just have to pretend to be competent. Shake the needle, "This won't take a second, look the other way," and you usually make a botch of it.'

MARIUS, A STUDENT: 'Yeah. Once in Truro, the consultant was operating and he was looking at this bloke's stomach, because he had cancer of the stomach, and he walked out of the theatre, and he said, "Right, finish him up. Finish him up"' and there was this gaping hole, in his wound, and I didn't know what to do at all. And the sister, who must have watched hundreds and hundreds of operations, knew what to do and told me what to do. It was quite useful, that.'

VIRGINIA, A STUDENT: 'I was doing obstetrics, and this patient wrote a letter saying she didn't want an electrode attached to the baby's scalp for continuous monitoring, and she didn't want to have an epidural, she didn't want to have an episiotomy. That was the big apprehension, because a lot of the women have been told that they get it done anyway. If the baby's head is too big to be delivered you have to make a small incision, or it may tear and have to be sutured afterwards. And it happens quite commonly. But lots of women have been told that they get it done routinely which is not true at all, because you wouldn't do it – I certainly wouldn't do it because I'm the one that would have to sew it up. And the fourth thing was that she didn't want to be sutured by a medical student. And I was supposed to deliver. But she was going to accept to be delivered so I said 'Fine.' I agreed.

'So she delivered and inevitably it didn't go as well as it should have done and she did run into a bit of trouble and she did have a tear. And I said, "I'll see you in the ward afterwards and I'll get the SHO [Senior House Officer]" – you know, the doctor – "to stitch it", and the midwife interrupted and she said, "You're negligent to leave your patient without having stitched her." And I said, "No, I'm going to fetch the SHO to stitch her because she's requested that." And she said, "Oh, the SHO's far too busy. I'll tell her that she'll have to wait an hour and a half, lying in the dirty bed and she can't go to a ward unless she's stitched." And I said, "She doesn't want me and I'm not going to bully her." But you see, there it was, the medical student and they didn't take any notice – so they bullied her, and I was told to do it. Effectively by the midwife.

'And it all blew up, because the midwife went to the consultant and told him all sorts of crimes, and he chose to shout at me in the foyer where all the mothers were. So then I did sort of have to explode and he eventually climbed down and said, "Well, I'll have to go and talk to them."'

ALAN, A STUDENT: 'One's encouraged to behave disgustingly from the start of the career really. There are rugger matches or something, it comprises junior doctors as well, responsible chaps, and they come back to the bar and they all get pissed and have a sort of dustbin in the middle and are all just sick into it. Or there are competitions and people who can't drink a pint in one swallow have to do things like literally drink a pint of urine. They're just *made* to and you cannot get out of it.'

MARIUS, A STUDENT: 'I suppose we get pretty drunk once a week.'

JILL, A STUDENT: 'Twice. And *very*.'

MARIUS, A STUDENT: 'Yeah. But then there's hecklings – a sort of initiation. Silly things like putting squash balls down people's pants. One of the girls was tied to James Davis and given a diuretic, fastened together and she had to go to the toilet every five minutes, just having met James Davis ten minutes beforehand. Another is assessing people, isn't it? Assesses blokes. A girl comes along and puts her hands down his Y-fronts and feels each ball and goes "Ah, 2 out of 10, 3 out of 10, no, 4 out of 10."'

DR WARFIELD: 'You regularly see in the BMJ that the alcoholic doctor started with heavy drinking as a medical student. I think this is probably true. I think in a sense it was drinking to relieve the stress of a fairly hectic life. Being pitched in at the deep end as a medical student where first of all you go into the anatomy lab where there are all these stiff people on a slab and many had never seen a dead body before, never mind having to dissect one. Then, later on, you're moved to a hospital and again there's a certain amount of stress in seeing people die, people who are in pain, people who are critically ill, people who are injured, people who have tried to commit suicide, people who are mad. I think this is perhaps one of the reasons why medical students have a reputation of fairly hard drinking.'

DR JUNE EDSTONE: 'I was still frightened of illness, I think. I know I couldn't read a medical textbook – or a surgical one – I would turn over two pages and the next horrific thing I saw I was dying of myself. As students I think it was taught rather badly. Our introduction to the wards was wards of people dying of cancer and other horrible diseases. I used to see people being appalled by having a terminal carcinoma being examined by an apprentice.'

MARIUS, A STUDENT: 'A burst aorta, in Truro. It's this thing called an aneurism – the aorta, which is the big vessel that comes out of the heart, and it was bulging and the wall was very weak, and the surgeon put his finger on the top and the whole thing sort of exploded everywhere, covered everyone in blood. He lost about three litres of blood in five seconds. Everyone's faces were covered in blood and that really made me jump. You could see the consultants were really worried as well, and they really pulled themselves together and tranfused him and tied off all the arteries and they sewed on a trouser graft, which is an artificial aorta, and he survived. And the nurses were literally scooping up the blood – ugh.'

STUDENT'S MOTHER: 'It seemed to me they got really quite *fiercely* drunk twice a week. I'm not surprised. I mean, Simon described some project he had to do which meant he spent a *long time*, several weeks, sitting in the mortuary and examining them – body after body after body. A man of twenty-seven had been declared redundant and flung himself off the suspension bridge. A boy of sixteen was brought in. "Too young to die," sang the mortician, working away.'

DR LUCY VERYAN: 'If you protect yourself totally you may not be able to care adequately, if you don't protect yourself at all, then you succumb.'

DR MICHAEL VERYAN: 'I remember when we were students, it shows you how hard-bitten we were by the time we got to the wards, after three years of basic stuff we actually got to see the patient. One of the girls on the ward had to clerk a patient – a woman who had to have open heart surgery – and this was in the very early days of open heart surgery and it was really quite a decision to make and she was in hospital for a lot of investigations beforehand. It was a woman of about late thirties – and she got to know her over a couple of months or so and became quite close friends. So when she went up for her operation the student went with her to hold her hand, to be there at the anaesthetic; and the woman died on the operating table, and this girl was really very, very upset and we were very cynical about it all. We would tell her, "For goodness' sake, you shouldn't have got so involved." It was really quite early on in our career but the message had come across.'

The Teaching

From the 1858 Apothecaries Act for about 100 years until the 1950s, the idea of a doctor's preliminary training was to produce, by means of being taught on patients in hospitals by doctors skilled in the various branches of medicine, a sort of utility doctor who could then take full clinical care of patients in general practice. Only thereafter – and increasingly as each specialty grew more complex and the specialties themselves more numerous – would the student choose some more esoteric and, almost by definition from this process, more important aspect of medicine.

It gradually became clearer and clearer that there were considerable disadvantages and inaccuracies in this system. For one thing, 95 per cent of all disease is treated in and from the home, and only 5 per cent in hospital. Yet the 40-50 per cent of students who would become GPs had no idea of the circumstances of the life they would lead until they entered it, and the potential specialists and consultants no idea of general practice from which everything they saw would initially derive. The diseases they were trained on were different. Many GP illnesses – children's diseases, many infectious diseases, pneumonias, and all the common complaints of mankind – never see a hospital at all. The bias of the training was rigidly scientific and medical when many doctors were arguing that general practice, indeed all medicine, should become more 'holistic' – that is take account of the social, psychological and familial circumstances in the ways we observed when we studied the consultation. Yet psychiatry and psychology were largely based on animal studies; to such a degree that a senior professor could say as late as 1969 that a psycho-behavioural approach to medicine was all very well for a vet but quite pointless for a GP. And, finally, the authoritarian, rigid, goal-directed style of conducting a consultation that hospitals taught was quite unsuitable for the much more subtle consultations being suggested by men like Michael Balint.

Many people didn't agree (and many still don't) with these ideas. From 1950 there was a continuous battle between those trying to introduce more general practice into medical training and those fighting to keep it out.

1982 might have seemed to mark some sort of victory. The vocational year's training, which had been going for some fifteen years, became mandatory for all future GPs. With that came acceptance that general practice was a specialty that could be and had to be taught like other specialties.

Yet how much of a victory was this? How fundamental was it? What you might call the advanced conservative view was put to me by the same dean whose forthright views you may recall on women's place in medicine. His views – I paraphrase because they were put at considerable and highly articulate length – were as follows:

The basic medical training at a teaching hospital was required to do just that – to teach the basic medical facts, to produce a 'basic' doctor. It is easiest to do this in the wards of a hospital. During this period the student will be making up his mind what sort of doctor he wishes to be – surgeon, radiologist, obstetrician, etc., or GP. He must therefore see enough of each to be able to make up his mind – but he is not being taught to *be* one of them yet. That comes later. There are arguments put forward that students should become involved with patients earlier on. The dean would disagree fundamentally with this. He believes that it is pointless them seeing patients until they understand health and ill health, until they have the elements of anatomy, physiology and biochemistry; until they have learnt how to examine, make a diagnosis and suggest a treatment, or at least have some idea of therapy – can consult in fact. Once this is learnt, it can be modified later to suit the very different and very difficult circumstances of general practice. There is also an idea that they should see patients to keep them interested, to arouse their interest. 'Well, hell, if they can't be interested in their careers just because they're not seeing patients, then there's something wrong with them.'

This last consideration is in fact fundamental, and is where the real battle is still being fought. All the objections to the earlier teaching of medicine remain if no real difference is made to the curriculum and its teaching, if general practice is just tacked on at the end or the side, as it were, if the departments of general practice do little more than let the students see – half-way through or at the end – a day or two or three in the lives of a few doctors Ivan Denisovich. And since general practice is, as is now abundantly clear to us, entirely to *do* with patients – in all their complexity and not isolated into specific diseases as they are in a hospital – then the most effective way general practice could influence student training would be to introduce as much of this involvement – helped by attendant and relevant studies – as early as possible.

The degree to which general practice has been *incorporated* in this way varies widely. In a few medical schools it is considerable. At Newcastle, for instance, they start off almost at once seeing a GP patient or two, as it might be a man with rheumatoid arthritis, whom they can be attached to, get to know, to see how he feels about it, what it's like to be a *patient*; they see an early model of what a GP is like with a patient he knows well. Later, as the course develops, it is related again to reality – at obstetrics they will be attached to a single, real pregnant woman. They may see the baby born. Their lectures on child development, on the reflexes, tie in with this baby. Later still, they see a chronic – perhaps their rheumatoid arthritic again; and finally in their fourth year – and so answering one of the dean's criticisms – they sit in on surgeries. They do now have considerable medicine, but they can see styles of consultation, types of presentations, quite different from hospital. Southampton is radical as well, and on the same lines.

There are other schools doing the same sort of thing, though one should perhaps note that it is not a simple thing to organize – nor infallible. The GPs chosen, or who choose, to help are very variable.

GIRL STUDENT: 'Well, I can't say I like him. He's very rude to his patients. He's got pretty strong political and religious ideas which he lets infiltrate into his practice. For instance with contraception he says things like, "The pill hasn't reduced unwanted pregnancies whatsoever over the past twenty years," which is obviously totally false. He just says that because he's against it, you know. He's very narrow-minded about I suppose the normal affairs of people, like extra-marital affairs or whatever, you know. He sort of *condemns* them when really they're none of his business.

'We go round to houses and quite a few people have very large families, you know, seven, eight or nine kids and he says to this woman, "I really think it's time you came along and got yourself sterilized." She had no wish to really. She just wanted to keep going the way she was and you can't really blame her for that. I mean, you can't just say to somebody, "It's time you got yourself sterilized," you really can't. It's like talking about the family cat. He's just so awful.

'He turned to me the other day and said, "I'm sure that boy's a real psychological problem. I think he's a homosexual." And I said, "How on earth can you say that that guy's a homosexual?" And he said, "Well, I think he is because, to start with, he's a hairdresser, he's got a pierced ear and smokes cannabis and he's moving to London."'

But in fact in the majority of medical schools the seeing of GP patients is perfunctory, happens seldom and is left till the end of the course. In many, where it is allowed at the start, it is only a few hours in the entire year. In some of the London hospitals they see no outside patients at all. And this is not a question of backward hospitals slow to catch up with progressive trends. One ex-professor told me that many consultants still deeply resent general practice being considered a specialty and, whenever there is a cut, make sure it falls on that department. Studies at Edinburgh, Manchester and Aberdeen, reinforced by other work, suggest that quite a number of students not only have a number of qualities trained out of them, but had adverse attitudes trained in. For instance, a high proportion left Edinburgh with views that at the least indicated insensitivity towards, and at the worst a positive hatred of, people and patients. Elsewhere, students have shown insensitivity to mental illness, suicides and the old; this last soon to be 20-25 per cent of their practice.

I talked to students who had come into medicine eager to learn to help and cure people and had been so bored by the first two or three years they had nearly given up. 'It's like learning to drive a car by reading about it.' Quite a number do drop out. A Professor of General Practice at a medium-sized university medical school said, 'The students are still starved of patients and in that milieu some are destroyed. I use the term advisedly. They are switched off completely. We call them drop-outs, but I think we have considerable responsibility for that.'

What should be done? The most radical solution would be to design a curriculum specifically for future GPs. Although, clearly, some form of 'basic doctor' concept is inescapable in any system of medical training, if this scheme were adopted much detailed learning could be cut out, particularly in biochemistry, but also in anatomy and physiology. Relevant subjects like sociology, psychology and psychiatry would be much more extensive and given from the point of view of general practice (and not, as is frequently complained now in universities or schools where these are already given, from the standpoint of the disciplines themselves). Relevant subjects not now taught would be included: sexual counselling, marriage guidance, all the consultation, communication and psychotherapy skills which now, if learnt at all as a trainee, have to be learnt from scratch and often in the teeth of previous conditioning.

Ideas of this sort are in fact being tried – at Bersheba in Israel, for instance. The serious drawback to them was fundamental in the paraphrase I gave of the dean – medical students don't enter medicine knowing which branch of it they wish to end up in. They decide during the initial five years (given not the slightest help, one might note).

There are powerful arguments, as we'll see in a moment, for suggesting that some sort of rough pre-selection for general practice would be a good thing. Nevertheless, so radical a pre-selection and training as I propose (while undoubtedly producing better GPs) would require not one but several earthquakes under the medical establishment. Probably the most one can hope for is that the early integration and involvement with general practice pioneered by places like Southampton and Newcastle become still greater and are taken up by every medical school in Britain.

PROFESSOR LAUNTON (a Professor of General Practice): 'How else can you get across the needs and wishes of people as people? If you lecture students on that, they'll be bored to death. If you do your role-plays they think this is just great, but it's not the war. Put them into a situation and make them think, confront them with a breathing person and give them an opportunity of working through their difficulties – personal difficulties – with humans. That's a different ball game. Put them in a situation where they don't know what the hell's going on and yet have to make some decision for that patient and then put it in the sort of situation that the decision they make won't harm the patient. That's what I'm talking about. Not learning the names of the branches of the nerves or the origin and insertion of the lumbricals, say or a trapesius muscle, although that's important too. But to do that to the excessive extent they do in this school is beyond belief, and then finding at the end of the day that a student can't even tell you where a supra-condylar fracture of the humerus is.'

The Problem of Selection

General practice is not a science; it is the application of science to people.

DR WHEATACRE: 'You don't need to be a scientist at all. There's very little science in medicine now. You've got to be able to *work*, you have to memorize a certain amount. I *know* that in certain diseases the potassium goes *down* and so on. Anyone can learn this. I just apply it. I take the blood and the potassium. The students sometimes say, "How does this work?" and I say, "I really can't remember. I knew once; but it's important to give this chap potassium. It's what one expects in his condition."

'The qualities you need are quite different. You need to have patience with people. You need to be prepared to go on with your neurotic old so-and-so for years and finally come to like her. Before you do, to be *interested*. You can't fake an interest. If you're not interested you can very quickly suppress all thoughts of Mrs So-and-so, who *needs* you, perhaps only as a listening ear. You must be interested, not put out, if a patient unexpectedly moves. You can look at it and say, "Why? Why has this patient taken against me?" And sometimes you can say, "I see, yes. I was very abrupt to him one morning." '

The model taken by Dr Wheatacre and those who think like him is that offered by Liam Hudson in *Contrary Imaginations*. Essentially, this discovered two sorts of ways of thinking and looking at the world. There are convergent thinkers, who like logic and certainty; they like converging in on specific points. Scientists are prominently and essentially convergent thinkers, who require system, things to be settled, to lead to rational ends. Convergers are uninterested in personal relations and limit their involvement with people, taking refuge from them in things. Opposite to these are divergent thinkers, who move out, who enjoy speculation, who are tolerant of uncertainty, indeed stimulated by it. They are interested in the human aspects of their culture and enjoy personal involvements; they take refuge from things in people. Artists and writers are usually divergent thinkers. (And many people, of course, have elements of both – Liam Hudson found 40 per cent were an equal mixture.)

General practice, in this scheme, is essentially an occupation for a divergent thinker – with sufficient of the convergent to take on board the necessary science.

Medical students are selected almost entirely on the basis of their performance in 'A' level science or maths; usually two or three As or Bs in physics, chemistry, biology or maths. Many schools don't even interview. (Not that you learn a great deal from a half-hour interview; still less from a headmaster's reports, which are also relied on.) Such a scientific bent is fine for what one might call the science-orientated branches of medicine. These are essentially all the branches which are not general practice. But general practice is *fundamentally* antithetical to the convergent qualities desirable in all, or most, other medical fields (which reinforces my suggestion for a quite different form of training).

Here, then, is another explanation of the high stress, alcohol and suicide figures found in medicine: a number of people are being chosen for a profession to which they are totally unsuited.

DR WHEATACRE: 'I've just had a particular case. A girl who is the daughter of an accountant; she was exceptionally clever at one of the Scottish primary schools. She wanted to be a children's nurse. But they said, "You're far too clever for that – you'll get three 'A's in science. You should do medicine." She went into medicine, reluctantly; it was expected of her. She qualified. I remember interviewing her for vocational training and her academic levels were so high, though she was not particularly pleasant, that we took her. She completed her vocational training, she went into a rather tough general practice in Sunderland, she took to the bottle and ended up by committing suicide. Now she was quite unsuitable; she was a very converging type and she couldn't *stand* the rough and tumble.'

Certainly the three GPS I saw who didn't like their work bore out this analysis. You will remember it was precisely the 'divergent' quality of GP life – its unsettled, surprising, open-ended elements – which caused Dr Yetts finally to defect. Dr Simon Kibane was a highly trained scientist and was quite clear that he would have been happier in that sort of medicine. Dr Axmouth was less clear-cut, but I suspect something of this sort was at least part of the trouble. (It was revealing that he saw himself in positions of power, able, that is, to control events.)

Convergent/divergent combinations are not rare; nor is a concern with, an ability to be fascinated by, people. Studying the problem of suitability over many years, Dr Wheatacre says that in the university where he works at least 50 per cent of students chosen for their science abilities alone have both qualities sufficiently to make excellent GPS. What is needed is some system to steer these people into general practice; or more particularly keep out those students who do not possess them at all.

In fact, in theory this could be done quite easily. Vocational psychologists are perfectly able to devise tests which would detect such qualities or their lack. Not only that, they could also detect a high proportion of those psychological factors which we suggested probably contributed to the too frequently catastrophic reaction to GP stress.

I put this to the forthright dean, Professor Chardstock. He looked at me blankly. Such tests take about two and a half to three days. His university got 2,000 applications a year for places. And apart from the time, the cost would be astronomic.

But from those 2,000, they select about eighty a year. To ask these to take out three days in their first term to undergo such tests does not seem excessive. It would then, at least, be possible to select out candidates unsuitable for general practice; or anyway suggest to them they would not find it suitable or congenial – something which, once pointed out, they would be likely to find inherently acceptable. As to cost, training a medical student costs the country about £100,000 as it is. The extra £100 or £200 each this would involve would be irrelevant. If it did something, which it would, to cut the suffering and inefficiency represented by the appalling alcohol and suicide figures it would be cheap.

The modest change proposed by those who agree with Dr Wheatacre (the entire faculty at Southampton, for instance, who have adopted it already), is that a sufficient increase in divergent thinkers could be obtained by allowing students into medical schools who had one arts 'A' level, in addition to their one or two science ones. Just *one* arts 'A' level, so that a scientific aptitude would be proved, and the student would not find it too difficult to compete with the all-science students.

Even this may be difficult to achieve, not to mention my own almost equally modest proposal.

MR ESTON (on the selection board of a London medical school): 'The consultants in the medical school to which they will be going are essentially uninterested in these issues. They're not going to conceivably further such an expensive test. They don't ask, and if you suggest, as I did, that English lit. would help, or art history or something, you see them bridling in an old-fashioned world: "What, those long-haired pansies . . ." and that sort of thing. Very much conformist and one sees why, because they are very busy and they do come back much more physically exhausted than, say, I do, and they come back and they've got a groaning table, and a lot of silver and a lot of oak and there's the portentous wife who knows her role as being a pillar of the local society and a few daughters who go to pony club and in for dinner their guests, the bank manager and a few other conformist, conservative figures in the local establishment. Not only are they too tired to bother, they don't go to theatres or ballet. Heavens! The idea! Too tired. And the wife doesn't encourage it. She was a nurse before. And so the cycle continues.'

Trainers, Trainees

Trainees are fully qualified doctors, who are now training to be GPs. They will either be spending six months with a GP, for instance Dr Trimdon below, or doing one of the hospital courses, when they might go out and attend one of the courses which Dr Blairhall has been running since 1972.

A trainer is a GP who, for £3,000 a year, trains a newly qualified doctor in his practice. These trainer doctors now attend a comprehensive and fairly arduous course; this was not always so.

DR TRIMDON: 'Well, they need to have basic grounding in the administration of general practice and we have a check list which we go through, starting with how to register a patient, how to do immunizations, how to make appointments, which consultants to use in a hospital, which ones you think are good, how to deal with mental illness; lots of tasks which are not encountered in a hospital environment.

'They've been taught everything but they haven't experienced it. And they forget. You've got to put them through the thing again. And then, of course, there are clinical conditions which are common to general practice which are not seen in hospital. Well, unless they've done a paediatric job, they won't know what a sore ear looks like, the various rashes in children; adults – bronchitis – well, they'll have seen that. The acute coronaries seen in a home setting without intensive care backing; they've got to be taught how to deal with these dire emergencies on their own. They won't have a sister filling up syringes of this and that and saying, "There you are, doctor."

'And they know nothing about skins. They know nothing about psychiatry. You can see that they are in a strange world and it's quite bewildering. But after you've shown them a few measle rashes, and dermatitis, athlete's foot, they really pick it up quite quickly.'

DR BLAIRHALL: 'I had to think of ways of explaining general practice to them, getting them *involved* in it. We had Geests, the hauliers. And we had a couple of drivers along to tell them what their job was like, and the strains of the job, and we had the transport manager along to tell them about *his* job, and they brought along one of these big forty-tonner vehicles and one by one the trainees were put into this and they drove it for a quarter of an hour. It was a fabulous educational experience. The next time a driver comes in with backache, they'll know what the pressures are of having forty tons at your back, and this is something that we've done every three years ever since.

'Another time we were discussing alcoholism and my partner had got an alcoholic who ran a pub, and he came along and he held the trainees, and the trainers that were there, absolutely *spellbound* telling them what alcoholism meant for him. And he didn't pull any punches about what he thought doctors ought to be doing for alcoholics, in particular. And, you know, at the end – and he was questioned, and he parried and it was a *first-class* session and, you know I went away from it – well, honestly, this video tape and stuff; it's a load of codswallop. Doctors learn from patients, and what we want to do when these boys come here, is to expose them to patients and let the patients teach the doctors.

'My next try was the evolving mother. And I got a girl that was newly pregnant, I got a girl that had just got a new-born baby, I got a girl with a toddler, I got a girl with a secondary school child, I got a mother with a teenage son, and I got a mother who'd just become a grandmother. I got six of them – the different ways that a mother changes her life – and I put one trainee to each of them so that the six different trainees got six different pictures of what motherhood meant to a woman, and then the intention was to send the patients away. The trainees would meet with their trainer and we'd discuss motherhood and how it evolves. The interesting thing was that the mothers wanted to come into the discussion too, so I said, "That's fine." There was a group of twelve or thirteen of us, and the six doctors gave the pictures that they got, so at the end of the day, they all got a direct picture of one and pictures through one of their colleagues of another, and we found it turned into a counselling session. Because the mother with a teenage child was having teenage problems and was finding her son unbearable. It was the elderly grandmother who told this mother, and counselled her. It was *marvellous* counselling. It was good for the patient; it was *wonderful* for the group.'

The other method Dr Blairhall used – as do many trainee course organizers – is role-play, in which trainees and trainers take the parts of the participants in various common GP situations. complaining patient, tearful patient (male), girl of thirteen wanting the pill, etc. Surprisingly, this method does seem effective in getting doctors to actually experience something of what those involved would feel. I said it was like war games.

DR BLAIRHALL: 'It *is* war games. And the other one that we did was putting the doctor into court. I persuaded some of my friends who were magistrates, to sit and have a session to hear conflicting medical evidence, and at that time my son had a good friend who'd just become a barrister and he came along, and a solicitor friend in the town came along. We sat round this table one evening and we had four cases prepared with conflicting evidence in each and the young barrister and the older lawyer sort of worked out between them which they would take, and then when they each got these doctors in court they'd give them *hell*. They'd cross-examine them and the chaps when they came out of the box said, "My God, if that was just a run through, it can't be worse than the real thing!"'

DR KIBANE: 'I went to the conference at Exeter in 1981 after it was announced that vocational training was to be mandatory. There was an absolute *explosion*. They all said they weren't being 'trained' at all. No teaching, no seminars, just greedy, lazy GPs eager to get an extra pair of hands to take surgeries, do night calls and weekends and pocket masses of cash as well.

'This caused uproar and since then things have improved a bit. My trainer went to Borneo for two months of my six months' course. I just took over his job. I mumbled about it to the course organizer but what else could you do? Actually, I was quite pleased. I'd been qualified for longer than some of the partners and would have felt a bit demeaned to be a "trainee".'

DR BONBY (TRAINEE): 'Looking back, my education in terms of psychotherapy was about zero. It's really far, far too late when you do your GP training because you've been so conditioned to doing things in a different way.

'The first two weeks I spent here, I sat with all the partners and saw their techniques of consultation. I then started off having long consultations, some of which my trainer watched through glass – being allowed to take much more time. And some were put on video – that's very, very useful. You can look at it and say, "Heck, I shouldn't have said that," or "Yeah – there I am just getting easily into the doctor's role."

'That is, it *can* be taught. But why not earlier? The basic difference between the hospital approach and the general practice approach is that in general practice you've really got to sort out the problem, and there's a whole barrage of things it could be. In hospital it's either one thing, a medical problem, or one of several – medical, surgical and gynaecological. And if you understand – OK. If not, well, you'll have to see someone else.

'My trainers are very supportive and understanding. They encourage you to talk it all out and understand the pressures and what your feelings are – what the patients make you feel about them, which is one of the key questions.

'Sometimes the trainers exploit trainees. It's difficult to know what to do. I know of one case where in fact the trainer was officially reported by a trainee. That usually cools things down because the trainee is worth £3,000 a year and if you're exploiting someone, well you might as well be nice and take the £3,000 or you'll lose the lot.'

DR THRIPLOW: 'Well vocational training really has been the greatest spur I think. We have regular meetings – trainees and partners – argue a lot. Often about cases in the week – like the case of swollen ankles. You've really got to read to keep up with them and explain your ideas to them and it makes you rethink your ideas and sometimes really good ideas, you may not have really thought them out, but you find they are really quite good when you think about it.'

It is probably still too early to say what effects the GP training scheme will have on general practice. Cartwright was disappointed to find no improvements in those areas she clearly regarded as indices of 'the good GP'. GPS who'd been trainees were not more likely to think personal problems the sphere of the GP, nor enjoy GP life 'very much', nor did they think fewer consultations were trivial. She hoped the main impact of the schemes lay in the future. I would agree. I don't see how they can fail to do *some* good; and I would expect much more than this.

But as regards the trainers, Ann Cartwright did find marked differences. They all scored much higher on the 'good GP' scale.

I found the same sort of thing. The arrival of a trainee galvanized jaded middle–aged GPs into exhilarating activity – chaotic old notes were culled and sorted, age-sex registers compiled and massive screening initiated. Under the shafts and questions of beady-eyed, articulate young doctors old minds began to work again.

Dr Nyewood was about to take to training in search, in part, of stimulation. So was Dr Kibane. The eight or nine GPs I saw who were already trainers had clearly been considerably stimulated. Whatever else it does, the vocational training scheme will certainly revitalize the increasingly numerous practices upon which it will depend.

40
THE FUTURE OF GENERAL PRACTICE

There are other things in the future about which one can also be certain. There will be more old people; the progress from acute to chronic will continue. Health centres and group practices will go on spreading, eating up single-handed practitioners. I do not see single-handed practice disappearing. In some places it can't, as with the inducement areas – unless helicopters and helicopter training become part of the inducement. General practice will always attract a number of people who want to be single-handed. Deputizing for night visits will also grow. To make sure it is of the right standard it will have to be integrated into the NHS GP system and be properly monitored by the BMA.

We can speculate. As the hospital side of the NHS continues to totter and groan under financial exigencies, it might suddenly be realized that truly enormous sums – billions of pounds – could be saved by channelling more money towards the GP system – which currently deals with about 95% of *all* medical problems for 5·2% of the total NHS budget (1980–81 figs). One GP I spoke to estimated that nine tenths of what he now sent to hospital he could, given fairly small increased resources, do himself in the surgery. Another GP said three quarters. All GPs agreed they could do a large proportion.

This would mean reviving and evolving the old cottage hospital/local surgery system; increasing surgery facilities somewhat and developing health centre and group practice little hospitals (nor is there any reason for these to be purpose-built – a modern mania). The main hospitals would be truncated and cater for serious illness and major surgery only. Because the infra-structure of the big hospitals is so enormously expensive, all minor operations and 'procedures', now mostly sent away, are far cheaper done on a local basis; as are the short-stay hospital visits for which GPs so often desperately need access to beds, as we saw with Dr Bilsby for example. Such a move would also allow GPs to retain interests and expertise which atrophies once they finish their hospital training.

More old people will mean more home visits; we have already discussed the question of who will do the visiting.

There will be further developments in chemo-therapy, and other dis-coveries. Among these, geneticists will enable far sharper prognoses to be made and preventative treatments to be initiated. Genetic predisposition has already been suggested for ulcers, diabetes, arthritis, heart disease, flu and skin cancer.

With the concept of the preventative we enter a future not so much of speculation as of hope. In his book *The Doctors*, published in 1965, Paul Ferris spoke of 'the radical new medicine of the future'. This was, in essence, preventative medicine. It hadn't taken place by then, although the ideas of social and preventative medicine were not new, because they had coincided with the drug revolution which began in the late thirties. These had made it possible to cure diseases once they had developed. 'Preventative' lost its urgency.

It still hasn't really regained it. As we saw, when you talk to doctors the same small basket of measures comes up repeatedly – immunization, testing for hypertension and diabetes, smears, advice on smoking, etc. – of which the implementation is very varied, the efficacy sometimes questioned, the onus still often left to the patient.

Yet it is, both in essence and particularly in its latest vaguer but thereby still more exciting development, a glorious ideal – never more exhilarating than when expounded by one of its most radical supporters, Dr Julian Tudor Hart, a passionate man who, like several idealistic GPs, struggles to subdue a powerful and highly authoritarian character. But many doctors would agree, at least, with some of what Tudor Hart says. Indeed, I don't see how one could, in theory at least, disagree.

The phrase is 'anticipatory care'. This means, In Hart's words, that GPs must 'become the active guardians of the health of our registered populations.' It means the GP must change behaviour, by an active, intense, violent programme of lobbying, education, and example.

'Active guardians' naturally includes the basket of measures with which we are familiar. Here the *efficient* application of known techniques would make a lot of lives far better. A survey of epileptics, for instance, showed 15 per cent had not seen their GP for a year, 5 per cent with frequent seizures were on the wrong medication, 9 per cent were overdosing, 70 per cent needed dosage adjustment.

But Hart doesn't just see the GP going out and seeking that 'iceberg of disease' we looked at. The range is far wider.

DR TUDOR HART: 'It is being quite specific and finding out, you look for the beginning of an alcohol problem, which is very common. You ask direct questions because people don't offer them to you, they come with "missing work on Mondays" and "vomiting in the morning" or being nasty to their wives. It is easier to control obesity before it becomes severe. We have to move over to the ideas of looking after people in an active way and worrying about them, not only when they come and complain to you, but worrying about them because they are your patients. You find 5 per cent or 8 per cent don't consult. Some are very healthy, but there is also a group who have problems like schizophrenia or alcoholism or even a lump in the breast which they are afraid to present to the doctor.'

And here the trivia which people often present becomes a tool – they bring the patient into the surgery and allow the GP to search. The GP is an agent of social control, of behaviour.

Nor, of course, can he do this alone. Such an extension needs an extended staff.

DR TUDOR HART: 'I need a dietician in my practice. We have a major problem of obesity which kills a lot of people indirectly, but that's the root of it. It causes a great deal of advanced arthritis in the knees and hips. A joint replacement for a knee, I don't know what it costs, but it must be a couple of thousand pounds; it is a very expensive operation and yet overwhelmingly the people who need it are people who have been very obese for about twenty years. That is a preventable condition, but it means that we have to not have thirty seconds and give people a diet sheet and tell them to get on with it; they have got to be taught about the nature of different foods.'

The primary care team would be expanded in order to search. 'Physiotherapy in general practice is very important. We need people who can take people swimming, who can get them riding bicycles again, who can take fat middle-aged people out and put them back into production again.'

Many doctors would agree with this, at least as an idea. In certain respects some would go further.

DR RIARD: 'I've been enormously impressed with a man called Graham Curtis Jenkins, by the way in which he used the occasions of developmental testing to teach the mother about what her baby can do and to enhance that relationship. To show her how by creative play she stimulates the child and develops a relationship with it. It's the most exciting thing to watch.

'I think what I'm saying is that when you're doing arithmetic about anticipatory care there are so many other factors other than simply the finding of disease. There are far more subtle things, like how do you maximize the potential of growth of the individual? In Mazlo's terms, how do you help to achieve self-actualization, self-realization? These are enormous goals of a very affluent society – perhaps more affluent than we are yet.'

We shall return in a moment to the cost. There is another response – is it worth it medically?

DR TUDOR HART: 'I don't think it is necessary to prove that. I think the truth is that for the great majority of people, the kind of care that they either want or actually think they are already getting from their GPs is anticipatory care. I think when they go to the doctor saying, "I have a pain in my ear, doctor," they want him to deal with that, but they also welcome it if he then updates, if he looks at his summary sheet and says, "Do you still get that pain in your back you complained of six months ago?" That is, it is this type of medicine people want, care and attention to this degree, to realize positively the full potential of medical resources and medical discoveries to make people happier and healthier.'

Now this would be extremely expensive in time. It has been shown that to achieve high quality control of diabetes requires about four hours teaching of patients; and discovering, teaching and controlling diabetics could be anything up to 10 per cent of a GP's practice. To do this and the rest adequately Hart would roughly halve the present list size – giving each GP about 1,000, 1,200 patients. This would take care of another future certainty – medical unemployment. In January 1983 the Government was predicting 8,000 unemployed doctors by the year 2,000. The BMA said it could be as high as 20,000, the number of GPs at the moment. Halving their lists, doubling the number of GPs, would be a neat way of solving the problem – and doubling or trebling the quality of care into the bargain.

The same is true of unemployment generally.

DR TUDOR HART: 'I think the hold-up is in people's political and economic ideas. Doctors would say generally, yes it would be very desirable in an ideal world, and as soon as people use that phrase you know they are going to start back-tracking. Well, what about this world? In this world here (Afan Valley, South Wales) we have over 40 per cent unemployed. A lot of those are very intelligent people who would like to work in the Health Service. It has always been labour intensive, and people like working in it because it is creative and people feel it is socially useful. They like doing that. Well, why shouldn't they?'

Most people would say it was a political decision, ultimately one which society must make itself. Thurston Riard points out that it is significant that the Government began to take medicine seriously when it started to show it could actually affect the productive capacity of the nation. With Lloyd George, but still more so with the implementation of the NHS, it became economically important for a modern industrialized state to service its workers right across the spectrum. And there is little doubt that full-scale anticipatory care would still further increase the productive capacity. But does this argument still have the force it did? When you can't even find enough work for the productive force you have, do you want to make it bigger still?

Or you could argue that anticipatory care *is* just an ideal; but it is best to have the highest ideals possible. Aim for this one, and you might just get most GPs carrying out that little basket of preventative medicine efficiently and conscientiously. That alone would be a large improvement.

I think Tudor Hart would go far further than this. He would argue that there is a moral issue here. It is not a question of profitability, but of what is necessary. Not to cure people when you can is immoral. And it becomes much more so when there comes a class or wealth divide. In the past, to give a great deal of time to a duchess and finally take out her large intestine, while you spent three minutes with a dustman and gave him a laxative didn't matter. Both actions were more or less illusory. But now the strict control of diabetes takes time but it does work. And the same is true of all that we have described, and much more – which money can still buy. 'To give just one other example, coronary by-pass graft is now probably *the* commonest single operation done in the United States. It is more common than appendicectomy. That is not the case here. The public are going to know eventually; you can't keep it secret for ever.'

In fact, unlike education, the logic of medical care is always to expand. If it does not expand, if the Welfare State is cut back, then the doctors are set on a collision course with the Government – one much sharpened if 20,000 of them are unemployed.

It is still further sharpened by a curious anomaly at the heart of the Health Service itself. Doctors are, by temperament and role, on the side of authority, they are conservative (we saw 75 per cent said they would vote Tory). And the Health Service is Britain's biggest single industry. But embedded in the Service, the idea upon which it was founded, was the principle of to each according to his need (the people), from each according to his ability (the doctors); not a socialist principle, that is to say, but a Communist one. Tudor Hart's medical objectives are therefore inextricably bound up with his political views. Explicit and implicit in what he writes and says is the expectation, it almost seems the hope, that conflict between doctors and the State is probably inevitable.★

There are two last, slightly contradictory things that may happen in the future. As jobs grow scarce, candidates for them seek to become better qualified. There is already a tendency for young doctors to take the exams of the Royal College of General Practitioners and add MRCGP after their name. As GP unemployment grows, so will this tendency. The Royal College very much favours the Balint-orientated, mini-therapy view of the consultation and this, too, will therefore increase.

This will draw GP and patients closer together. But there is also the suggestion that GPs are less close to their patients than they once were, and may move even further apart. Certainly this has been a trend. The medicine we saw in the twenties and thirties – the medicine of delivering babies, of endless home visits and succouring by the GP because he could not cure, the

---

★For a fuller account of Dr Tudor Hart's views see the *Journal of the Royal Society of Medicine*, vol. 74, December 1981.

fact that GPs were usually single-handed – all this made for a closeness, which grew less as all these factors ceased to operate. Thurston Riard sees all the analyses and research into GP-patient relationships, the arts of consultation and so on, as a symptom of this decline. He compared it to writing about the British Raj. People write about what they've lost. The evidence that this trend is continuing is more contradictory. Cartwright certainly finds fewer home visits, and there was a decline of 8 per cent in those who saw their GP as a personal friend. There is always the possibility that, if the primary health team is enlarged along anticipatory medicine lines, the patient becomes lost. His concerns are shared – or divided – among too many people.

But if we get significant anticipatory care, GPs will have half their present number of patients; indeed the point of such a move would be, precisely, that they should be able to devote more time to them. Cartwright also found that young GPs do visit more, and wished to do so. She found that more families had the same doctor than ten years before. As for *personal friendship*; that is asking a great deal, certainly more than all the GPs I spoke to expected, or wanted, whatever their age. The close relationship of a patient and his GP goes beyond friendship and is different from it. My own feeling is that it will remain, now, much as it is – the fairly complex factors working in both directions are approximately equal.

41

'*THAT* IS THE FASCINATION'

After all – how distant can you get? The historical accident of the rising apothecary needing to make money rooted the GP, from the 1850s on, in local communities with stable populations; an extension to the whole population, in fact, of something which most of the middle and upper middle classes had enjoyed for 100, 150 years with their physicians.

But this means the GP and his patients are locked together, in most cases for life; at least for many years at a time. And how strongly both want this can be demonstrated if one considers any alternative. A Brighton GP told me it would be far more efficient if primary care was hospital-based. You could cover the entire Brighton area with ten GPs working in the hospitals and immediately referring to nurses, specialists and whatever; 'But the idea makes me shudder; I expect it makes you shudder too.'

Any country can train medical men. It is the knowledge based on this long and intimate association with his patient, his family and their community which is the source of a GP's most important insight and one which cannot be taught – an importance which increases as we once again begin to appreciate the essentially 'holistic' nature of medicine. And as the source of his power it explains the ultimate focus of his interest.

Indeed, it is natural enough. It has been interesting to compare the various practices in this book: the barely converted tobacconist, the fortress slum, the slow, nineteenth-century pace of the Highlands, the glades of glass of a great southern county health centre. The growth of the chronic, or the chemo-therapy revolution are interesting as well. But surely what remains in the mind are the people. The GPs: Dr Kelling with his gongs, shaking with rage, shaking his notes over his desk; the Chaucerian description of Mrs Locking and the blood in the wee, or Dr Locking himself, sitting for an hour beside the corpse in his car – 'Bugger off, Jock'; Dr Jane Edstone with the nets of her poacher lover. The GPs – and their patients: the old man whose feet were raised step by step up the stairs by his wife and sister-in-law; the woman who said, 'My husband and I have been having an argument without words'; the old lady weeping when Dr Chathill told her her husband was dead, the tears running down her face 'leaving white trickles as it washed the dirt away'; Sassall's 'wife' who was really a man.

'You must love your patients,' said Dr Wheatacre. Yet it isn't quite that.

Chekhov, Maugham, Cronin, Munthe, Conan Doyle, Céline – it is no accident that a good many novelists have been doctors. A novelist becomes involved with his characters, he may even 'love' them in some sense, but he has to remain detached from them – Graham Greene talks about the necessary amount of ice in a novelist's make-up. Only thus can he analyse, dissect and put them together again – or bring himself to destroy. And novelists, like GPs, function over time – time, what one might call the 'narrative' element of a GP's life.

There are, of course, novelists whose main concern is not really with individual character. So too with doctors. But the best doctors, like the great novelists, find a profound fascination in human beings. And it is right, therefore, to end a book about GPs on this note, since their lives *are* people – and this is true of the whole range, from the brief appearances which flash and make moving or surprising a turbulent inner-city practice, to the long narratives of a settled GP in the country.

DR KINSHAM: 'Talking of worst cases, that girl is Australian and she mixes in a circle of mad Australians, one of whom is the worst case of shop-lifting, he tells me with some pride, *ever*; £250,000. He got £8,000 to £10,000 a week. But he hasn't done it for two years now. He went to prison. He came to see me, signed on, and said, "You've got to do something about this. It was so ghastly in prison. You must help. I know you helped Doris." '

'Well, yes, Doris was another of these mad Australians, a very *large* personality, enormous hats, and she had carcinoma of the clitoris. She's twenty-eight and the normal treatment of that is to have a wide incision of the area of the clitoris and the leg – you cut away everything around there – terrible. Worse than those female circumcisions. She came to me and said, "I want to see a female gynaecologist" – with which I finally concurred, but they all – she saw two more – all said she would have to have this operation. So I said, "Look, there *are* some anti–mytotic drugs. Look in the *Indexus Medicus*" – I showed her how to use it – "in the Westminster Library and tell me what you find." '

'She came back with some papers on Chlorambucil, an anti–mytotic drug which had been used. I got my favourite gynaecologist (*not* a woman) and he used it. And she's been fine ever since. Back to Australia, still with her clitoris, married. She gave me a crate of Dom Perignon champagne in 1967.

'Anyway, in came this chap. I couldn't think what to do, but I had a long talk with him and he was violently against his father and society and we went into it. I chatted about it to some patients of mine who are psychoanalysts etc. – one very well known. He said, "Really, you know, it's all a defence against depression." So, on the theoretical basis it might be, I started him on anti-depressants in small doses, And that stopped him. He hasn't done it since.

'Interesting. But he'll go off. I shan't see either of them again. It's very different from the country. Different type of case. But you get a variety and strangeness.'

DR WHEATACRE: 'You'll get a girl, a depressed girl; only last week, a girl looking rather like an ordinary teenager came in and her periods were irregular. I said, "Is there any possibility of pregnancy?" – she's eighteen. "No," she said, quite confidently. She came back two weeks later and said, "You know, I've just got one of these pregnancy tests you buy, and I'm pregnant." She said, "I wasn't trying to deceive you – I was trying to deceive myself because I couldn't believe I was." They'd used a sheath – nothing wrong. "But I'm pregnant." So I asked her what she wanted to do and she said, "Well, my boyfriend", and she's had a boyfriend, steady relationship with this chap, "my boyfriend wants me to keep it." And I said, "What do you want?" And she said "I don't know." "Are you going to marry him?" "Well, I hope to marry him." "Does that mean that you're not sure that he wants to marry you?" "No, no, no, no," she said, "we're going to get married, but there's my career." And she's a very clever girl. A very good shorthand typist. She went straight into that. She's got three interviews: one at the university, one as a medical secretary and one somewhere else, pending – you know, in the next week or two.

'So I had a long talk with her, but this was fascinating. I wouldn't have guessed that this, well, fairly ordinary, one might almost say cheap-*looking* teenager, sitting there. I knew her mother and knew she existed, but she herself had never been here. I then, in the course of the three days, came to realize that this is a very mature young woman. And I'm fascinated to see what's going to happen. I'm sure she's going to keep the baby. But she's still got her father to face. So I said, "Well, I'm on your side. It's your choice, not mine – not the doctor's, not your mother or father's. If you like, ask them to come and talk to me and I'll explain to them." I'll be very interested in what happens to this girl. I don't know now. But I will know eventually.'
[I had to leave Dr Wheatacre for ten days while I journeyed north. He kindly asked me to stay the night on my way back. I did so, and he resumed his account.]

'She came back; she came back on the Monday, or three or four days later and when she came she was quite different. Not so hesitant and frightened. And as soon as she sat down she said, "I'm going to keep it." I just said, "Yes, and what do your parents think?" And she said, "Well, my mother says that it isn't fair on them to have to look after this baby while I go out working and my father is just horrified with the whole thing because he just thinks I'm a little girl. I'm an only child and he's absolutely horrified, but my boyfriend wants me to have the baby and I'm going to have it." I said, "Well, what do you know about having a baby? What do you know about preparing?" And she said, "I know I shouldn't smoke and I don't smoke anyway. I know I shouldn't drink and I don't drink much and I won't drink any more, and I know you shouldn't put on weight."

'So she'd really thought it through, you see. I mean, most eighteen-year-old girls don't know this. She'd obviously been thinking about this, or talking to friends, or finding out and I said, "Right, OK, where do you want to have the baby?" and she said, "Oh, well, I don't know. I'll leave that to you." And I could sense slightly that she was a bit unhappy about her parents, and I said, "If they are being difficult about it, ask them to come and see me (because I know them both) if you like. What do you think?" And she said, "Oh, I'd like them to." And the days have gone by and they haven't appeared and I have thought to myself, "Well, obviously, they have come to terms with it", and she rang up this morning and said, "You said you wanted to see me in a week or two to discuss where we have the baby. When?" I was so interested and I hadn't got a Saturday morning surgery, but I said, "Well, come tomorrow morning and I'll be in."

'And the interesting thing about this girl is what seemed to me an ordinary only child from lower-middle-class parents - he's some sort of small businessman, nice, not very broad – and yet she turns out to have got quite a bit of character. She comes. She doesn't know me. She's frightened that she can't get a termination and because I've sort of treated her as a human being she now talks to me rather as a girlfriend of my sons would do. I mean, she spoke to me quite confidently on the telephone whereas initially she just sat quietly. She realizes that I'm on her side and that's very pleasing.

'And you see, I know her family, her father and her mother. And the interesting thing, of course, looking at it from the point of view of general practice, in the next ten years we will see what happens to this girl and I bet she does well. She'll learn more than she thinks in one of those jobs, she'll get on and they will get married earlier than they think they can afford. And she'll then take over the baby, or perhaps grandmother will have got so attached she'll act as a kind of mother surrogate, which works very well. I think that's probably quite likely. But I don't know, and I'm going to see the dénouement, well, not the dénouement, the maturing of a girl, you know, continuing. And it's there – *that* is the fascination.'

LIST OF DOCTORS

DR WILLIAM ABBERLEY, 60. Single-handed inner-city practice in the South.

DR HENRY ABNEY, 52. Large eight-doctor rural/urban Buckinghamshire practice operating from a spanking new health centre.

DR PETER AXMOUTH, 30. Two-doctor practice in an overspill New Town in the South.

DR DAVID BILSBY, 35. Four-doctor Lincolnshire practice. Married to Janet Bilsby.

DR ANTHONY BLAIRHALL, 58. Home Counties six-doctor practice in a health centre.

DR FRANK BONBY, 27. Trainee GP in inner-city group practice.

DR TIMOTHY BRANE, 66. Three-doctor inner-city group practice, largely private.

DR TIM CERNEY, 46. Northern industrial three-doctor practice.

PROFESSOR JOHN CHARDSTOCK, 48. Dean of a northern medical school.

DR JAMES CHATHILL, 52. Six-doctor group practice in a large West Country health centre. Married to Mary Chathill.

DR JAMES COLKIRK, 44. Single-handed Highland inducement practice. Married to Elizabeth Colkirk.

DR JUNE CRESSING, 30. Part-time married GP in four-doctor East Anglian practice.

DR IAN CULROY, 47. Three-doctor practice in Sussex, urban/rural.

DR MALCOLM DOLWAR, 34. North-country rural four-doctor practice.

DR JULIAN EASTCOURT, 62. Four-doctor rural/urban practice in the south of England.

DR JANE EDSTONE, 58. Three-doctor practice in the Midlands.

DR CLARA ELLON, about 70. Single-handed East Anglian city practice.

MR ESTON, 63. Consultant surgeon at large London teaching hospital, and on its selection board. Active in medical politics.

DR SALLY FINSTOCK, 35. Two-doctor egalitarian practice in the North.

DR SUSAN GLYNDE, 55. Part-time married GP in five-doctor group practice in the South.

DR HAMSTALL, 39. Three-doctor practice in Norfolk town. Friend of David and Janet Bilsby.

DR JOHN HURY, 67. Single-handed inner-city practice.

DR MARY IFFORD, 65. Three-doctor practice in the West Country.

DR MIKE KERRIS, 35. Northern industrial practice run with his partner Nick Trull on egalitarian lines.

DRS SIMON AND JANET KIBANE, 35 and 32. Sharing the position of one GP in a six-doctor practice in Cornwall.

DR PHILIP KINSHAM, 52. Three-doctor group practice operating from a large inner-city health centre.

DR LANE. Author of an amusing and moving account of general practice in the thirties: *The Diary of a Medical Nobody*.

PROFESSOR LAUNTON, 59. Professor of General Practice at a Midlands medical school.

DR SAM LOCKING, 54. Two-doctor practice in Cumberland. Married to Polly Locking.

DR HARRIET LYNSFORD, about 50. Three-doctor rural/urban practice in Yorkshire.

DR JOHN MARTHAN, 55. Single-handed south of England practice, nephew of old Dr Simon Marthan. A very interesting man, whose tapes, due to recorder malfunction, were infuriatingly four-fifths inaudible.

DR SIMON MARTHAN, 84. Qualified 1921, went for a cruise to Australia, then joined his father and brother in their half-rural, half-urban Midlands practice.

DR HENRY MISTON, 40. Rich, single-handed private practitioner in Scottish city.

PROFESSOR D.C. MORRELL. Wolfson Professor of General Practice at St Thomas's Hospital Medical School.

DR TREVOR NYEWOOD, 65. Three-doctor Berkshire group practice operating from a new custom-built centre, leased to them by the Parish Council but occupied only by them.

MR POYLE, 44. The chemist who largely served the Three Elms surgery of Dr David Bilsby's four-doctor Lincolnshire practice.

DR GEOFFREY QUAINTON, 94. Inner-city single-handed practice.

DR THURSTON RIARD, 49. London group practice. Active in GP and College politics. Ex-Professor of General Practice.
DR RUSHDI, 49. Single-handed inner-city practice.

DR SALEBY, 53. Single-handed inner-city practice in the Midlands.
DR SASSALL. The name John Berger gave to the doctor in his book about a Welsh GP: *A Fortunate Man*.
DR JOHN STANE, 81. Practised in Glasgow in the twenties, then in Fife, finally, and for most of his life, in Lincolnshire.
DR GEOFFREY SUGNAL, 43. Five-doctor practice in the Midlands, urban/rural.

DR ANDREW TELSCOMBE, 49. Large eight-doctor East Anglian group practice operating from a big converted private house.
DR PHILIP THRIPLOW, 58. Welsh rural five-doctor group practice. Married to Alice Thriplow.
DR HENRY TRIMDON, 56. Senior of three partners in large urban practice in West Scotland.
DR MARY TRIMDON, 45. Wife of Dr Henry Trimdon. Large slum practice in West Scotland.
DR NICK TRULL, 28. Partner with Mike Kerris in northern egalitarian practice.
DR JULIAN TUDOR HART, Afan Valley group practice, South Wales.

DR ULLEY, 55. Four-doctor group practice in Berkshire.
DR ANNE UPLEES, about 43. Three-doctor practice in a large West Country river-sea town.

DR THOMAS VELLING, mid 60s. South African. Practice on the outer fringes of South-West London. When I saw him his partner had just departed.
DRS MICHAEL AND LUCY VERYAN, 47 and 40. Old county town five-doctor group practice in the south east of England.

DR FRANK WARFIELD, 50. Five-doctor city practice in the south-east. Two of the doctors are women, each part-time.
DR WASING, 89. Had practised during the twenties, thirties and forties in a large southern coastal town.
DR WATTS. GP in the twenties and thirties.
DR JOHN WHEATACRE, 75. Senior Partner in five-doctor Midlands industrial practice, from a health centre occupied only by them.
DR WYRE, 60. Describes his father's rural practice in Northumberland. He himself was in a three-doctor group practice in Wales.

DR TIMOTHY YETTS, 44. The 'drop-out doctor'. Had been for eighteen years, and until just before I saw him, one of five GPs in a North London group practice in a health centre.

SHORT BIBLIOGRAPHY

This is not even remotely a list of all the books and articles I consulted. It is certainly no indication of all the books that could be read about General Practice. The literature is enormous. This is simply a short list of works that anyone interested will find expands or explains some of the topics touched on in the book itself.

Balint, Enid, and Norell, J.S., (eds) *Six Minutes for the Patient – Interactions in General Practice Consultation*, Tavistock Publications, 1973.
Balint, Michael, *The Doctor, His Patient and the Illness*, Pitman Medical, 1968.
Beales, G., *Sick Health Centres – and how to make them better*, Pitman Medical, 1978.
Bennet, Glin, *Patients and Their Doctors*, Balliere Tindall, 1979.
Berger, John, *A Fortunate Man – the story of a country doctor*, Allen Lane, 1967.
Byrne, P.S., and Long, B.E.L., *Doctors Talking to Patients*, London HMSO, 1976.
Cartwright, Anne, *Patients and Their Doctors*, Routledge & Kegan Paul, 1967.
Cartwright, Anne, and Anderson, R., *General Practice Revisited*, Tavistock Publications, 1981.
Ferris, Paul, *The Doctors*, Weidenfeld & Nicolson, 1965.
Fry, John, (ed.) 'Trends in General Practice', *British Medical Journal*, 1979.
Hudson, Liam, *Contrary Imaginations*, Penguin, 1967.
Huntington, June, *Social Work and General Medical Practice – Collaboration or Conflict?*, Allen & Unwin, 1981.
Illich, Ivan, *Limits to Medicine*, Penguin, 1976.
Inglis, Brian, *Drugs, Doctors and Diseases*, Mayflower Dell, 1965.
Inglis, Brian, *A History of Medicine*, Weidenfeld & Nicolson, 1965.
Jarman, Brian, 'A Survey of Primary Care in London', *Occasional Paper 16, Journal of the Royal College of General Practitioners*, May 1981.
Jones, W.H.S., *The Doctor's Oath – an essay on the history of medicine*, Cambridge University Press, 1924.
Lane, Kenneth, *The Diary of a Medical Nobody*, Corgi, 1982.
Paine, Leslie H., (ed.) *Health Care in Big Cities*, New York, 1978.
Pritchard, Peter, 'Patient Participation in General Practice', *Medical Annual 1983*.
Working party of the Royal College of General Practitioners, *The Future General Practitioner*, British Medical Journal, 1972.